THE WEB OF LIFE

Life Force:
the Energetic Constitution of Man
and the Neuro-Endocrine Connection

John Davidson M.A. (Cantab)

SAFFRON WALDEN
THE C.W. DANIEL COMPANY LIMITED

First published in Great Britain in 1988 by
The C.W. Daniel Company Limited
1 Church Path, Saffron Walden, Essex CB10 1JP, England

ISBN 0 85207 199 X

Production in association with
Book Production Consultants, Cambridge, England
Typeset by Cambridge Photosetting Services in Bembo
Printed and bound by Billings, Worcester

Dedication

To all my teachers
Whether they knew it or not.

But most of all
To my Spiritual Teacher
Without whose inspiration
Nothing would have happened

The most beautiful and most profound emotion we can experience is the sensation of the mystical. It is the power of all true science. To know what is impenetrable to us really exists, manifesting itself as the highest wisdom and the most radiant beauty which our dull faculties can comprehend only in their most primitive forms — this knowledge, this feeling is at the centre of true religiousness.

Albert Einstein, *Ideas and Opinions.*

Of how it is that the soul informs the body, physical science teaches me nothing; and that living matter influences and is influenced by mind is a mystery without a clue. Consciousness is not explained to my comprehension by all the nerve paths and neurones of the physiologist; nor do I ask of physics how goodness shines in one man's face, and evil betrays itself in another.

D'Arcy Thompson, *On Growth and Form.*

The life is not a function of the form, the form is a product of the life.

Will Durant, *Mansions of Philosophy.*

Acknowledgements

To all those who have gone before,
And to those who will follow

It would require a history of one's life, and of previous lives too, if one were to acknowledge all the influences which have gone into the shaping of one's vision of reality.

Such a thing is clearly impossible, for, if we are honest, we will realize that we have come to where we are with very little intention, forethought or planning, and indeed with practically no memory of the continuum of events, thoughts and experiences that have made us what we are. We have simply followed the pattern of our destiny.

Bearing this in mind, let me thank the following people. Firstly, my spiritual Master, Maharaj Charan Singh Ji, whose profound mystical teachings and practical instruction in meditation have provided a foundation upon which the whole of life's experience may be understood, whether spiritual or mundane. These are universal teachings and a spiritual practice beyond all human divisions of nationality, religion or idiom of thought. They are as old and as man and as deep as the Source itself.

Secondly, I must own my indebtedness to Dr Randolph Stone and to discussions of his Polarity Therapy with many students of his methods. He was really the first in the modern era to combine the science of healing with the Eastern wisdom within a paradigm of energy.

Then, I must thank Stephen Arroyo for his insight into the emotional or psychological aspects of the *tattwas* or elements. His book, *Astrology, Psychology and the Four Elements* has been most revealing for me.

Whilst in India, immediately prior to the typesetting of this book in December 1987, I had the good fortune to meet Dr James Said – a quietly spoken and gentle man of deep scientific as well as mystical understanding. We had many fascinating discussions concerning his work and discovered that we had independently arrived at many of the same conclusions. As a result of these discussions I was able to augment some of the sections of this book and he very kindly agreed to write an introduction. He has dealt specifically with what I have tackled in only a broad or general fashion.

Dr Andrew Rawlinson, lecturer in religious studies at Lancashire University kindly went through the manuscript checking my Sanskrit transliterations and making other valuable suggestions. An exerpt from one of his papers has also provided an excellent insight into the nature of the *devas*, for which I am grateful.

Dr Robert Greaves, a medical practitioner in Shropshire, also read through the manuscript, making some useful suggestions.

On the more mundane level, Sheila Clarke did most of the word processing and Dennis Halls did nearly all the drawings. Such help is essential!

For the poetic interludes and other quotations, I must gratefully acknowledge the following authors, translators and publishers.

Ideas and Opinions, Albert Einstein, Souvenir Press.
On Growth and Form, D'Arcy Thompson, Cambridge University Press.
Mansions of Philosophy, Will Durant, Ernest Benn Ltd., 1929.
Al-Ghazali the Mystic, Dr Margaret Smith, Luzac & Co.
The Living Flame of Love, St. John of the Cross, translated by David Lewis, Thomas Baker.
Lines composed a few miles above Tintern Abbey, William Wordsworth, Oxford University Press, 1944.
Gilbert Keith Chesterton, Maisie Ward, Sheen & Ward.
Poems of T.E. Brown, Vols. I and II (My Garden and Indwelling), T.E. Brown, University Press of Liverpool, 1952.
Miracles, Walt Whitman.

Amongst the illustrations, although almost all have been redrafted to provide one continuous style throughout, I am thankful to the following authors/publishers for permission to draw upon their original work:

Essential Endocrinology, Laycock and Wise, Oxford University Press, for figure 6-3.
A Histology of Body Tissues, M.Gillison, Livingstone, for figure 6-1.
Hormones, Messengers of Life, Lawrence Crapo, W.H. Freeman and Company, for figures 5-1, 7-2, 10-2 and 10-3.
Mind, Body and Electromagnetism, John Evans, Element Books, for figures 4-4, 7-1, 10-2, 12-2, 12-5 and 12-7.
Polarity Therapy, the Complete Collected Works of Dr Randolph Stone, CRCS, for figures 4-2, 4-3 and 10-1. These three figures are Dr Stone's originals and have not been redrawn, although the text has been typeset.

Contents

Foreword

by Dr James Z. Said

Dr James Said is a naturopathic physician with a deep interest and understanding of the human system as a multi-dimensional, integrated web of complex energy patterns, energized by consciousness. His study and research cover both the life sciences, as well as advanced modern physics, whilst his therapeutic techniques have resulted from a fusion of many disciplines, including chiropractic, Polarity therapy and other forms of energy medicine. He is highly respected in the U.S.A. and elsewhere for his teaching, research and therapeutic skill.

Science is experiencing a fundamental transformation. The basic tenets that describe science's underpinnings are being challenged and re-thought. This shift in paradigm encompasses the scientist as much as it does the body of knowledge being organized.

The scientist, from the standpoint of classical dynamics and thermodynamics, was a dispassionate, uninvolved observer of physical phenomena. His world was mechanistic and knowledge was required to fit the scientific theories of the day in order to gain acceptance as legitimate observation.

With the advent of particle dynamics, relativity theory and quantum mechanics, the scientist had to modify his observational status. He realized that the observer himself altered the outcome of the phenomena being observed. The scientist's observational role could no longer be regarded as purely objective, but rather became empassioned and raised to the status of participant. His theories had to account for his own role, as much as they did the experiment or phenomenon he sought to understand.

Today, field dynamics and vacuum state phenomena are further altering our view of ourselves and our world. We now recognize that a fundamental matrix, or substrate, of energy underlies all physical phenomena, including ourselves. The once observing, then participating, scientist is now as much a part of the study as the event or system he is in the process of understanding. In this paradigm, the scientist acknowledges a unity to all function and structure. The forces that create anything from within this vacuum state, create everything from within it. These same forces that maintain and evolve our world, operate identically on, and within, each of us.

Every physical system that manifests out of the zero-point energy, or vacuum state, appears outwardly to be different from every other physical system. As each system oscillates, or vibrates, it generates a unique waveform, or vibrational signature, which describes the fundamental make-up of that system.

When analyzed, the waveform can be seen as a composite of energy, generally characterized as 'light' and 'sound'. As light, the waveform describes electromagnetic energy with frequencies in the visible part of the spectrum, yielding the colors we register with normal sight, as well as frequencies elsewhere in the spectrum. This includes ultraviolet, infrared, radio or microwave, for example, which yield 'colours' in those parts of the spectrum to which the eyes are not sensitive. As sound, the waveform describes the modulation of energy, with frequencies that are sonic, and thus heard, as well as both subsonic and supersonic frequencies, beyond our normal auditory range.

The vibrations of modulated electromagnetic energy outside our normal visible and auditory ranges can be detected with appropriate instrumentation, enabling us to perceive a much broader range of physical phenomena. When the human body, for example, is viewed as an energy system, we derive a much deeper and more subtle understanding of what the body actually looks like and of what it is made, how it functions or malfunctions, and how it interacts with its environment both externally and internally.

By observing the human energy field and its dynamics, as well as the corresponding structure and motion of the physical human form, we can more specifically research and more clearly appreciate the body's response to both coarse and subtle events. What effect, for instance, does a thought, or a feeling have on each system, organ, cell or molecule in the body? What are the interactive dynamics between our individual energy fields and another's or our pet's, or the foods we eat, or the medications we take? And what of the field effects of the clothes we wear, or the music we listen to, or the structures or places where we live, work and play?

Research to date demonstrates that these questions can be, and are being, answered. The directions for research are virtually inexhausible in their diversity, but in each case they put the researcher himself central to the questions being asked.

We are, after all, an energy system of sound and light interacting with and within a world of sound and light, all vibrating atop a universal vacuum state substrate that supports the manifestation of our being! This is equivalent to a pond supporting the vibrations, or ripples, of a pebble being thrown into it. The event, the toss of a pebble, is recorded on the two-dimensional surface of the pond. Our entering the physical arena is, likewise, an event, but now recorded as oscillations, or ripples, on a multidimensional surface of space-time. And the event, as well as the surface of space-time itself, emerge for a vacuum, or zero-point energy state – a state of essence, or latent being, which carries the blueprint, or primary template of physical phenomena and experience.

Already much research has been conducted leading to a greater understanding of the essential energy state of our being and our worldly experience. The beginnings of this research perhaps even predate recorded history, but, at least, much of this knowledge has been preserved in some of our earliest documents delineating human understanding. John Davidson has combed a large body of literature, both ancient and mystical, as well as current leading-edge science, and has synthesized similar understandings that are both historical and cross-cultural. The resulting manuscript, *The Web of Life*, is a provocative venture into the correlations of many seemingly diverse ways of viewing ourselves and our world as dynamic systems of energy.

John Davidson's work begins to explore the language and conceptual framework that are emerging as a wholly new paradigm of understanding our life experience. His concepts are equally well grounded in both current scientific thinking as well as the more esoteric and equally sophisticated paradigms of the ancient philosopher-scientist and mystic. In both cases, man's understanding of himself is central to understanding his world. And, as both systems acknowledge, with ourselves as the laboratory, the extent to which our understanding can develop and evolve truly has no limit or bound.

Dr James Z. Said
Merlin, Oregon, April 1988

Introduction

In my first book on these topics, *Subtle Energy*, I attempted to paint a universal picture in which all aspects of existence and philosophy could meet in understanding and harmony. In particular, I concentrated upon those aspects of energy within our human experience which are more readily accessible to our conscious and sensible intelligence, that is: the 'outer' physical world, together with its more subtle factors, the energies of our human mind and emotions, as well as the dense and subtle energies or matter that envelop our inner consciousness and which we experience while being corporeal human entities.

Specifically, I tried to demonstrate that the principles of modern western science are quite compatible with the ancient wisdom of the east and that really, we are all trying to achieve the same objective – namely to make some sense out of the human situation in which we find ourselves. The manner or idiom of our expression may vary according to culture, but the same essential factors always manifest themselves. I did also point out that the eastern wisdom – especially of Indian and Sanskrit cultures, with which I am personally most familiar – can provide a far deeper underlying conceptual, as well as practical framework on which to understand both mystic, human, biological and outward physical phenomena.

In this present book, *The Web of Life, Life Force – The Energetic Constitution of Man and the Neuro-Endocrine Connection*, I would like to expand on the relevance of the eastern understanding of the energies that give us physical life and indeed provide the controlling, organizational and adhering factors that mould inert matter into the form and shape of a living body in which the soul or consciousness may temporarily reside.

This means, once again, a fusion of eastern understanding – worked out in personal, subjective inner experience by centuries of yogic and mystic practice – with modern biochemistry, physiology, physics and western concepts or descriptions of the world and the bodies we inhabit.

In particular, I would like to describe the parallels and interconnections between (on the one hand) polarity or duality as a universal and essential principle; the five *tattwas* or elemental conditions or fields of energy; mental energies; the *pranas*; the *chakras* or centres of pranic energy distribution in the body; the human mental, emotional and subtle apparatus, and (on the other hand) modern discoveries in neuro-endocrinology, genetics and the peripheral and central nervous systems.

Finally, I would like to suggest some ways in which the integration of this knowledge can be used for further research and in the formulation or development of therapeutic practices that can use this knowledge for human betterment. For knowledge needs manifestation in practice for its fulfilment.

I must, I think, apologize if my style of writing is sometimes overly forthright and spells out theories or concepts as if they were proven realities. For myself, many of them make such good sense that I go along with them wholeheartedly. I am, for example, fully convinced of the mystic expression of life as an experiencable reality and it is from this that the concept of energies "being created or manifested from within themselves" takes its shape. But some ideas are just ideas, part of the adventure of life.

However, I do not in any way feel that any of the ideas expressed herein should be shared by all. All I can suggest is that each one of us must always encourage and keep fresh their awareness of being alive and, according to his or her own predisposition, make whatever attempt they can to unravel the mystery of their own life, for themselves.

I am, therefore, fully aware that these concepts are only *possibilities* for some, while remaining sheer nonsense to others. But rather than continually break up the text with such comments as, "it seems to me", and "I think that" or even "according to my perceptions", I have ploughed on regardless and trust to my reader's goodwill and understanding. Maybe that is naive, but life requires exuberance for its full outward expression. It is not a game for the lily-livered and the faint-hearted. One cannot always be looking over one's shoulder. So I simply invite you to join in the fun, but not necessarily to agree with any of it. That is purely your own choice. But keep an open mind. One has nothing to lose, and life is definitely a mystery that requires *some* answers and consideration. And one cannot simply leave such a search to others.

A book of this nature is necessarily incomplete in the sense that much detail, especially upon the western analytical side, has to be condensed. The intricate mapping by research scientists of biochemical pathways and interactions in all bodily mechanisms, not just in the cellular synthesis of hormones, is a work of laborious skill, much of which, though fascinating to me personally, needs to be omitted in order to concentrate on the principles to which the book is addressed. If this book has an audience amongst some of these scientists, its final practical outcome may be the seeking for even more fundamental patterns and interactions underlying those already revealed. For therapists and physicians of all callings, I hope it provides an insight into the life energy principles and their relationship to modern methods of scientific explanation. To the 'general reader', if such a term has much meaning, I hope it will stimulate and perhaps clarify some of the puzzles we all face as part of being human.

Reading the conventional accounts of biochemistry, physiology and the intricacies of life forms, it is very clear that the essential difference between inert matter and matter that has been woven into a unique and complex tapestry in the body of a living creature, is not fully appreciated for what it is. Existing scientific paradigms maintain that life itself is nothing more than inert matter in complex patterns. The ancient wisdom of all cultures, however, has pointed out that consciousness is prior to matter and is the essence of life. Life and consciousness are ultimately synonymous and it is the presence of life within the physical body of a living creature, even a lowly plant or bacterium, that maintains the scientifically observable complexities of life processes. When the life departs, the complexity *immediately* begins to decay. This is a subject I return to many times during the course of this book.

For this reason, therefore, I maintain that *the LIFE FORCE needs to be 'discovered' in the same way that Newton 'discovered' gravity*. It is the key that will enable students of the life sciences to gain a deeper perception of what is going on. It is the missing factor that must be accounted for in all biological theories, including Darwinian ideas concerning evolution.

It provides the link for understanding the relationships between brain and mind. It is the bridge that allows the neuro–physiologist and the psychologist to talk to each other coherently.

All these topics are discussed, often in detail, in the appropriate sections of this book.

I have, in places, delved in some little detail into biological processes, but, in every instance, I have only used scientific terminology after first defining it. If, even then, you find yourself a little out of your depth, it does not matter. Because this is not a textbook on such subjects and you only need say to yourself, "Ah, what he is trying to point out is that its biochemistry and physiology is both beautifully organized and complex" – and then skim through to the end of that section.

The scientific detail is interesting to myself because it exemplifies the basic principles of the life force and of energy in action, and in each one of these instances only enough detail is given to indicate the pattern by which things happen. But if you find it difficult, then just read those paragraphs very lightly. Also, there is absolutely no need to memorize facts as you go along, and there is an index to help you refer back to things if need be. Knowledge is to be enjoyed, not made an object of agony!

When I first began to write this book, I had no idea of the excitement and adventure that lay before me. I had long studied eastern philosophy. I was trained in the life sciences and I had worked in Cambridge University's famous Department of Applied Mathematics and Theoretical Physics, (but not as a physicist), where Professor Stephen Hawking and the theoretical physics group have done all their work on the theoretical basis of black holes and grand unified theories. And although I knew that the yogic way and the scientific way had both to be looking at the same reality, though from different points of view, I never realized how exactly these approaches would marry.

Every part of scientific knowledge fits within the greater framework of the inner wisdom. The problem with this book has become not one of finding material to include, but of deciding what to exclude to prevent it becoming unwieldly and bogged down in details, especially those of a biological nature. Yet it is essential to put enough in to demonstrate to many different kinds of people, with a wide variety of backgrounds and personal philosophies, that there is a correlation and a deeper paradigm in which to view life and science, if one is interested in looking.

It is said that history repeats itself, meaning thereby that patterns re-occur in all things. This is true, but certainly within recorded history our present situation has never before been documented. We are at a crossroads, with the potential to follow paths to disaster or betterment. It is time, therefore, to drop our prejudices and to realize how insignificant are our personal egos, desires and ideals. Modern communications and science have stirred up the energies of our planet so that the cultures are mixing in ways never before imaginable. "We already have enough information to transform our lives", wrote Simon Martin in his foreword to *Subtle Energy*. This is also true, but we must develop the consciousness, awareness and desire to make that synthesis of information and knowledge take practical form. This book is just one adventure in that direction.

John Davidson M.A. (Cantab)
Cambridge, September 1986

Poetic Interlude

*Ask that I may be forgiven if my pen
has gone astray or my foot has slipped,
for to plunge into the abyss of the Divine
mysteries is a perilous thing and no easy
task is it to seek to discover the Unclouded
Glory which lies behind the veil.*

Al-Ghazali

CHAPTER I

The Human Constitution

A Mystical Synopsis

All the mystics, in all the ages, have expressed the same truth. Man is a soul. In his inner being, in his essence, man is a drop of the Divine Ocean, the Supreme Being, Universal Consciousness. Travelling outward from this Source – outward, not in terms of space, but rather in the quality and complexity of vibration and manifestation – the soul becomes clothed in bodies or vehicles of increasingly complex and dense energy patterns, his attention becoming more and more outward. In the human condition, this outward direction of mental attention has become habitual to such an extent that at this far pole of the creation, the physical universe, he is so encumbered and entrapped in the outworking of the attributes of Universal Mind and matter that he is quite unable to know who or what he is. Indeed, in the majority of cases, he is hardly aware, in a real sense, that he is alive. The central, burning question as to what he is and what he is doing in this world is smothered by the incessant demands of his senses and his involvement with the outward show of motion and activity.

More specifically, in its descent, the soul first encounters the Universal Mind, where the qualities and attributes of energy and matter as they appear in our familiar physical world are first manifested. Sanskrit, as well as modern mystical understanding, talks of three sets of energy plexi related to qualities within the vibrational fields of existence. These qualities are also known as the *tattwas*, roughly translatable as the *elements*.

They are, in descending vibrational fineness: *akash*, *air*, *fire*, *water* and *earth*.

These five tattwas first arise in the *Causal region* of the Universal Mind, where they are the highly subtle essence or blueprint of those found in the true *Astral region* or region of *Sahans Dal Kanwal*. This is the *Thousand Petalled Lotus* or *Sahasra*, the glittering and entrancing powerhouse from which all creation below takes its existence and form. These five states then reflect once again within the physical form with which we are familiar, though indeed I would say that we are only partially aware of its real constitution. Man's physical form is thus constructed of the five tattwas in both their gross and subtle aspects.

The naming of these tattwas by their material, outwardly physical manifestation – though common practice – can be misleading. So let it be said right away that all energy substance is of the tattwas. This we *experience*, through our physical form, not only as the material phases of matter, but also as the energetic substrate of our emotions, our sensory perceptions and our motor responses. This will be discussed more fully, as we progress.

As in all coherent energy systems, order and organization is required for its maintenance and existence, and this we see most clearly in the superbly structured, yet adaptable, nature of living organisms, where these tattwas are merged one with another into the highly intricate matrix of interconnections that is observed from without by western biological science. One should not, however, make the mistake of discounting these eastern ideas as quaint, but possessing no practical application, for reasons we shall discover in the ensuing chapters. They represent a fundamental and essential understanding of energy interchanges within both inert matter and living organisms.

Indeed, while western science has no fundamental answer as to how a body holds together and why it should suddenly die and its processes almost immediately cease, the eastern wisdom is replete with understanding that is in no way incompatible with scientific descriptions. Eastern wisdom, does in fact provide an underlying conceptual framework, without which much of western science appears haphazard and almost meaningless. Certainly, the intense analysis characteristic of our western idiom holds out very little hope of providing answers to the fundamental questions of life, consciousness and what happens before and after death.

Pranas, Chakras and Tattwas

Our living human form, then, is constituted of an intricately woven fabric of the five tattwas in gross and subtle state. The weaver and integrator of this fabric is ultimately our soul, our consciousness or real life, deep within, but in physical manifestation its cohering and life-giving power flows out as the vibration that patterns and organizes these tattwas. The Sanskrit term for this subtle, vibrational pattern-maker is *prana*, roughly translated as *life energy* or *life breath*.

Flowing like a complex wave through water, prana flows through the tattwas in their subtle state, creating the energetic blueprint out of which the gross physical body is formed. This subtle blueprint has been called the etheric body and contains within it six major centres of resonance, organizational plexi, five of which relate to the energetic density and quality of the five tattwas in their subtle form, plus one higher control point.

These six plexi are known as the *chakras* and the pranic vibration, being modulated by the quality of the tattwa within which it is vibrating, also takes on the appearance of possessing five states. The pranas are therefore also stated to be five in number.

Because of the life-giving qualities of the pranas, related to the higher intelligence or consciousness within, these chakras are more than just the primary nodes in a wave-form, but are spinning wheels of organizational power.

The Indian yogis and mystics, therefore, describing these centres in the way attuned to their own nature and according to the understanding and idiom of their culture have ascribed a named, controlling deity or *deva*[1] to each chakra and it is from here that the thousand lesser 'gods' of *Hinduism* have come into being. *Brahma*, for example, is the deity of the watery quality or state of matter, expressing itself in the physical body at the sacral or sex centre, responsible for the creation of physical bodies and the control of the watery 'humours' within the body. The embryo, for example, develops in the amniotic fluid, while the kidneys – part of the water controlling system of the body – are also partly under its influence.

[1]See over page for footnote

The pranas, flowing out from the level of the physical mind, just above the sixth chakra at the eye level, provide the energy and organizational qualities required to weave these tattwas into a functioning living body. Impressed from within by the energy of our *karmas*, the effects of previous actions, thoughts and desires etched into the fabric of the *Antashkarans* or organ of physical mind and thought, and enlivened by the higher mind and soul, the pranas are the life-giving vibration that intricately moulds the tattwas into the form of our physical body, familiar to our senses.

[1] Andrew Rawlinson Ph.D., writing in a 1986 edition of *Religion*, provides an excellent appreciation of these devas and subtle tattwas when he writes, "The physical world is a coagulation of subtle or essential elements. All physical forms are as they are because they exist within, and are held together by, these subtle energies. 'Physical forms' here means not only the properties of individual things (for example, the shape of a tree or the behavioural pattern of an animal) but also the characteristics of physical locations (eg. a pool and its banks, a forest on a hillside). There are in fact no individual entities as such; they only appear individual when the field of which they are a part is ignored.

"This worldview, however, is not quasi-scientific. That is, it does not attempt to relate individual things to their environment as if all the factors that are being related are on the same level. On the contrary, it is a heirarchical worldview. The elements or energies which imbue, or give rise to, physical forms exist at a higher level. And more than that, they are both living and intelligent – in a word, they are conscious. Or, in the terminology of Indian religion, they are *devas*.

"Let us restate this principle – and then extend it somewhat. The physical universe cannot be understood apart from the living, conscious forces – the devas – that have given rise to it. A deva is therefore both a being and a principle. The word 'being' implies a personal force and word 'principle' implies an impersonal force, but there is no real distinction between the two. A deva expresses itself (both consciously, which is the 'being' side, and automatically and lawfully, which is the 'principle' side) according to its place in the hierarchy of devas. Thus a 'high' deva has a large range of influence and a 'low' deva has a more restricted range. Whatever exists within a deva's range is in effect under its protection and control.

"Now we must link this hierarchical model of devas with the idea of the elements that make up the world. Different devas have different qualities. When they 'express' themselves, so to speak, they naturally give rise to different physical forms (in both the senses that we mentioned earlier) that embody these qualities. The Indian religious tradition has a number of terms for these subtle qualities: *guna*, *dhatu*, *bhuta*, *tattwa*, *rasa*."

This physical mind (antashkarans), the subtle organ of thought, is found in a sub-astral chakra, the lowest of the astral set, located above the six physical chakras.

In this respect, it is easy to see how, at death, in the absence of the complex, vibrational pranic patterning, containing a reflection of the higher creative life principle of *Shabda*, the subtle and gross tattwas that once constituted a living body, degenerate into a far simpler form of manifestation. Complex molecules break down, integrated biochemical networks lose vitality and coherence, electro-biological activity ceases and – given time – the five basic elements or constituents merge back and separate out into the relatively still and simple tattvic reservoirs of inert matter.

Just look about you at the non-living substance of the physical world. See how, in the absence of an inner life force, its molecular structure has simplified and become, comparatively speaking, still. How earth, water and air have largely separated out. Perceive the sharp demarcation in vibrational and energetic quality between your living body and the dead matter surrounding it. Being aware of your own being, mind and consciousness, expand your understanding of how life is not just a fortuitous and temporarily self-sustaining conglomeration of molecules and electricity, but has inner dimensions beyond the most powerful of microscopes. And how that inner life force is the most important aspect of your being.

Prana, however, is not consciousness itself, but a step-down or derivative, thereof. In addition, consciousness or soul is entangled in the human being with the physical mind or organ of thought. Mystics describe the soul and mind as being "knotted together at the *eye centre*" – the two-petalled lotus of the ajna chakra. Consciousness, in its pure form, does not descend below this eye centre. We experience this mixture of mind and soul as our *attention* and without deep meditation and mystic experience, it is not possible for us to know easily which is which, with the exception that it is the mind which pulls us out to the senses and the physical world and it is the soul, together with the higher aspects of the more inward mind – beyond thought processes – which draws us within.

In subsequent chapters we embark upon a specific description of these chakras and tattwas, but firstly let us continue with certain fundamentals of universal philosophy.

A considerably fuller description of the higher mystic energy patterns is given in the book, *Subtle Energy*, as well as other literature. I am attempting here simply to introduce the concepts of the tattwas, the pranas, the chakras and the antashkarans, as the primary energy patterns covering the soul and higher mind in the human constitution, so that we may later see how they reveal themselves in the discoveries of modern physiology.

But first we need to examine some fundamentals.

Polarity and Duality

The great, essential principle underlying all energy manifestation in the universe, both within and without, is that of duality or separation. Every aspect of life, every pattern of creation, every particle of matter, every movement of energy is held in existence by duality or polarity – by fundamental and opposing forces. There cannot be an 'up' without a 'down', a 'yes' without a 'no', a 'left' without a 'right', a 'positive' without a 'negative'.

In nature, we have a continuous panorama of patterns, of ebb and flow. Growth gives way to decay as spring and summer move into autumn and winter. Energy turns from the outward to the inward. Who has not experienced the sweet indrawing nostalgia of the first autumn days? Wet and dry, heat and cold, light and darkness all alternate and while nature is able to adapt itself, the changes become the basis for continued life cycles amongst the species.

In science, we have electrons and protons, acceleration and deceleration, anabolism and catabolism. Whenever a force is found either in physics or the life sciences that performs one function, scientists know that there has to be another equal and opposite force for the maintenance of balance and equilibrium. And this is true at the more outward grosser levels, just as it is true in molecular, atomic and subatomic levels. There is acid (H^+) balanced by alkaline (OH^-), which together form the balance in H^+OH^- or H_2O, water, the universal substrate of organic life on earth.

There are molecules which are the mirror image of each other, left and right-handed molecules so to speak. In nature, for example, almost all amino acids (of which all proteins are made) are *laevorotatory*, while artificially produced, laboratory amino acids are both *dextro-* and laevo-rotatory. The DNA helical molecule, the genetic encoder itself, is only found in a right-handed form, though there is no known scientific reason why this should be so. In many instances, the two kinds of otherwise apparently identical molecule have different properties, even experienced as sweet and bitter, in flavour. The exact role played by this aspect of polarity is not by any means understood, but their effect on electromagnetic radiation, such as light, is to rotate its plane of vibration – hence the terms laevo- (left) and dextro- (right) rotatory.

Male and female aspects are polarized, sometimes into separate bodies, as we find in humans and mammals, while some of the lower species are either hermaphrodite or can even change sex according to the needs of their community. Certain fish, for example, are led as females by one dominant male. But when the male dies, one of the females becomes male, complete with a change to the brightly coloured, outward male characteristics and social role. The social factors here stimulate, via endocrine secretions, or hormones, a change in basic sexual polarity.

Psychological traits amongst humans are also understandable in terms of their essential polarity, which is usually complex. Thus the characterization of *all* aspects of male and female as opposing polarities is incorrect. The man may not be the positive, outgoing, expressive partner in a male-female relationship, nor may the woman play the passive, receptive, indrawn role. But what is required for harmony is *balance*.

In Indian thinking, the polarity or dualism inherent in nature is expressed as the *gunas* or attributes of mind and matter. In Chinese Taoist philosophy they are thought of as the balance of *yin* and *yang*. *Rajas guna* or *yang* is the positive, outgoing, expanding polarity while *tamas guna* or *yin* is the negative, receptive, indrawing, cohesive quality. The balance is the *sattvas guna*, also known as truth or harmony. It is the zero point of origin from which arise the plus and minus of rajas and tamas. In place of the sattvas guna, the Chinese simply talk of the balance of yin and yang. This zero balance point is, however, a real state, with the constituents of the substructure which result in the zero or balanced condition being of great importance in influencing the nature of that balance. In more general terms, the same harmony can be achieved in many ways.

In any rajas or yang activity there comes a point where the outward energy is expended and an indrawing must occur. Thus the tamas or yin state is a time of consolidation, of building up of resources, of apparent inertia and decay. After which the energy is reversed in action and flows outward once again.

On the downswing of a pendulum, for instance, energy is being expended and the motion is rajas or yang. Then on the upswing, energy is conserved, condensed and stored. When the 'storage' is complete, then this potential energy is expressed outwardly once again – and down falls the pendulum in its arc. These cycles may be long or short; and there will be cycles within cycles, within cycles, too, almost ad infinitum.

This duality and cyclic patterning is apparent in all the universe. The evolution of the Big Bang and the Expanding Universe concepts into one of an expanding and contracting universe would mirror exactly the ancient Sanskrit writings concerning *pralaya* or dissolution. Everything comes into being (rajas, yang) and goes out of being (tamas, yin) and in the process provides the framework or the energy for the next becoming. How avidly we gardeners spread the rotten, dead remains of plants onto the ground so that the new generation of plants may be strong, healthy and vibrant. But how does the dead give rise to life? Because energy is conserved and recoiled, ready for the next spring into existence. And so it is with universal activities – our bodies, too, undergo pralaya or dissolution after their alloted span.

Planets and suns coalese, providing the warmth and nourishment necessary for life, and then expand and explode. Then, once again, they condense (it is said) even to the extent of becoming a black hole from which little, if anything, can escape. But ultimately, even the intense concentration of energy in a black hole must give rise to an instability and a need to move outward once again. That is unless a black hole ultimately becomes a point of suction or dematerialization of energy back into the subtle state, part of the mechanism of pralaya. Nothing in the universes of mind and matter is eternal. Ebb and flow are an intrinsic part of the pattern.

In the world of subatomic energies, we find the same principles at work. Within the atom, electrons are paired with protons, 'up-quarks' with 'down-quarks', and so on. Electrons, too are paired with each other in terms of their equal and opposing spin, making an effective zero or balance in their magnetic field. And all other characteristics are balanced, so that existence may continue.

At subtle levels of energy, in pranic, tattvic, emotional and mental energies, the patterning of polarity is also intrinsic and essential. There must be a point, therefore, where the subtle becomes the physical. And this point will lie in the movement, the charge, the mass, the electromagnetic force and other properties of both subatomic and subtle energy. The subatomic, being created out of the subtle, will carry the polarity aspects through the 'curtain' into physical manifestation. And the harmony or balance of these energy fields will be of great importance in the overall balance or harmony of the gross physical matter thus projected or manifested. In our environment therefore, we will perceive good and nourishing vibrations or atmospheres, whilst in our bodies we will experience them as good health and harmony.

The world of the subatomic, therefore, being so close to the subtle, carries within it the necessary seeds of energy which, when rearranged correctly, can bring about a cure of both simple and complex disorders.

Life Patterns and the Chinese Elements

The Chinese understanding of yin and yang is further expanded in their system of elements. Unlike the Sanskrit and tantric descriptions of the tattwas, which represent real energies, the Chinese elements are understood as the manner of expression or essential attributes of energies in manifestation. They represent the patterning and mode of activity of energy, like an analysis of waveform according to polarity.

Thus their elements of *water, wood, fire, metal* and *earth* can best be understood through the example of the seasons, through the swing of a pendulum or through the process of purification of metals – a process known to Chinese chemists long before it was discovered by our European ancestors.

Water energy is winter, the extreme of the yin condition. It is full of stored, potential energy, the dampener of all activity, the receptive medium of all substances, the universal solvent. It is the resting phase of in-drawn tranquility, the meditation before action, the point of motionlessness at the highest level in the swing of the pendulum. It is the potential in a seed, the core of being, ready to expand into life.

Emotionally, and mentally, water energy is our centre point, our inner potential, our will to continue in existence and to care for ourselves; it is our point of stillness and balance, of quiet self control.

Physiologically, it is the power inherent in the sperm and the ovum, the biochemical potential locked into the DNA genetic coding, significantly coiled, potential energy ready to spring.

It is physical strength and endurance, representing the solids and fluids of our body, where energy is condensed into material form. It is the strength of the spine that gives the body its focal point of energy distribution. Upon the spine, the head and major sense organs are situated; within the spine lies the bodily messenger system of the nervous system and subtle energy administration centres of the chakras. From the spine are articulated the arms and legs which permit us movement in the physical world, without which we are paralyzed. And from the spine are 'hung' all the major bodily organs, while along its length runs the aorta – the conveyor belt through which blood and nutrients are passed to the vibrating tissues of our physical being.

When in balance and conserved, water energy provides the springboard for the next cycle of activity; when deficient, the next cycle lacks tone, quality or flair. It goes off with a fizz, not a bang. A hard, dry winter brings a vibrant and glorious spring, while a warm, wet winter allows rot and disease to penetrate. Low water energy results in physiological, emotional and mental insufficiency and weakness – fear, suspicion, lack of resistance, premature aging and a general absence of vitality. Vitality itself is not of the water energy, but its expression requires the cyclic indrawing and potential coiling of the full yin condition.

This potential for energy storage is dissipated by unbalanced activity in the yang phases – excess in all its manifestations, emotional, mental and physical, such that it becomes difficult to withdraw into a resting or water condition. The key to health and happiness lies in balance and a control of the mind and senses by the inner essence of our soul or consciousness.

Water energy, then, represents the state of rest, the full height of the pendulum swing, the quiescence of winter. Quite suddenly, however, movement occurs. The inner potential seeks expression and a new cycle of being manifests. This is the energy of *wood*. Wood is new yang, the first flush of coming into being. It is Spring and Birth. It is the rapid development of the embryo and the newly-born, the first irrepressible growth of green shoots and leaves from root or branch.

It is the energy of the first movements from rest, the initial acceleration of the pendulum, the expansion into being. Life flourishes carrying all of nature with it. It is the energy behind the procreative urge, the vital power in the early period of creative thought or action; the elation of new growth, the bursting forth of potential, the reawakening of our inner beings. It is both vigorous and invigorating. Who has not felt the special joy of Spring, the energy of new ideas, the expansive expression of freshness? Even the birds sing as they do at no other time and the spring pageant of flowers seems to have a vibrancy of life and colour that passes after the first buxom flourish of the early rise to life.

In desert climates, it is the rainy season when all of life, forced into quiescence by the heat and dryness of high summer, is suddenly released. Here we see that the term *water* can be misleading if taken literally, for it is absence of the watery substance that forces the withdrawal into the yin or resting state. Similarly, with all the other descriptions of the Chinese elements, one has to perceive the meaning through relation to one's own experience. Over-intellectualism and conceptualization will prevent the deeper understanding from breaking through.

Suppression of our woody nature leads to frustration, anger, and even violent emotion manifesting ultimately as dullness, lethargy, depression and toxic conditions within body tissues. Dammed water becomes stagnant. Energy needs to flow for its healthful expression in all the phases of life, or else it becomes destructive. This we see in sociological circumstances where a person's creative talents remain unutilized. One whose work does not permit their expression must find an outlet for them in other areas of their life if their emotional and physical well-being is to be nourished and remain truly healthy. This is the energy patterning and manifestation inherent in 'job satisfaction' and in feelings of fulfilment in one's daily life.

Different natures and personalities have tendencies at various points on the swing of the elemental forces of yin and yang. Some are more 'watery', stay-at-home, quiescent, receptive, sensitive, placid; some are more active, creative, 'woody' or 'fiery'. Each of us is endowed with all of the aspects, but we manifest more of some parts of this spectrum than others. And this is essential for the balanced expression of life: together we make one whole, and life continues. There are those who are meant to be the creators, those who sustain and those who take apart or condense, bringing activity to a state of rest once more, before its energies are dissipated and lost. Nature has places for all the fine divisions of activity within this spectrum, all of which are necessary for the continued well-being and balanced life of our planetary ecology. The diversity of species is, energetically speaking, quite essential, one of the reasons why destruction of natural habitats and species will sooner or later rebound back upon us with an equal and opposite force. It is inevitable, though it may be channelled, if action is not left until it is too late.

After spring, comes deep summer, full yang, *fire* energy, the on-going outward expression of growth and life. It is the summer garden of Delius with the constant and busy hum of insects, the vibrant flowering and growth of plants, the waving grasses, the joy of being alive, the fullness of being. It is cooperative and balanced interchange; the busy market place; the urge to give, to care and to love. It nourishes our beings, as well as our biochemistry; it is the full flood of life – peaceful, flowing activity.

When inhibited or blocked it leads to tension, manifest-ing itself in emotional and bodily disorders. Energy is often blocked in the neck, shoulders and head leading to soreness; the mind is unquiet and runs riot. It is the tension and over-excitement of the creative person who either cannot give, or is blocked in his giving by a refusal to accept in those around him or her. It can be a direct personal selfishness or an obstruction in the need to give. More frequently it is a combination of both. Giving is thus its own reward, for we thereby nourish ourselves, in a very real and energetic sense. If the full and wholesome cycle of our fire energy does not find adequate expression, then hyperactivity and a tendency to overextend ourselves is the end result, with symptoms of sleeplessness, hysteria and emotional problems, with a feeling of the head about to burst. Physiologically it is 'living on adrenaline', a hyperactive metabolism, an acid system and much more besides.

The solution lies in balancing one's life, finding ways to give of oneself, of cooperative activity with one's family and associates, of finding points of harmony and expand-ing them across the structure of one's life. And physiologi-cally one can give release to pent up energies by taking exercise, seeking appropriate therapy, careful adjustment of diet, modifying one's living patterns and, if one can, meditation.

The high speed and the pressures of our modern life have made imbalance in the outgoing expression of the 'fire' energy, a symptom of our times, something we all need to be aware of and bring into balance.

Metal energy is the time of fruitfulness, of harvest, of the achievement of objectives. In ancient Chinese chemistry, gold and other metals were first subjected to fire, to intense heat, in the process of their purification. Fire itself is created out of wood, which is burnt. As the metal runs out into ingots, it is cooled with water, thus stabilizing the metal energy. So this cycle, common to the ancient Chinese mind, may perhaps be the basis for the terms used to describe the changing flow of yin and yang.

Metal is the nostalgia of autumn, when energy is moving inwards once again. There is an automatic shed-ding of that which has served its purpose. The leaf has drawn the energy of sunlight into the heart of the plant and now dies. The seed and fruit come to fullness, potential energy for the next cycle. Frequently, seeds require the hard frost of winter before they can sprout: the cycle has reached completion, but the energy needs deep recoiling and maturation before it can burst forth once again into vigorous new growth. The time of metal energy allows us to draw in our resources, letting go of what is useless – discarded autumn leaves – before entering the water phase of deep stillness, receptivity and potential. If we are not nourished by our activities, we become tired and lacking in energy. Neither our mental, emotional nor physical life possess vibrancy or tone. We drift from day to day, feeling over-stretched by our creative, yang or busy phases and depressed or lethargic during the quiet times. If we better understood the patterns of our life, we would respond with greater awareness to the processes and live in harmony with the changing seasons of our being.

Similarly, would we better understand both nature and our fellow humans, allowing life the space it needs when called for and being on hand to provide support when our own input is required. Blind adherence to conditioned, sociological patterns and expectations leave us without the inner strength of adaptability to changing circumstances and moods, and lacking in intuition, finesse and timing in our most essential interactions and activities. Metal energy allows us to let go of emotional attachments that no longer carry meaning or relevance. Autumn, therefore, holds the pangs of nostalgia, even occasioning fits of grief or melancholy as we try to hold on to what is passing from us; but this mood, when correctly understood, can lead to inner sweetness as we follow the current within, without resistance, to peaceful receptivity and calm.

Often, we are afraid to enter within ourselves in meditative repose, but keep ourselves unnecessarily occupied, frittering away our precious life in trifles, failing to follow the call of our inner being as we follow the ingrained habits of a million or more lifetimes. Perhaps we think that 'life' will pass us by, if we take time out for achieving inward composure and letting go. Tensions develop as we hold onto what is gone and the frustrated emotion is stored as blocked energy patterns in the chest and upper thoracic areas of our body and spine, causing pain and respiratory difficulties. Over-release is exemplified by a flood of self-indulgent emotion, often accompanied by sobbing. These are the tears that are a part of the drama of the emotionally insecure, peeping through weeping fingers to gauge the effect of the scene.

Within all these four major phases, there lies a balance. Each one, when manifest in harmony with the others and in its due season, fulfils an essential role in the outworking of life's energies. This essence or balance is known to the Chinese as the *earth* element. It is akin to the sattvas guna of Indian thought. It is that which maintains all that is positive and healthful in each of the four phases. It is the centre of being within each, where energy in not wasted but used or conserved according to the best requirements of the moment. It is a pendulum in regular swing, not disturbed, wobbling or out of synchronization. Rigorously, it is the still point of suspension which permits the pendulum to swing in harmonious activity and without which tamas and rajas, or yin and yang, oscillating motion cannot arise.

Earth, therefore, is the energy of healthful ease, the bodily harmony that manifests as well-being, at all levels. It is a well-toned musculature, a clear mind, a vibrant circulation of blood and body nutrients accompanied by the easy elimination of waste products. It is the steady in-breathing and out-breathing that accompanies a peaceful heart. The earth energy gives one a broad and tolerant outlook on all of life, a balanced perspective that sees one through the changing tides with an easy and understanding mind. Overabundance of apparent balance leads to nit-picking and obsessive concern over detail in an egocentric attempt to achieve equilibrium, while under-activity is manifested in an over-tolerance to that which is clearly unhealthy or incorrect.

It is quite clear, therefore, that these Chinese 'elements' represent very real states of life, a more intricate mapping of the ebb and flow of yin and yang than is expressed in simple terms of duality. Within all life and energetic processes, these patterns are inherent; the one is present within the other. All energy is movement and all life is energy and consciousness. Creation means activity and polarity, and these elemental patterns are found as the intrinsic, essential 'beingness' of motion, from the smallest particles of the subatomic realm, to the in-breathing and out-breathing of the universe; from the inner regions of the higher mental domains to the vagaries of our human thought and emotion; from the primal, first created energy to the subtle essences that maintain our bodies as expressions of that inner life force.

Sattvas Guna – The Zero Point of Balanced Potential

It may need to be emphasized that the nature of the sattvas guna is not exactly that of the harmonious sum of the rajas and tamas aspects. Rather, it is the point of balance that gives rise to these creative and inertial principles. It is not so much the product or result of the combination of the two, but more the balanced potential out of which tamas and rajas both manifest. The harmony of sattvas is therefore more real than the activity and inertia of rajas and tamas, though it is itself created – and therefore ultimately unreal.

In the step-down process of creation from within, the sattvas guna is seen in the zero points of the inner skies, or akash, which we find as the physical vacuum giving rise to the grossly manifest physical world. It is also the point of suspension in a pendulum and the fulcrum of a balance or see-saw.

In mathematics, it means that the zero occupies a more primary point of reality than its expansion into those factors which *arise* from that zero. In science and electronics, it tells us that balanced potential energy of any kind occupies a point of creation for many possibilities and that if we can draw on that potential directly – without the need to first express it in action – then our system will provide us with cleaner and finer energy. It would be akin to extracting or transforming the potential energy present in a body of water because of its height and gravitational attraction, without adopting the grosser approach of pouring it down a hole to drive a turbine, (ie. hydroelectric power stations). It also means that we could extract energy directly from the creative vacuum rather than naively wasting a difference in electrical potential to pump electrons along wires, (the flow of current electricity).

In this regard, one can see that the yin (tamas) and yang (rajas) of the Chinese must be understood within the context of Tao as the inward creative essence. Tao – when expressed as the balance point in the world of duality – also represents the same as the sattvas guna. It is only when balance exists as something underlying and relatively more real that the play of duality (yin-yang or tamas-rajas) can be manifest. The important presence of this balance is often forgotten or misunderstood in modern Western interpretations where yin and yang are seen in a more conceptual fashion. The three gunas are three real energy currents in creation, not as rivers of moving substance, but as patterners of the Divine, Uncreated potential into the worlds of form, both within and without. The primary creative principle being that of the Word, the Logos, the Name or the Shabda.

Thus, in the Chinese elemental model, the sattvas guna is also expressed as earth, the balanced potential within all states. Actually, Chinese mysticism is said to have been derived from Indian sources, just as Buddhism was adopted in China and modified according to their local idiom. This explains why the Indian manner of understanding is (generally speaking) more deeply mystical, because it relates directly to the inward energetic structure of things, while the Chinese manner of thinking is more conceptual.

Karma, Energy and Reincarnation

Everything is created from within itself. The ancient Hermetic[2] axiom: "As above, so below", holds true under all circumstances. 'Within' and 'above', are equivalent, both meaning the same: vibrationally and in essence, closer to the Source. The Source, being one, is beyond duality. It is eternal, complete and self-existent. The idea of causality is totally absent, there being no differentiation. In all lower or outward manifestations, however, the prime law is of cause and effect – both horizontally at the same level of energy vibration and vertically from within to without, and without to within.

---

[2] *Hermes Trismegistus* is a Greek name for the Egyptian god, *Thoth*, who is credited with various mystical works.

This law of cause and effect is known to Indian philosophy as *karma*. Karma means 'action' or 'doing'. Concomitant with duality and polarity is motion and difference, and in the causative links between all motion and action lies this law of karma. Karma is the 'interstitial' law governing all activity and inherent in the manifestations of all matter and energy, which exist only because it is moving, causally, between opposites. Even apparently motionless matter around us is known by modern physics to consist of moving 'particles' and vibrating energy fields.

In our life, we perform actions, both physical and mental/emotional. All our actions make a groove or impression upon our organ of thought, or antashkarans. Severe actions make a strong groove; minute and inconsequential actions make a groove of a light nature. Our thoughts, emotions and desires – fulfiled or unfulfiled – make a similar mark upon our mental apparatus.

When we die, this record of our life – impressed upon our mind – remains with the soul. The body returns to the earth, the pranas and subtle energies 'evaporate' like waves from agitated water when it becomes still; but the record remains, a unique fingerprint of all our activities, thoughts and desires.

This 'black box', the energy plexus, then becomes the energy centre out of which our next life is fabricated. It is the source of our destiny, our *pralabdh* karma, the inner design of our outer life. At our death, if there are too many seeds of actions from the past life to be accommodated in the next lifetime, then the resultant energy or karmic pattern is transposed to a higher level of energy within the higher mind structure. It becomes our store of karmas, our *sinchit karma*. Thus, in future lives, our destiny is drawn partially from the immediately preceding life and partially from the sinchit karmas, being the sum total of unworked-out karma from a multitude of previous lives.

As life succeeds life, the complexity of this energy patterning becomes so immense and so clouding to the higher energies of the Universal Mind and hence of the soul deeper still within, that we become slaves of our karma, our destiny. Contrary to much western thinking upon this subject, this does not imply a fatalistic approach to life; quite the reverse. Man is given arms and legs and is 'expected' – has the capacity – to act according to the highest ideals, but behind it all is a deterministic order and patterning.

If man really had free-will, this world would be utter chaos. Every desire and whimsy would be fulfiled without delay. We would be masters of our lives. Nothing would be unexpected – no illness, no unhappiness, no death – at least not for ourselves! What we may wish upon other people would be another matter! We appear to have a free will because of our illusory sense of ego, of self, and as long as that sense of self-identity remains, then we have to make decisions according to our best discrimination. This world is the plane of action, and act we must, whether we like it or not. And somewhere within the plexus of action and reaction, we have enough conditioned free-will to be responsible for our actions and thoughts, which – making new or *kryaman* karmas – provides the mechanism for rebirth on this plane of existence, after our death.

This subject has innumerable ramifications, beyond the scope of this book, but the aspect which interests us here is that all our health and state of bodily harmony and disharmony is conditioned, through our mental apparatus, into our emotional and physical layers of being. It is destined. And we are also destined and meant to struggle with it. This is a part of the game of life.

So, all our illness or health, come – in a very real sense – from within ourselves. The vibrations of our karmas are reflected and moulded into every cell of our body and every action we perform. Not only that, but everything that happens to us is a manifestation of what lies within our minds. *We* have created the pattern of our so-called outer lives. Our lives reflect our mind and personality in exact detail.

How often do we observe that the same patterns happen to ourselves, our friends and associates, time and time again? Some are born lucky, some contented, some are driven, some always attract misfortune. How? Psychologists are right when they say that it is the function of our personality and subconscious mind that makes things happen to us. But without an understanding of the inner processes of karma and its outworking through the energy fields of the physical plane, the picture is incomplete.

Our bodies and state of health, therefore, are vibrationally patterned by our inner karmas, or the energy patterning which provides the character of our life, from within. All understanding, therefore, of these processes must bear in mind that the underlying pattern which makes an individual unique cannot be totally changed (unless that is also destined, karmically!). It can only be brought into a greater or lesser degree of balance, also according to the destiny of that soul.

All approaches to health, therefore, are those of the philanthropist who attempts to make life better for the inhabitants of the prison. They are attempts to achieve balance. This effort is of great importance, to relieve suffering in the world and in one's own individual life. But the greatest philanthropist of all is the one with the key to the prison, who lets all the prisoners escape from harsh justice. But this is the role of the deepest mystic and its discussion is, once again, beyond the scope of this small volume.

CHAPTER 2

Eastern and Western Idiom

Observation of Life Processes – From Within or From Without

It is well understood by both traditional eastern philosophy and western science that in all nature, there is order and structure. Their views on the origin of all we perceive may be at variance – or at apparent variance – but the yogic and mystic practices of the east as well as their approach to the healing of human ills presumes a cosmic pattern, just as much as western science seeks for essential patterns or natural laws within the universe.

The inherent difference of approach lies in the direction of the search. In the east, man looked within himself by means of specific spiritual exercises in order to discover by personal experience the laws and patterns of nature. The macrocosm is reflected within the microcosm of man, say all their sages. Look within yourself and there you will find the key to all mysteries, whether spiritual or physical. All of life manifests outwardly from within. If therefore one travels inward along these inner pathways, the answers to all questions are found. These answers, however, are not couched in intellectual concepts – the intellect is, after all, only another energy pattern – but the intellect is illumined and able to express its experience in more cogent fashion. The inner experience is then described in the best possible language, without recourse to discursive philosophy and intellectual entanglement.

Traditionally, in the east, the healers of men's physical troubles were also practitioners of yoga and other spiritual practices. They were wise men (or women) whose understanding of human and spiritual mysteries was greater than most. They were respected, even venerated, in their community and their influence and justly ascribed reputation were such that people would travel hundreds of miles to consult them.

Given a universal concept of energy, manifesting itself in multitudinous forms, it becomes easy to understand the two approaches of eastern and western philosophy to the same problem. While western-oriented science tends to analyze the structures and patterns from without, discovering thereby an ever increasing diversity in some aspects (e.g. biochemistry and the life sciences) and an increasing fundamentalism and unity in basic forces (i.e. modern physics), the eastern approach has always been subjective.

The problem, says the eastern philosophy, is life. We do not understand it. However, we are alive, so the study must begin within ourselves. Our own body therefore becomes the laboratory in which the search must be made. To the easterner this means meditational and yogic practices to "enlarge the space within" and provide "room" for our attention to penetrate into the depths of our consciousness. The results are personal and highly satisfying in many ways, but quite unprovable or demonstrable to anyone else, in an outer sense. But this does not make them any the less valid. Indeed, since life is lived, willy-nilly, personally, it makes the approach highly meaningful.

The process, however, reveals not only the inner workings of one's own mind and the universal mechanisms of our subconscious and emotional energies, but it also permits the inner eye to be brought to bear on the mechanisms by which the body functions – that is: its physiology, biochemistry and much more besides. Even in western psychology, one of the greatest thinkers of our time, Carl Jung, was deeply imbued with eastern concepts and drew his psychological writings largely from personal adventures into his own being, also reflected against his professional experience with patients. His approach was therefore largely subjective, but the impression of truth shining through it, is enough to override the normal western objections to this methodology.

The nomenclature, terminology and methodology of the subjective study of physical energy patterns are necessarily different from those of the objective approach, but since they are essentially approaching the same energy complex, the parallels will always be there. What is required is an acknowledgement that the inner approach can greatly enhance the meaning of the outer analysis and even give it new life, energy and direction.

Indian and Chinese Approaches

In India, yogic philosophy became manifested in the healing arts as *Ayurvedic* medicine, which includes the basic philosophy and understanding of energy patterns within the human constitution, as well as practical methods of cure. This includes *hatha yoga*, *pranayama*, herbalism, dietary considerations, conduct of life and various naturopathic practices. Hatha yoga uses specific exercises and stretching postures to enhance the flow of energy around the body, thereby creating more balanced and harmonious body function.

In modern times, the effects of hatha yoga have been researched by a number of yoga practitioners using conventional western techniques. Blood flow and pressure, body biochemistry and general health is definitely improved to a considerable degree. Hatha yoga also contains within its repertory certain exercises to increase energy harmony (and thereby eliminate disease) in particular organs and systems of the body.

Pranayama aims at controlling the flow of pranas through control of breathing and other inner meditational exercises. The pranas, being part of the subtle energy blueprint that controls the organization of body function, are primary in physical health. Pranic balance and well-being precede physical health and conversely, physical health and well-being can be achieved by creating balance and integrity and increasing the 'amount' or intensity of vibrant activity of prana within one's body.

Ayurveda understands the manner of working of the tattwas or elemental states and their control points in the chakras. Ayurvedic herbalism, dietary regimes and naturopathic principles are based upon an understanding of the balance of these elemental fields within the individual patient. Thus, a person lacking in the nourishing energy of the fire element exhibiting itself perhaps as digestive disorders and inability to assimilate food may be prescribed herbs, diet and so on to bring this aspect of their physiology and emotional-mental life into greater balance. The approach is, of course, automatically holistic in the sense that the practitioner immediately seeks fundamental causes rather than merely treating the patient symptomatically.

One may think that treating the balance of the elements for a patient with stomach ulcers and digestive disorders, for example, sounds almost like 'witchcraft', but then the symptomatic approach to the same conditions of painkillers, anti-acid pills and surgery sounds so superficial that one wonders how intelligent human beings got involved in such sorcery! Ultimately, the cause within the individual's life has to be treated – not the external manifestations of inner imbalance.

Traditional Chinese and Far Eastern philosophy pursue a very similar line of practice in the healing arts. The Chinese healing philosophy sees everything as a manifestation of *Ch'i*. Ch'i means energy at a subtle level. The ancient sages, seeking ways of balancing this Ch'i, according to its yin and yang characteristics, evolved healing techniques that included acupuncture and acupressure massage, as well as the more traditional practices of herbalism, consideration of diet and other natural methods.

In fact, the Chinese materia medica contains some of the most powerful herbs known to man. Some of these have even been researched in modern medical institutions where they have become known as *adaptogens* – substances which significantly enhance the body's adaptability to stress, biochemical or otherwise. An aqueous extract of *Astragulus membranaceus*, for example, has been shown to restore immune function in ninety percent of patients with depressed immune response, a characteristic of cancer, as well as AIDS[3].

Traditionally, these herbs are administered according to their specific effect on the bodily organs and systems, encompassed within a philosophy of yin and yang harmonization. And this is not primitive – it is deeply fundamental and requires a degree of spiritual and human understanding that was essential for any neophyte to develop if he

---

[3] *Astragulus* further strengthens adreno-cortical function, also depressed in cancer patients, and ameliorates the negative effect of radiation and chemotherapy on bone-marrow, gastro-intestinal and immune function. For a fuller description see *Radiation* by John Davidson and *Chinese Tonic Herbs* by Ron Teeguarden.

were to serve his fellow human beings in the capacity of physician.

Education and Understanding in the Healing Arts

This disregard of education in true spiritual and human values leaves many modern doctors lacking in any basic framework or paradigm within which to perceive and understand their patients. Those who have developed a higher understanding have done so quite independently of their medical education. The result is a generation of technically trained specialists who may have little or no sensitivity to what is really going on at a deeper level. Even the most obvious and basic perceptive skills and human understanding are lacking in many instances. Treatment is done by the book, by the symptom and by the laboratory test, not by an integration of these symptomatic indicators with a personal knowledge through long consultation between the patient and a doctor whom he trusts, and who understands the basic principles of spiritual and human life.

Teaching in the east was traditionally performed on a personal basis of guru and disciples. The student was not given knowledge until his inner wisdom could accommodate it. The result was that humanity, understanding, compassion and perceptive abilities were developed as primary faculties, which was infused with a specific knowledge of healing techniques, the outcome being a true healer, someone whose very presence had healing qualities.

Modern medical students are fed almost entirely with 'facts', with the result that, since knowledge without inner wisdom has a tendency to increase ego, many people feel upset by the demeanour of their doctor and by his (or her) inability to communicate anything to them that is of real value in their total life. This is, of course, quite dependent upon the human qualities and understanding of the doctor involved, factors which are not related to medical knowledge.

It is for these reasons that people are instinctively seeking out practitioners of the so-called alternative healing arts. Probably the one greatest difference between conventional and alternative practitioners lies, very generally speaking, in the quality of their spirituality and humanity. This greater inward wholeness reflects automatically in their more holistic understanding of nature's processes. This is generally why such people choose holistic rather than allopathic techniques. It is, for example, far more satisfactory, as well as practical, for a patient with heart problems to be advised gently, but with strength, to calm down and change dietary and life patterns, reinforced with treatment and practices that help him in this objective, than it would be for him to be given pills to take whenever an attack is felt.

Many medical people see the wisdom in this approach, but very few are able to bring these methods into a conventional hospital or medical practice. The structure of modern medical practice and theory almost precludes it.

If one examines it dispassionately, one finds that allopathic medicine is completely empirical and reductionist in nature. Conventional medicine is entirely devoid of any theoretical model of what a human being actually *is*. The result is that an analysis of the parts is conducted according to standard laboratory procedures, providing observations which are thought to be objective, but like all experiments in physics or biophysics, represent only the outcome of the interaction between the observer, his equipment and the thing observed.

Furthermore, the experiment, or observation, having been designed according to certain preconceptions, only 'sees' events within the context of these preformed ideas and the highly specialized instrumentation resulting therefrom. Consequently, we only see what we are looking for and medical science proceeds in a blinkered fashion, seeing only that which it sets out to see. This fact concerning scientific observation is well understood in the world of quantum physics, but is almost totally ignored in medical, and indeed most other areas, of science.

I am not suggesting that a reductionist analysis of the parts has no value at all. But we must understand that allopathic medical science and, indeed, much of alternative medicine, too, actually has no model of a human being into which such elements of analytical and experimental processes can be fitted and understood. The result is that an incomplete analysis of the parts, according to only a specific point of view, is considered to be the nature and best description of the whole. This is because there is no fundamental paradigm through which the nature of these parts, *as a whole*, can be understood. So apparently logical conclusions are drawn which, as complete perceptions, are fundamentally flawed, for the underlying preconceptions are, at best, fragmentary.

Thus, for example, the observation that "DNA *relates* to form", or is involved in the process by which form comes into being, is taken to mean the same as "DNA *originates* form". In reality, such a supposition is unjustified. For although part of the relationships may be observable, *it is still quite unknown how the genetic code results in the overall form of the body*, including such 'simple' features as distinctive skin, hair and eye colourations, the shape of the nose and so on. Not to mention its role in intricate biochemical relationships and transformations.

In fact, one can apply this to all medical 'explanations', including such observations as "some viruses and bacteria cause disease," or "some drugs or herbs can cure disease," and so on. Such statements are not wrong, but they are amazingly incomplete and with their accompanying analysis of underlying 'mechanisms', they relate more to our divided, human mental condition which finds it so difficult to understand things as a whole, than to real knowledge of the one, whole, integrated energy of nature.

To really understand, for example, how aspirin, a herb or needling an acupuncture point affects the whole human being, we would need to possess an understanding of the total human energetic constitution and be able to see how our treatment or interaction has modified the condition of the whole. And at all levels, too, physical, subtle, emotional and mental. Just like adding a drop of coloured dye to a glass of water, the influence spreads throughout and a new equilibrium is reached. But an understanding of human energetic structure is not reached by an analysis of all the parts, for what we decide are 'parts' is according to our own preconceptions and theories, and in any event no analysis can ever constitute an understanding of the whole. Neither is there is ever an end to analysis – one can always analyze the 'parts' in greater detail.

So there are many ways of considering this whole

structure. However, since energy is all that *is* in nature, a model of a human being as a multilayered energy structure is the most appropriate image to hold in one's mind. And this is the common denominator in both eastern approaches where we talk of ch'i, meridians, yin and yang, pranas, tattwas and so on, as well as of western approaches where we consider molecules, electromagnetism, electrons and a world of subatomic interactions.

Nature is what she is, and we tend to look at her through the window of our own mental conceptions. So the more we can remove these constraining and largely subconscious conceptions – which condition what we see – the more we will have direct perception and consciousness of what is going on.

Even within the paradigms of current, western scientific knowledge, to approach an understanding of human structure in a reductionist way would require a full comprehension of the body as a subatomic energy dance. This would need to be based more upon our (limited) understanding of energy interrelationships according to quantum and relativity theories than upon the study of molecular interactions, as it is at present. We could no longer, for instance, consider our molecule without also examining its continuous infrared 'emissions'. We may call them emissions, but that is only a convenient handle by which our mind can divide up the observable processes into manageable chunks. But to nature, the molecule and its emissions are all part of one integrated, energetic process of interconnection and relationship. Indeed, the molecule itself is only a convenience of our thought, a way of considering just one part of the overall dance.

The body is really a shimmering sea of energetic movement, an energy dance, a web of interconnection. Molecular and atomic changes take place in nanoseconds, billionths of a second. Molecules, atoms, electrons, subatomic particles, electromagnetic radiation, gravitation – all these are our appreciation of recurrent themes within this dance. They are *our* analysis, nature herself knows nothing of such things. In her workshop, there are only the patterns of duality, relationship and movement. But more of all this later.

So if, therefore, we are to practice the healing arts for the benefit of our fellow humans, we must become open-minded enough to concede that in reality we know very little – that we have a lot to learn. And that the learning may come from a quarter we never previously suspected.

This Little Kingdom – Man

Our human body, made of flesh and bones, is not what we think it is – something solid and ultimately real. It is only the outer skin of a multilayered, multifaceted structure, created from within-out. In our deepest place lies our soul, a part of the Uncreated God. This is our Source. Around Him, lie increasingly complex patterns of energy which we call the creation. These comprise His game, His play, His projection.

Each soul is a drop of this Uncreated Ocean. Around each soul lies a multi-layered web of energy patterns, relating to the layers of the creation. They are a projection from within-out. A microcosm through which we may contact the macrocosm. The human, physical body is the outermost layer of this cosmic onion.

So our body, which appears so real, is just a shifting, moving pattern of projected energy. It has the relative reality of only a projected image upon a screen. Our subtle body, our human mind, our astral and causal bodies, these are the more inward layers around our soul.

What is without is formed from what is within. And when a nearly-outer layer (our human mind) tries to unravel the mystery by looking yet further outward at the most superficial layer (our physical body), then we can understand why there is such human confusion and ignorance. The way we perceive ourselves depends upon the level at which our attention is focused. If we only see the outer layer, then we take the body as the ultimate reality of life. But then we are also confused and cannot make head nor tail of it. If we go within, then we can see that we were only looking at a surface phenomenon.

Subtle physical energies, human mind and higher energies of the mind worlds within, these all lie as the creative pathways through which a human form comes into existence.

And within it all lies our soul, our real life, our consciousness, a spark of the Divine Flame, into which we have the capacity to merge.

Poetic Interlude

Rapt in oblivion, the soul
Doth in a single moment, learn
More than the busy brain and sense,
With all their toil, could ever earn.

Mirrored within its God, it views
Today, tomorrow, and the past,
And faith sees here, in time, the things
That through eternity shall last.

St. John of the Cross

CHAPTER 3

Yogic and Mystic Perceptions

Introductory Concepts

Much of the detailed literature on yoga is written in the Sanskrit language and is therefore inaccessible, not only to most westerners, but also to the majority of Indians, too. Moreover, the writings come from a variety of sources, from yogis and mystics of varying degrees of attainment, and were certainly never put together as a coherent body of explanatory literature. They are rather the outward manifestation of ages of deeply spiritual tradition within the Indian culture, a tradition expressed through innumerable systems of practical spiritual exercises or forms of yoga.

This apparent confusion is not, however, a real drawback, because, as all the texts agree, every aspirant must have a personal *Guru*, or spiritual teacher, to instruct him or her in the spiritual exercises. Just as in all matters of life, there is no substitute for a real, living teacher, the same holds true in an even deeper sense where spiritual and yogic practice is concerned. Moreover, the real aspirant or seeker will automatically be drawn to a guru of the spiritual height to which he inwardly and sincerely aspires. In the same manner as the super-talented musician will automatically find himself in the master class, so too are we drawn to a guru who can satisfy our spiritual needs. This is a law of nature.

The seeker, therefore, will be taught by word of mouth and personal association with his guru. To attempt to learn meditational and yogic practice from a book is never a good idea, however advanced the writer. And because the guru teaches by expression of his own personal experience and requires no book, he is able to make everything clear to his disciple. Any reading that is then done is supported by the transmitted understanding of his guru. Prior to this, the aspirant's reading is a part of his seeking – which ultimately brings him to the feet of a master. "When the *chela* (disciple) is ready, the guru appears," says the ancient text.

I am personally fortunate in this respect that I have been the disciple of a mystic adept of the highest order since the age of twenty-two, after an early life of constant seeking and enquiry, and I can state quite truthfully that all my small understanding of things mystical is due entirely to his unceasing care and attention.

In this book, however, I am in no way attempting to describe the full mystic philosophy, but simply to give some understanding of the human constitution as seen by eastern mystic and yogic spiritual science. I use the word 'science' advisedly and correctly, because science means knowledge and since the aim of mysticism and yogic practice is knowledge of one's own inner being and source, yoga is indeed a true science, though the techniques and paradigms are fundamentally different from those of western approaches to knowledge and understanding.

So, in this attempt to familiarize western readers with traditional Indian and yogic concepts, we must first describe some of the Sanskrit terms which are essential, a few of which have already been used. Language is a means by which we understand concepts and convey our meaning to each other. Thus, if someone describes an object as red, or more precisely, let us say, as vermillion, our up-bringing and education permits us to appreciate a quite exact idea of their meaning.

But suppose that there were no red objects in the English-speaking world and therefore there was no word 'red' or any of its subsets of vermillion, crimson, scarlet and so on – if we were then confronted in a foreign land with both our first experience of red and a range of words to describe it, we would have severe difficulties in our translation and conveyance of the meaning of these new words, to English-speaking people.

Similarly with terminology used in Sanskrit and yogic literature. The attempts to translate words into the nearest similar in the English language immediately requires a re-definition of the English word, such that it now has the meaning to which we are conditioned, plus that which we are now attempting to ascribe to it. The result is a confusion in the mind of the reader or listener.

It seems better, therefore, to say: "Here is a concept with which the English language is not familiar and rather than attempt to translate it into a concept or word which already carries a high degree of conditioned understanding, it would be better to use the Sanskrit word itself and attempt to endue it with the meaning it has in its original language." This, indeed, is how languages evolve, drawing in new words wherever required to enhance communication.

That is all, perhaps, somewhat long-winded, but it is important for us, when understanding new concepts, to know that *we have to step outside what we think we already know*, to countenance something quite completely new and different in our approach to our experience of life. Parallels there will be, but we must try to prevent ourselves from taking an 'alien' concept and insisting that it must fit into one with which we are already familiar. If we have a certain finite number of shapes into which we fit similarly shaped objects and we are suddenly faced with an object that does not fit, we are more likely to appreciate this new shape for what it is if we admit its essential difference and study it, rather than doing our best to compress it into the nearest best fit or discarding it altogether.

In this respect, therefore, we need to understand certain basic concepts and their associated terminology before we can approach the meaning and reality described by their use. Perhaps I should point out at this stage that as far as possible I have returned to exact Sanskrit translations as well as consulting other living practitioners of the mystic path, for clarification of these terms, rather than relying on less immediate interpretations either by western or even Indian writers. The early theosophical writers, for example, were particularly prone to using Sanskrit terminology in their own and often confused manner, sometimes consciously and sometimes, I believe, unknowingly redefining certain Sanskrit terms according to their own understanding.

These early theosophists themselves pointed out that they had no established doctrine. However, the force of personality of some of the early founders has effectively resulted in what is today often considered as established occult or mystic fact, although the degree of spiritual enlightenment or instruction of these writers was not that of the yogis, sages and mystics who originally wrote the Shastras, Vedas, Samkhya and Tantras of Sanskrit literature. In fact, the occasionally hectoring and even arrogant tone of some of their writings is so far removed from that of true mystic literature that one wonders as to their personal motivations.

Indeed, these theosophical writers have themselves stated that they may have made mistakes unintentionally and in some instances even intentionally, a fact which means that while we may profit from their writing in a general inspirational way, we are under no obligation, nor is it necessary, to come to grips with their specific doctrinal presentation or cosmology, since it may be either incorrect, incomplete or a misconstruction of true yogic or mystic philosophy and cosmology. I mention these points of view because of the wealth of theosophical writings and their influence upon modern times including a number of sincere writers and researchers into these and allied subjects. Theosophy is only a very partial presentation of true mystic philosophy and (most essentially) practice.

Some Sanskrit Concepts – Tattwas, Maya, Purusha, Prakriti

It was in the first chapter that the *tattwas* were initially mentioned. In its widest sense, tattwa means something like 'essence' or 'quality of form.' It is most frequently translated as 'element,' but with the immediate qualification that it is not to be confused with our established meaning of that word. Let us therefore call it tattwa and circumvent the problems associated with mistranslations.

Tattwas are 'real' energy in both gross and subtle material and materio-mental realms. They are not concepts or intellectual abstractions, but are real fields of vibrating energy.

Nature's cycles and patterns frequently express these phase or quantum jumps, rather than smooth gradients. At a physical level, we perceive this in the *sudden* molecular or atomic rearrangements which occur when substances move from solid to liquid to gaseous. The same pattern is seen in all events that occur when a certain constraining threshold is reached – whether it is falling over the edge of a cliff, turning a key in a lock, or a crash in the stock market.

There are, as we have said, five such primary tattvic phases. The Sanskrit literature does, however, use the term in more general ways, too. According to descriptions in the Shastras and Tantras, there are three categories known as *Atma*, *Vidya* and *Shira Tattwas*. The *Shira Tattwas* are described as the *pure* category. They relate to changes in consciousness that take place as the soul when first separated from the Source, sees itself as both 'I' and 'That', as a part of one's self or being, but with attributes. These pure tattwas, therefore, relate to the first manifestations of duality within the One.

The *Vidya Tattwas* or *pure-impure* category are those of *Maya*, the weaver of illusion and limitations (called the *Nanchukas*), whereby, for example, the all-knower becomes limited in knowledge and the all-mighty becomes unable to perform all actions – the soul in essence being a drop of the One, perfect, unlimited, almighty and all-knowing Being. Here, the dualism of separation is such that the original acceptance and knowledge that 'That' is a part of oneself is lost and experience becomes that of an 'I' perceiving objects which are separated from oneself. Each soul is therefore also separated from the other, whilst the tattwas, through the agency of Maya, begin to weave the web of bodies, (vehicles or energy systems required for communication and functioning), around the ever-darkening soul. To begin with, the soul knows itself as separate and yet within the object perceived, but, as the coarsity of vibration deepens, it loses even this consciousness and the lower vibration of tattwas are thus categorized as of the *impure* variety, or *Atma Tattwas*.

In our description, the five tattwas are thus Vidya Tattwas in their causal form, at the level of the Universal Mind, but have become Atma Tattwas at the point at which we presently experience them in the physical realm. For they have obscured not only our awareness of our soul, but frequently that of our mind as well. This is why many people think that their mind, thoughts and emotions are due purely to biochemistry and bioelectrical brain activity. They think that mind and body are the same. They have no real awareness of their own mind, consciousness or inner life whatsoever.

To begin with, the pure Being or *Purusha* understands and experiences the universe as created, but homogeneous. He is both consciousness and *Prakriti*. Prakriti means 'primal energy'. Prakriti is then diversified and manifests as mind and matter and the multitude of beings in these universes. This is the region of Universal Mind where the gunas also first arise.

The inner power, then, manifesting at first through Prakriti in the causal realm of Universal Mind, and subsequently via the intermediate agency of the *Sahasra* or *Sanhans-Dal-Kanwal* – the thousand petalled lotus or energy transference power-house in the astral region – then results in the creation of the human mind (*Antashkarans*), the senses (*Indriyas*) and the five tattwas of our physical universe, with which modern writers are most familiar.

Prakriti is the prime cause or essence of material substance. Matter, in the scientific sense, is its final outward expression. Prakriti is that which gives form to the creative power of the One, known as the Shabda, when it reaches the realm of Universal Mind. Form is, in a sense, the result of stress or strain arising within the primal Prakriti under the influence of the three gunas or modes of duality.

The Five Tattwas

According to yogic and mystic understanding, the physical universe is formed from the subtle essence of the five tattwas. These are: *Akash*[1], often translated for want of a better word as ether, *Vayu* (air), *Tejas* (fire), *Jala* (water), and *Prithvi* (earth). It will become apparent from our on-going description that the tattwas are both the subtle essence and the material substance which constitutes their

---

[1] In general, I have used Sanskrit transliterations. In this instance, however, rather than the Sanskrit *Akasha*, I have used the Prakrit form, *Akash* which is used frequently throughout the text and rolls more easily of the tongue. Similarly, I have used *Antashkarans* (human mind), rather than *Antashkarana*, and *Ahankar* (ego) rather than *Ahankara*.

final physical reality as perceived by our senses, and out of which the physical condition is experienced.

These five tattwas are distinct in their individual natures and without the organizing role of life energies from within, these five modalities are inimical to each other. Earth and solids stay in one place, water seeks its own level, air reaches into the space above while the plasmic state of pure physical fire is found only in the sun and the stars, but manifests also in the heat and flame we know of in our daily tangible experience. Akash is the inner well-spring of the other four, the 'space' within which they arise.

In living forms, a most remarkable phenomenon takes place. These otherwise 'antagonistic' states or vibrations are woven into the most intricate and varied patterns, held together by the power of the soul or life within and formed into an organized and integrated whole by the activity of prana. This is the real *morphogenic* or *morphogenetic field* of such writers as Dr Rupert Sheldrake, whose first thoughts along these lines were crystallized into specific theories during his first stay in India, where he was no doubt exposed to Indian philosophy and yogic ideas. He was, however, not unaware of such concepts during his time in Cambridge, prior to his Indian departure. Consciously or unconsciously, spiritual, mystic and yogic science, whether Eastern or Western, have provided the well-spring of so much that is true and beautiful in human life. Indeed, truth, beauty and aesthetic appeal in human experience are simply reflections of the inner reality, which lies beyond all human divisions of nationality and language.

The interplay and fusion, then, of these five elements in our human form accounts for all the varied manifestations of structure and physiology, organs and systems as well as the variations in mood, expression, emotion, personality and thought to which, under the primary patterning influence of our karmas, we are all prone, as human beings.

Mind, Tattwas, Emotion and Personality

The word emotion means to 'move out'. Thus our mind, in its natural concentrated centre in the forehead, between and above the two eyes, moves outwards and downwards playing against the five subtle tattvic fields. This interaction we experience as emotion, our feelings, which find expression in the body. Inwardly, we try to control our emotions from the mind centre in our forehead. When someone is calm, concentrated and unemotional, we say that they are 'centered'. When our attention is spread throughout the body, and – via the senses – moves out into the physical world, we say we are 'scattered'. The scattered person has less control over his emotions. The particular variations of interplay between the human mind and the subtle tattwas therefore gives us an infinite variety of personality traits, with identifiable characteristics provided by each tattwa. This is what represents our unique, but identifiable personalities, the underlying patterns in which the mind and tattwas interact.

So, beginning at the base, the earthy, solid vibration of prithvi has its centre of administration in the rectal chakra, being responsible for the well-being of all the solids in the body – bone, hair, skin, fibrous tissues and so on. The sense of smell and the functions of elimination and excretion are also spun out from this earthy tattwa, whilst psychologically, the characteristics of earthy types are those of solidity, pragmatism and preoccupation with material existence. They are frequently of a more persistent and determined nature than wilful or inspired, relying more on 'hard work' and practical rationality than on intuition, concepts and ideals.

Conversely, from the airy tattwa is formed the respiratory system, controlled from the *hridaya chakra*, situated at the level of the heart. The lungs and heart are under its primary care, while the flow of oxygen to all bodily tissues also lies at the centre of its functioning.

Psychologically, the airy types are light and often ungrounded. Preoccupied with the ideas of things, they bring about actualization of their desires more by willing them into manifestation, than through the practical application of the hours of persistent work with which the more earthy nature is familiar. When a predominantly airy type makes friends with an earthy type, you will often find that while the airy personality has most of the ideas, it is the earthy one who brings about their actualization and does all the hard work!

However, we discuss the attributes of each tattwa in turn in ensuing chapters and my interest here is in introducing these concepts, so that one may begin to understand that they are not just interesting curiosities from an antiquated and outmoded culture, but when fully understood represent a fundamental reality in the energy patterns which constitute our physical existence.

Since these tattwas are the root substance out of which our bodies and physical life are made, an understanding of their manner of manifestation and their particular characteristics as it applies to daily experience, allows us a deeper insight into how and why things happen in bodily, emotional, mental and outward forms.

For the purpose of study, one first needs to comprehend the individual characteristics and modes of expression, both subtle and gross, of each tattwa. In reality, of course, we are formed from a holographic[2] intermingling of these tattwas and in all but the perfect human, there is an imbalance, due to our karmic patterning, in their individual expression. It is this factor which results in the great variety found amongst humankind in both psychological and bodily manifestation. Certain aspects of particular tattwas find expression both outwardly in our physical bodies and subtly in our emotions and personal psychology, resulting in a blend of characteristics that are uniquely identifiable as the individual.

Similarly, the organs and systems of the body, while they may have one or more tattwas predominating above all others, are the result of a holographically patterned admixture of all the five tattvic states, thus relating all parts to each other in one vibrating, shimmering whole.

In Ayurvedic thinking, for example, there are three major combinations or basic constitutions (which are themselves also intermingled). These are *vata* (air and akash), *pitta* (fire and water), and *kapha* (earth and water), with the different bodily aspects being seen as manifestations of these three combinations.

In terms of the gunas, yin and yang, or polarity, the earth and water tattwas possess the tamas or yin aspects of inertia, compression and receptivity, while air and fire are of the outgoing, expansive rajas or yang nature. Between them, when in balance, they form a harmonious, balanced

---

[2] In a hologram, each part contains an image of the whole.

and healthy individual. When one or more of these tattwas are out of balance, then we experience physical, emotional and mental disturbance.

This understanding of the tattwas and polarity provides, therefore, a deep and real framework into which western scientific knowledge can be placed and readily understood. It also suggests new ways forward in a more holistic approach to the scientific method, for it gives us a containment and an understanding of the strengths and intrinsic limitations of the scientific method. One could start by seeking out more subtle wave-like patterning, vibration or oscillation at molecular, sub-molecular and subtle levels that relate to the organizational patterning of the pranas, whereby the activity of every molecule and subatomic particle and force is maintained from within in designed, rather than fortuitous or random existence.

Akash, Vacuum, the Brain and Modern Physics

While modern science recognizes the gross, outer forms of the four tattwas, it is only recently that the gross aspect of akash has been 'discovered'. In fact, it has even been contained within mathematical and conceptual formulation. At this point, you may like to have a look at chapter twelve, *Life Energies And Modern Physics*, which goes into this subject in greater detail. But in general and brief terms, the gross form of akash is the all-pervasive vacuum, within and from which all subatomic particles and the fundamental forces of nature come into being.

Contrary to previous scientific thinking, vacuum is not 'nothing with dimensions', but is actually a balance point of ultra-high potential energy, infolded and locked-in to itself. It contains waves, oscillations, vibrations and polarity as with any other energy manifestation, but because we have no gross physical sense organ with which to detect it, it appears to us to be 'nothing' or vacuum.

There are, of course, many energies already known to science for which we have no perceptual organ. This includes most of the electromagnetic spectrum of radio waves, X-rays and so on. These vacuum waves and polarities, then, in respect of their outward manifestation, mostly sum to zero and hence we cannot observe even their effects. *In places, however, the vacuum energy forms a spining vortex which, by causing stresses within the 'fabric' of the vacuum energy patterns, manifests the properties of mass, solidity and gravitation, electrical charge,* and so on. Such a vortex is a subatomic particle. And the 'fundamental building blocks' of our physical world *are* subatomic particles. Everything consists of subatomic particles and the forces between them, forces being due to different forms of 'stress' or energy interchange and relationship within the vacuum state.

In conventional quantum physics, these fundamental forces are seen as interactions involving the momentary existence and 'exchange' of 'virtual' particles. In general terms, we can say that the forces are simply a part of the way in which the energy patterns of the vacuum are interrelated, bound together or interact.

Thinking (incorrectly, in fact) of subatomic particles as little solid blobs of something, physicists tell us that if all the subatomic particles comprising our earth were compressed so that no space or vacuum existed between them, they would take up no more volume than a pin-head or perhaps an orange. That is, our apparently observable physical universe is mostly space or vacuum and the manifested objects consist of widely spaced spinning vortices of energy (subatomic particles), thereby trapping the energy of vacuum in manifested form. These vortices are automatically connected with each other through the stresses and patterning that are responsible for their formation within the fabric of this energy-rich vacuum. These are the forces of nature, of which, scientifically, there are thought to be only four; they themselves also being interrelated. They are the electromagnetic, the gravitational, the weak and the strong forces, (see figure 3-1).

We are already familiar with electromagnetic (e.g. light, radio waves, X-rays etc.) and gravitational forces. The *strong force* is said to be responsible for binding quarks together into protons, neutrons and other heavy particles, the residue holding together the protons and neutrons themselves, within the atomic nucleus. The *weak force*, on the other hand drives particle transmutations, rather than exerting a pushing or pulling effect in a strictly engineering sense. It is the weak force, for instance, which provides

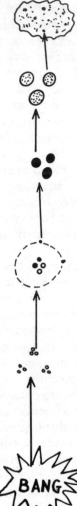

OBJECTS
are mostly comprised of NOTHING,
within which exist:

MOLECULES,
(e.g. water)
which consist of

ATOMS,
(e.g. Hydrogen)
which are made of

SUBATOMIC PARTICLES,
(e.g. Protons, electrons)
which are formed out of

EVEN SMALLER
SUBATOMIC PARTICLES,
(e.g. quarks)
which came into existence out of

NOWHERE
in a Big Bang,
a long, long time ago.

Forces and interactions between the particles or objects are said to be due to other particles (described by quantum theory) or stresses in their geometrical arrangement within space and time (relativity).

Gravitation *is the attraction of objects at a distance.*

Electromagnetism *is represented in the force of electrical charge and magnetic polarity.*

The Strong Force *holds subatomic particles together and forms them into atoms.*

The Weak Force *provides the energy required to convert one subatomic particle into another.*

Figure 3-1. The 'conventional' understanding of material substance, according to current modern physics.

the energy for a neutron to decay spontaneously into a proton, an electron and a neutrino. Because the weak and strong forces act over incredibly tiny distances their effect is felt only within the atomic nucleus itself and though both these forces are far stronger than gravity, it is the latter's long range which makes it the most powerful cohering influence in our macroscopic world.

In the more conventional concepts of modern physics everything is reduced to the existence of particles described by various aspects of quantum theory. Because the vacuum is really conceived of as nothing – and cannot therefore transmit forces within itself by 'pushing' or 'pulling' – it becomes necessary to describe forces as particles. Even gravity becomes reduced to *gravitons*, electromagnetic vibration to *photons*, the weak force to *W* and *Z particles* and the strong force to *gluons*.

However, when the intrinsic nature of particles is understood to be that of energy patterns, observable focuses of the vacuum energy matrix, we see that describing forces as the 'interchange of particles' is the same as saying that it is all one web of interconnected energy.

It is not surprising, therefore, that the theory, as it is presently formulated, does not quite fit all the facts. On the other hand, Einstein's theory of relativity and of gravitation being caused by stresses or curvature within the fabric of *space-time* due to the presence of *mass*, also explains some of the observed facts – but not all. However, within the context of vacuum state theory, both 'stresses to space-time' and 'interactions between particles' are seen to be the same thing, but described in different ways. For 'stress' is itself an energetic interaction and space-time is one aspect of the vacuum or akashic state itself.

There is also a further fundamental philosophical dichotomy between the two theories, for while Einstein's approach assumes a deterministic order in the universe, the theories of quantum mechanics and particle interaction are approached in a basically probabalistic manner.

Understanding of manifestation out of a vacuum which is a real energy field provides the unifying factor between the two concepts for *both particles and forces are due to various kinds of activity within the vacuum state.* Some of this activity appears to our instrumentation as spinning particles which create the illusion of mass, whilst other aspects are observed as forces or relationships between these spinning vortices.

Actually, the conclusions of quantum theory that the basic structure of the physical universe is inherently probabalistic and non-causal in nature relates to a confusion between the realization that we can only ever observe our *interaction* with a nature in whom we are embedded, and an inability to deal with the wealth of data concerning subatomic particles in any other way than statistical.

In addition, our understanding of the nature of causality also needs to be extended. But a considerably fuller discussion of this topic is required to give it proper justice and this I have attempted to do in the next book in this series, *The Secret of the Creative Vacuum*.

So we can readily understand, from this discussion, how gravity can be seen as either space-time, curvature in the fabric of vacuum, relationships within an integrated medium driven into complex but ordered manifestation by higher cosmic forces, expression of an implicate order, or as 'particles' or 'waves' flowing between objects. They are all alternative and complementary ways of perceiving the same phenomena, different facets of the same diamond. Similarly, the strong force can be seen as due simply to vacuum interaction between the spinning vortices of energy responsible for the creation of protons and neutrons, for instance, whilst the weak force, which is involved in the transmutation of one particle to another, is a part of the energetic activity which permits the change of one kind of vacuum activity into another.

All particles and forces are thus the interplay of a supremely organized pattern, spinning bubbles and blips upon the surface of vacuum, the ultimate driving force for this play of energy patterns being the Shabda, the mystic sound, the Creative Word of the Supreme, (see figure 4-5).

The gross form of akash, then, *is* the vacuum state. In fact, in mystic cosmologies we frequently encounter descriptions of these 'skies' within. The inner 'sky' of the body, for example, is comprised of the subtle form of akash. And it is this energy of akash that gives us our intelligence, with the brain thus being perceivable as a physical integrator of subtle energy activity, with pathways leading both from without-in, as well as from within-out. For the outflow must be balanced by an inflow to complete the circuit of creation.

In fact, I believe that with the emergence of a vacuum state understanding and technology, the brain will come to be viewed in a totally different functional capacity. Just as the advent of present computer technology was immediately applied to brain function as the most advanced concept we could imagine at that time, so too will an understanding of how energies come into being out of energies deeper within themselves – to begin with, out of the vacuum state – give us a far deeper model and visualization of brain activity and, indeed, all bodily activity.

The neurochemical system that uses sudden reversals of polarity across cell membranes, with the concomitant flow of sodium and potassium ions (electrically charged atoms, accumulations of subatomic particles), combined with the synaptic and neurohormone messenger and connection system is an ideally complex, vibrating medium for the encoding of life-process patterns from within-out and without-in. It also provides the means for the body to biologically engineer the vacuum and more subtle states. It seems quite clear that if nature had really intended our neurological system to be built like an enlarged domestic wiring system, we would in fact have been endowed with a system of straight-wire conductors.

Relating this thinking to our theme, in the higher astral and causal regions, we again find these skies, also spoken of as akash, which can sometimes cause confusion to a reader. But the inner skies are simply higher and more inward harmonics of the same kind of balance point or condition out of which the lower vibration is created. In just the same way, the first essence of the five tattwas is found in the causal region of the Universal Mind, where time also first arises. For a more complete mystic cosmology, however, which describes these inner 'mansions', I would refer you to my previous book, *Subtle Energy* or to the mystic writings referred in the bibliography.

The Body as a Tattvic Hologram

Our human body then, is patterned out of the five tattwas, under the influence of mind and prana. Now the principle of all manifestation is, "As above, so below." The One becomes two, but each part remains related to the other and to the whole. In reality, they are indivisible. In its descent, the two become the many, but always the relationship of all the 'parts' to each other and to the whole is maintained. Finally, it is crystallized in a human body, but each part is still related to each other part and together they operate as a whole.

This mechanism of manifestation is specific and should be capable of precise modelling, if only we had an exact understanding of energetic relationships at the subtle level. Probably the best physically understandable model we have at the present time of this manifestation process is that of a hologram, though I am always somewhat suspect of using man's latest technological invention to model the way we ourselves function. Such models have been shown all too frequently to be quite inappropriate in the light of greater wisdom.

A hologram is a means of storing an image by freezing the *interference* patterns created from two or more sources of coherent or laser light. There is no need to understand the actual mechanism here except to say that two or more waveforms or oscillatory patterns, when interacting upon each other, form such interference patterns. You get this effect when you drop two stones into a pool of water. The resulting concentric rings add and subtract against each other forming another pattern.

This interference pattern, when frozen into a suitable material is called a holgram and is unique in that *any small part of it can be used to project an image of the original whole*. This is like every cell in our body (the parts) containing the capacity within their identical DNA to represent the whole. This is discussed in more detail in chapter six.

The five tattwas, then, are interacted and interwoven under the patterning influence of prana and in a holographic fashion, so that all parts bear an imprint of the whole in their energetic substructure. The result is a human body which is perfectly formulated and can be described as a *tattvic hologram*. Within this hologram, the various parts reflect the whole in a multitude of ways. We have already mentioned the cell and its repeated DNA. There is also the repeating cellular structure itself. We also have five fingers and five toes which are spun out as an outward patterning of the five inward tattvic essences.

We also find that almost every organ of the body carries an imprint of the whole. The foot and hands in reflexology, the iris in iridology, the ear in auricular acupuncture, the tongue, lips and face in oriental diagnosis, the pulses in acupunture, and so on. They are all used as patterns for diagnosing or treating the whole body. And not only that but these sensory and motor reflex or holographic zones that reflect the condition of the whole body are areas for *input* of energetic nourishment (yin function), as well as output (yang) patterning.

This is why we need good lighting, accoustics and harmonious sensory input from our environment for maintaining good health and mental-emotional well-being. Poor energetic input through any of the senses results in the general feeling of malaise progressing to degenerative phases, according to other influences, that are so often experienced in our modern artificial environment. This is why people often feel tired, worn-out, depressed and finally ill in many modern office environments which are designed without any knowledge of human energetic or emotional requirements. In simple terms, ugliness tires us – ugliness in all its forms.

The tattwas, then, are woven holographically by the mind and pranas – modulated and constrained by our karmas – into the form of the human body which medical science finds so difficult to comprehend. This holographic model is extremely powerful for it reflects the universal pattern of cosmic construction itself. Man's individual human mind, for example, is a ray or reflection of the Universal, cosmic mind. It is a part of the universal hologram. But within this individual mind, within this part, lies the imprint of the Universal. Man is therefore the microcosm who can reach out to touch, experience and become the macrocosm. This is the secret of his construction and therein lies the gateway to the secrets of the Universe.

Man appears outwardly to be just a part of the universal, vibrant, integrated, living hologram. But when the light of consciousness shines and expands within him, his inner being – the part – can become the whole. Increasingly, his consciousness encompasses the whole of creation – inner and outer. And this is precisely the nature of a hologram. It is, after all, a uni-verse, not a multi-verse.

"As above, so below." This principle of reflection from within is the mechanism of manifestation, from the highest spiritual regions, right down to the detailed construction of a physical human body. Each cell, as we said, contains DNA, a pattern of vacuum manifestation running throughout every cell in the body. Patterned by the inward mind potential, this effectively means that every cell has its own cell 'mind' and its own cell karma – its own organization and patterning of mind and prana from within. This is demonstrated by the continual repetition of the cellular structure and the DNA molecule.

At the level of atoms, molecules and larger structures, with our limited minds, we think we perceive linear cause and effect pathways. But these, being reflections or effects are still parts of a more holographically structured energy system, the whole of which cannot be comprehended by our linear-style, conceptual thinking.

Indeed, as we move into the subatomic realm and thence through the curtain into the vacuum and deeper levels, *the laws governing energetic relationships change dramatically.* These laws are, in fact, more holographic in nature. Mind itself, for example, has the capacity to be 'everywhere all at once.' This we experience all the time in a limited fashion simply by our ability to perceive (with our senses) and comprehend (with our mind) many things, simultaneously. We also experience it in telepathic links that occur simultaneously across space, regardless of distance.

It should also be pointed out that this is quite contrary to the model of our brain as a computer. In a computer, there is only one central processing unit, only one point of logical activity. Our mind, however, impresses the brain and is itself patterned thereby in a holographic fashion. That is to say that energetic activity is both multitudinous, simultaneous and integrated, in such a way that all the various parts know what each other part is doing. This is the glorious and scientifically unrecognized function of prana, given existence by consciousness.

Returning, then, to our original thought, each cell of the body is both autonomous, and yet in contact and energetically related to the whole. And this holographic relatedness is still *present* within the world of effects with which our present science is familiar, but actually *lies* within the vacuum and more subtle states. So science has failed to perceive it, because the cause and effect laws governing the vacuum state are not understood or even suspected of existing, except by a few avant-garde thinkers.

Our present allopathic and linear paradigms are a reflection of a limited mental capacity. This is in addition to the intellect itself possessing intrinsic limitations, even when used by the wisest of souls. As we expand our consciousness by meditation, we automatically come to see that it is the whole which is important, not the part. That any body of scientific knowledge which is based upon analysis of the parts is working only with the bubbles upon the surface, while remaining unaware of the surging creative ocean beneath.

Similarly, we must realise that the tattvic patterning is also holographic and holistic in nature. The manner by which, for example, the fingers and toes reflect the activity of particular tattwas (see figure 4-1) is not linear but reflects the holographic energy-relatedness principle at work. This is why it often appears naive or odd to the linear mind. And why such people reject it.

This, too, is how the endocrine glands reflect the tattvic characteristics. Indeed, it is the mechanism of holistic integration by which all parts of the body whether organs, tissues, cells or molecules are all woven into one complete tapestry, one functional whole.

Allegorically, this is perhaps the meaning behind the tale of Humpty-Dumpty. For when broken into a myriad fragments by our human mind acting in a negative, outward mode[3], not all the king's horses and all the king's men can put Humpty back together again. Nothing earthly can make us perceive that he was just one great egg – the egg of the Universal Mind, along with the astral and physical regions within it.

We can also perceive within this holographic model the increasing tendency towards unity and oneness. As we move within, the parts relate more and more to the whole until there is no differentation at all. It all becomes One. So it is an expression of the Love of the Supreme. For if He is Love, then everything manifested must be an expression of that Love. All energy in creation is actually Love in

---

[3] Philosophically, this is known as *reductionism*.

action. So the very structure of creation expresses and proclaims the unity and supremacy of Love, the intense and increasing relatedness of the part to the whole, until the part becomes the whole.

As Juan Mascaro put it most succinctly in his introduction to the Bhagavad Gita, "Just as the mind can see that all matter is energy, so the soul can see that all energy is Love."

Tattwas, Personality and Astrology

As we said, psychologically, the interplay between our mind energies and the subtle tattwas gives rise to our personality characteristics. Thus an individual may have earth as a dominant keynote in his nature, expressing itself, for example, in practical skills, square hands and a consistent and reliable nature. And this, in combination with strong airy overtones providing a fleetness of perception and response, together with an ability to conceptualize, would result perhaps in an innovative and inventive nature.

An admixture of water is revealed as the sensitive response to events, so that a dominant, watery quality in a person is experienced as an intuitive, instinctive, and often deeply emotional approach to life. Watery types need the containment of earth, the conceptual, structuring of air or the impulsive drive of the fiery nature to bring them balance. They are easily led and moulded, but are often sought after by others because they are instinctively valued for their compassion and willingness to listen.

All natures and tattwas, of course, are themselves under the universal sway of the gunas or the swings of polarity. Thus the negative aspects of the watery type are a tendency to emotional self-indulgence, while the earthy type can be too solid, intolerant and unmoving for comfort. Air may never touch earth, and while getting along fine with other airy types, may be a source of continual frustration to their earthy associates who tend to see them as being too much up in the clouds. The airy ones, on the other hand, may consider their earthy counterparts as far too stubborn, dense and even boring, for their quicksilver minds. For what appears as persistence and pragmatism to earth is viewed by air as an unwillingness to adapt.

All combinations are possible and, as in many aspects of life, there is an external patterning that permits one to read objectively the combination of tattwas which are particularly active in each individual, both constitutionally, or within their basic being, as well as on a day-by-day basis. This manifestation of tattvic activity in both physical as well as psychological life, is the energetic causative factor underlying the readily observed phenomenon of a person's emotional and mental characteristics being reflected in both their physical appearance, as well as their state of health or disease. That is, both the subtle energies and their gross, physical actualization are built out of the same admixture of tattvic energies. Or, put more simply, we are each one person, one energy complex, all aspects of our life and being reflecting the content of that whole.

The science by which this patterning can be read is known popularly as *astrology*, but the underlying mechanism of its reality is little understood. The interplay of the tattwas lies at the energetic basis of the true science of astrology. But whether the stars and the planets are causative factors or whether, like a hologram, they simply bear the imprint of events, predispositions and patterns, is not understood. Perhaps the answer is both.

Clearly, the heavens are not the *primary* causative factor of life on earth, for they themselves are not self-existent, but subject to the same laws of cause and effect which influence all motion and existence. But all energy is interconnected, there being only one inner source, and therefore one would expect to be able to read the condition of certain parts of an energy system from the condition of any other part. The problem is one of technique and the ability to perceive and correctly interpret all the necessary aspects.

Astrology, in its most scientific respect, does just that, enabling one to read the patterning of the tattwas which are manifested in the individual from the patterning of the celestial and planetary bodies. The skilled astrologer is therefore able, not only to understand the nature of personalities and events, but also to note the underlying physical constitution of a person and to predict where the imbalances in tattvic combinations and polarity are likely to occur, and when. The significance of such diagnostic and predictive skills in the healing arts is quite clear, though such knowledge is only really appreciated in the context of a holistic approach to health. The symptomatic and super-ficial approach of papering over the cracks does not possess in its conceptual framework the depth of understanding required to comprehend the deep relevance of constitu-tional types and inherent propensities for ill-health or imbalance. But to understand the properties of the basic building materials of a structure is of immense value when dealing with the minutiae of its functioning, as well as its intrinsic strengths and its weaknesses.

It is clear to any observant and thoughtful eye, how different we all are, yet much of modern medicine ploughs ahead on the assumption that we are all the same. An understanding of tattvic constitution would provide a scientific framework in which to really use the scientific method to its full advantage, while side-stepping many of its insensitive and clearly non-common-sensical aspects.

Astrology is a remarkably detailed science and quite amenable to analysis by scientific method, though it requires, too, an intelligent, intuitive and lively grasp of its principles – as with any branch of scientific study. It is simply the study of patterns.

A really excellent book which describes the way in which astrology, psychology and the tattwas are interconnected is Stephen Arroyo's, *Astrology, Psychology and The Four Elements*. The fifth element, akash, is omitted from astro-logical study, for being the source of the other four, its effect is more universal than particular. Each of the four elements has three manifestations – *cardinal*, *fixed* and *mutable* – corresponding in some degree to the tamas, sattvas and rajas gunas or modes of being. The four elements, in each of these three manifestations, result in the twelve (four times three) signs of the zodiac.

Thus, for example, amongst the three air signs, *libra* (cardinal) is the balancer, the bringer of stability and har-mony; *gemini* (mutable) is the restless, changing mind with innumerable ideas, while *aquarius* (fixed) possesses the more detached qualities necessary to coordinate both people and concepts. But this is not a book on astrology and if you want to understand the patterning in a deeper manner, I would direct you to the very clear writings of Stephen Arroyo.

Serendipity, Precognition and Awareness of Patterns

Being the right person, in the right place, at the right time is an aspect of life we call serendipity. To those who have it, life is full of pleasant coincidence, accompanied by a sense of timing and finesse. Their energies flow in a comparatively effortless fashion as they weave their way through life. The perfectly serendipitous person is perhaps only a perfect mystic, whose vision and point of control lies beyond karma, but the rest of us definitely experience an admixture of serendipity and struggle.

It is in many respects, a question of attitude. The optimistic person is 'lucky', while the downhearted, pessimism of the Eeyore-type (a lovable, but down-on-his-luck character from *Winnie The Pooh*), draws down upon them negative events and the very objects of their fear.

Really, however, it is just a clarity of karmas and mind which permits one to both see into the future and to live with balance in the present moment. Foretelling the future is really an appreciation of *patterns*. When one catches a ball, for instance, one is really predicting the future from an intuitive appreciation of the present facts and past experience. One expects the ball to behave in a particular way. If the wind catches it *unexpectedly*, we may drop it. If we already know which way the wind is blowing, we will build that into our mental, sensory and motor processes that still permit us to catch it. If we start analyzing the mechanisms by which we will catch it, while the ball is still in the air, we will be likely to drop it. A smooth flow of energy is required, mental, emotional and physical.

Similarly, in life, the really successful people – in an outward sense – are those who appear to divine the future and always to be where the opportunity lies. And it stems from an appreciation – conscious, unconscious and intuitive – of the way things happen.

But there is a higher side to it, too. For happiness and an easy flow of energy will arise when we consciously or unconsciously tune in to our destiny, when we begin to work with the patterns and promptings of life, rather than to fight them. In this sense, it is possible that we are reading the mental akashic record in which our destiny is

77

written and are working with it in positive confidence, knowing that it is the way things are going to be.

Emotional Expression and Psychological Constitution

The karmic imprint of our mind energy and its outworking in the subtle tattvic fields gives us, therefore, our predestined and basic personality type or nature. So when people talk psychologically about discovering their true nature or finding out what they really think or feel, what takes place is a more or less truthful recognition or personal perception of this underlying psychological constitution.

Mostly, this more inward nature is overlain by the conditioning of our childhood and the habituation and crystallization that takes place as we unconsciously strive to handle our relationships with others and come to grips with our own thoughts and feelings. This conditioning and these behaviour patterns are still dominated, of course, by our more inward constitution, but may not be really representative of our more natural inward colour, were it given a more free-flowing expression.

As human beings, we will be comparatively happy and feel fulfiled when our energies flow freely from within and we possess a considerable degree of self-awareness.

With emotions bottled up and held below the threshold of consciousness or awareness, we will always be full of energy blockages, crystallizations and tensions. These will quite naturally be expressed in our outer life, behaviour and relationships, as well as within our bodies in our state of health and disease.

And it is this energetic complex which lies at the basis of all psychosomatic perceptions, as Archart-Treichel and many others have astutely observed.[4]

The solution lies ultimately in a very high kind of meditation and inner concentration. For while almost any form of meditation or even prayer will help to smooth out some of these tensions and blockages, helping us to feel better and permitting us to be more productive and

[4] *Biotypes*, by Joan Arehart-Treichel.

straightforward, this will only be in the context of the karmic mind patterns with which we were born and which are pre-destined to find expression. Meditation will therefore bring us into tune with our destiny, so to speak. But the highest solution is to be able to rise above the level of destiny or human life through deep meditation. Then we simply go through our life in the best way possible, without creating new entanglements.

The alternative approach of psychological therapy has only a limited value, relative to one's sense of personal well-being. For the inherent danger is that, like a man in a quicksand, every analysis ties us deeper to our problem – our sense of personal self or ego. To talk with friends and seek advice at difficult moments in our life, even to consult professional counsellors of a high order is a part of the natural flow of life. This would seem to be within balance, depending upon the individual, but to adopt the habit of psychologizing one's way through life leaves one with just one approach to everything and one topic of conversation – one's self – wherein lies the original source of the problem.

The Human Mind – The Antashkarans, the Indriyas and Tanmantras

The human mind is constituted of a four-petalled lotus or chakra above the sixth or *ajna* chakra of the physical body and known as the *Antashkarans*, the 'petals' of a chakra denoting its energy aspects or separate energetic functions. The four aspects are known as *Buddhi, Manas, Chit* and *Ahankar*.

Buddhi is the faculty of discrimination, of impersonal consciousness of the *Jiva*, or soul imprisoned in a human body. It makes decisions based upon the impressions gained from the manas and chit, mind-stuff and memory. But while buddhi is the discriminatory faculty, it has in itself no power to initiate action, being impersonal. Buddhi is the detached logic behind intellectual functioning. It is rationality, though infused with understanding of morality and the higher qualities of life, according to the degree of consciousness of the individual and his contact with the higher or inner energies and realms of his own being.

So buddhi itself requires a degree of personalization for it to find expression in an individual human being. This is the faculty of *Ahankar*, of personal awareness. It is ahankar which identifies with the perceptions of the senses and the subsequent responses. Buddhi and ahankar together, thus comprise the 'experiencer'.

Manas is mind–stuff, per se. It is the energy substance which registers impressions from the senses (indriyas) and its reactions are instantaneous according to its habits or grooves of previous experience. The faculty of enjoyment and of desire is also couched in manas. The experiencer is affected by the material world of the five tattwas in five separate ways, giving rise in him to the sensations of sound and hearing, colour and form and sight, touch and feel, taste, and smell, (see figure 3-2). These modalities are general essences of material appreciation, though all sensations are themselves of particular objects. These generalities are known as *Tanmantras* and it is from them that both the tattwas and the perception of individual objects becomes possible. The tanmantra of a sound, for example, is not that particular sound itself with its unique waveform and characteristics, but is the modality or essence of sound, the 'beingness' of sound as a perceivable quality of matter.

There are thus five tanmantras corresponding to the sense–objects or physical material things derived from them; these being sound, colour and form, touch and feel, flavour, and odour.

While tanmantras are both qualities of material substance and attributes of experience, the *Indriyas*, or senses, are closely associated with the faculties of the manas aspect of the human mind as it looks outward and interacts with the tattwas. They are the mental means by which the inner consciousness is aware of outer material vibration or energy patterns (which, in their universal aspect, are the tanmantras). The indriyas are not the physical sense organs themselves, but the mental faculty whereby the experiencer is conscious of the objects of sensation. They are ten in number, (see figure 3-2) containing both the receptive, afferent organs of perception or sensation – that is the ear (hearing), skin (touch, feeling), eye (sight), tongue (taste) and nose (smell) – and the five organs of action initiated by the mind in response to sensory input. These are thus the motor and efferent impulses of the mind, ultimately translated into efferent nerve impulses in the motor nervous system, together with certain specific endocrine responses. These five action-indriyas are the mouth, hands, legs, anus and genitalia, through which speaking, grasping, walking, elimination/excretion and the procreative functions are performed and by which means outward manifestation and actualization is given to the mind's desires.

An indriya being the mental faculty, operating through that sense organ, but *not the sense organ itself*, it is thus possible for the yogi to perceive without the aid of the physical sense organ itself. There is a good example of this experience quoted in *Subtle Energy* from Yogananda's book, *Autobiography of a Yogi*. In his expanded state of consciousness he perceives objects as if with his eyes, through the normally opaque atomic screen of the 'solid' objects of this world. This also happens during 'astral' projection, where the individual finds himself viewing his body *from outside*. Some people are able to do this at will, while others experience it at times of emergency – during an operation, times of emotional or mental stress or even during 'sleep'. Interestingly enough, it is also considered symptomatic of a schizophrenic tendency, though the mechanism, validity and reasons for the experience are usually misinterpreted by conventional psychiatry.

This so-called 'astral' projection is not actually astral at all but a temporary dislocation of the subtle physical body, away from the gross body which it normally inhabits, patterns and animates. It would more correctly be called etheric projection. The experience does, however, demonstrate that the mind, consciousness and indriyas are independent of the gross body – that they are not a function of brain biochemistry but exist on an altogether higher level of energy.

All the faculties of mind, being energies of a subtle nature, are open to perception by the inner attention of one whose concentration is focused within in specific meditational or yogic practices. Indeed, there are records of hypnotized subjects being able to perceive without the use of the physical sense organ usually required for that perception. Moreover, it seems that some switching of the subtle pathways between the physical sense organ and the mental indriya can take place, so that hypnotized subjects have been able to 'see' with their feet, 'hear' with their knees and so on.

While one is able to readily appreciate that there are indeed five major modes of physical perception, it requires some consideration to understand that all *actions* can be categorized into the five described. We again suffer from difficulties of translation here, because 'grasping' for example, contains within it all actions related to 'getting hold of' something, of physical manipulation. And although the hands are the major motor organ associated with the sense of touch and the airy tattwa, one may also use one's feet or head or other parts of the body in this process. Similarly 'walking' is the act of 'going', of moving one's body somewhere and just as one's perception of an scene is through a mixture of the five senses, so too do our actions contain a mixture of the five motor indriyas. These indriyas are once again mental faculties. They are the mental characteristic which makes the action possible.

So just as the soul is encumbent with vehicles or coverings that relate vibrationally to the realms in which it is functioning, just so do the individual tattwas or vibrations which make up that world have particular sense organs within that main vehicle, sensitive to or resonant with those particular energy fields, permitting perception of all aspects of that realm. For this reason, we have five senses, tuned to the grosser manifestation of the five tattwas. This is summarized in figure 3-2.

Tattwa	Tanmantra	Indriya of Perception	Organ of Perception	Indriya of Action	Organ of Action	Chakra
Prithvi (Earth)	Odour	Smell	Nose	Elimination	Anus	Muladhara (Rectal)
Jala (Water)	Flavour	Taste	Tongue	Procreation	Genitalia	Svadhishthana (Genital)
Tejas (Fire)	Colour & Form	Sight	Eyes	Walking/ Moving About	Feet & Legs	Manipuraka (Navel)
Vayu (Air)	Feel	Touch or Sensation	Skin, esp. On Hands	Grasping	Hands & Arms	Hridaya (Heart)
Akasha (Ether)	Sound	Hearing	Ears	Speech	Throat & Mouth	Vishuddha (Throat)

Figure 3-2. Tattwas, tanmantras, indriyas & chakras.

The indriyas, then, are an integral part of the operation of manas. We are persistently bombarded by sensory input, most of which is ignored, for we could not maintain sanity if we were continually and specifically conscious of all the sensations pouring in upon us. We must, therefore, first apply our *attention* to any sense perception before we can become aware or conscious of it. This attribute of attention is the function of manas, being the energy field in which sense impressions are registered. It is also the function of manas to make instinctive *selection* of sensory input as well as providing a *synthesis* of the input from the various sense organs such that we feel that our various sense perceptions are linked with regard to an object or scene. That is, the input from our eyes, ears, nose, tongue and skin are all synchronized and merged into one complete perception of what is going on. This, if you consider it, is no small task and requires the presence of innate or instinctive intelligence, or consciousness.

Manas thus receives sensory impressions from the 'outside', via the physical sense organs and thence through the indriyas, but it is itself quite automatic in its functioning and requires the existence of buddhi and ahankar to give it 'life' and for its activities to be experienced. Buddhi surveys the impressions gained by manas and makes intelligent selection and decisions thereon, while ahankar becomes the executive, personal faculty when any action is to be taken, passing its decision back through manas and the five motor indriyas, for the decision to be executed. Ahankar, in relationship with the other aspects of the human mind, is thus the primary source of personal 'motive'.

In fact, in all but evolved souls, the faculties of mind have become uncontrolled under the influence, primarily, of ahankar. Through ahankar, we have come to identify with both the sensory impressions of the 'outside' world and our own reactions to them. So ahankar has become our personal sense of human ego and we think that certain objects or people 'belong' to us, despite the fact that the attribute of belonging, in any true or permanent sense, is clearly quite impossible.

Looking out of the window into the garden I think of as mine I can see a robin who quite clearly feels it is his! There are neighbours' cats and dogs who patrol the area, too, leaving their marks of 'mine'. We also have badgers, squirrels and a multitude of other creatures, many of them with distinct ways of marking their own personal territory. And within not too many years hence, we will all be gone and some other group of creatures will be laying personal claim to this small plot of land. So how can I claim, in terms of the highest reality, that it belongs to me?

Ahankar, however, is a necessary faculty of a balanced and controlled human mind. Individuation is the nature of human existence, but it should be within our conscious control. And this can only be achieved by meditation over many years and most probably several lifetimes. It is not the work of a few days.

Ahankar, then, identifies with the sensory, enjoyment and desire aspects of manas. The process takes place with such rapidity that the buddhi or discriminatory faculty is severely curtailed in its functioning. The desire for personal self-gratification is too strong, so that our rational mind is frequently ignored, even in spite of its best intentions. Without buddhi and ahankar, therefore, the activities of manas and its associated indriyas are quite dead.

While manas is the immediate and present faculty of cognition and perception, the last faculty of the four-fold human mind is that of *chit*. Chit is memory. It is the storehouse of all the impressions gained by manas. Psychologists talk of short-term and long-term memory. If manas is associated with the functioning of short-term memory, then chit is the substance in which long-term impressions are lodged. Thus, ahankar and buddhi draw automatically on this reservoir of experience when making their decisions and actions.

There are those, for example, whose ability to remember is partially or completely lost. It means that their chit is not functioning correctly or that the linkages between the physical brain and the antashkarans have been disturbed at some point. Interestingly enough, amnesia due to brain injury does not normally effect the long-term memory, which is already lodged in energies beyond the level of physical functioning. Loss of short-term memory, however, is often disturbed including that of the events surrounding the injury itself, which means that the pathway of signals from the outward event through the brain mechanisms and into the higher levels of mental energy were disrupted – either temporarily or permanently.

Brain and mental functions are a fascinating topic and one we return to in a later chapter, but let us say here, that the existence of thought energies at a higher level than that of the physical brain explains quite precisely why research scientists have never been able to find thoughts by dissection. Furthermore, an understanding of the interrelationships between the brain, the chakras and higher pranic and mental-emotional energies in the body provides the basis for understanding all mental and emotional problems that arise in human beings. Any part of the mechanism, physical or subtle, can be disturbed for any variety of reasons, giving rise to the clinical symptoms of so-called mental illness, psychological imbalance or mental handicap. This we also discuss in a later chapter.

Some tantric descriptions of the antashkarans describe the functions of chit and manas as more interfused, ascribing the faculty of sight, for example, to chit, while in others the faculties here ascribed to chit are designated entirely to buddhi. Sometimes, the word chit is also used as a general term for the functioning, human mind and in that instance is more appropriately considered as synonymous with the antashkarans themselves. Since the mind, however, does exist as a real energy field, there is no doubt that these faculties exist as real entities, interwoven and working with each other at a vibrational level separate from and higher than that of the physical matter of which our gross bodies and the objects of the physical plane (*Pinda*) are composed.

The Subconscious Mind

The subconscious mind known to western thinking is comprised of the impressions upon the antashkarans, intermingled with the lower energies manifesting in the tattvic energy fields through the six chakras. But much of western psychological analysis is conceptual rather than relating directly to energy plexi or centres. As in most western thinking the approach is from without-in, being unaware of the manifestation of energy patterns and human constitution from within.

Jung's concept of the animus and anima, the male and female psychological aspects within the minds of all of us, points to the essential polarity out of which the Universe and its separate parts are all constructed. Understanding of patterns induced into our subconscious mind during childhood or as a result of the events of our life, and which mould our personality, are correct; but without the practical understanding of subtle human energies, they are left as a more nebulous and conceptual philosophy.

As stated earlier, the antashkarans contain not only a record of the events of this life, but also those of previous lives, too. These are our *sanskaras* or impressions of past lives, which provide our interwoven destiny and personality of the present life. Thus, as every parent knows, a child is born with a personality and innate talents, as well as inabilities. This is then modified by the processes of life, especially during childhood, when the mental organ is soft and pliable to impression and suggestion.

Experience, Matter and Consciousness

Note from the foregoing that it is more correct to perceive the sensory and motor indriyas as the result of the manas aspect of mind interacting with the five tattwas, the yin and yang polarity of energetic outflow and inflow resulting in the sensory input and the motor output. Manas is the attention and ability to perceive, which when directed upon the subtle forms of the five tattwas results in sensation and action. Thus, while the unconscious aspects of human biology are mediated through the pranas, the directed and conscious nature of our mind energy, both of which are enlivened by the soul within, results in a *personal sense of experience*, through our physical senses and actions.

These pathways, however, are by no means fixed, for it is also possible for the mind to consciously follow the pranic pathways and influence autonomic functioning and physiology. This dual pathway is already manifested, for example, in both our indriyas – where we are not consciously aware at all times of every action or every sensory input, but where we can be – and in such actions as breathing or walking, which can be carried on either unconsciously or under direct mental control.

This is only an overall control, however, for the biochemical and physiological processes are still outside our normal consciousness, maintained by the pranic current, and yet patterned unconsciously by the karmic imprint within the antashkarans. Actually, one needs to ponder this whole duality of form or matter and consciousness, for it is the interplay between the two, as the primal and original duality or polarization, which has resulted in all manifestation and existence.

Subjective and Objective

Note therefore, the essential difference between the tattwas, pranas and chakras on the one hand, and the ten indriyas and antashkarans, on the other. While the former are essentially 'objective' energetic substance or vibrations, the latter are 'subjective' aspects of the active human constitution related to our ability to experience changes and to function in the fields of energy substance. The tanmantras bridge the gap between the objective and the subjective. Colour, for example, is both inherent in the objective energetic structure of the thing itself and is a part of the subjective mechanism by which we appreciate it. It is the essence behind the indriya of sight, for instance, and without which sight would have no meaning.

But note, however, how there is always an energetic medium of substance through which subjective experience is felt. Thus, even the antashkarans and indriyas are themselves energy fields, but close to the subjective centre of personal attention or consciousness. Thought is a real energy, for example, whilst the indriyas are contained within substance close to the mental level, as well as in the gross physical manifestations as the sense organs with which we are familiar.

So the difference of objective and subjective is drawn only for the purposes of explanation and initial clarity, for in reality, we are (subjectively) an integral part of (objective) manifestation. It is ourselves, through our karmas, who pattern the apparently objective world around us. In a very real, energetic sense, we are all shareholders in this physical world and co-creators of its 'reality'. No wonder it has the superficial appearance of being in such confusion, while – on taking a more detached view – we can perceive order and organization in the movement of every particle and the interactions of every force. So we are not left to just muddle along, there *is* a guiding principle within it all.

Indeed, the truth is that there is no outside – there is nothing outside our consciousness. What we think we see does not really exist. It is a movie show played out from our human mind, within ourselves. The 'outside' tattwas are reflected from the inside subtle tattwas and appear to be outside only due to the outward direction of our attention. We, as the perceiver, are our mind and we are perceiving, *within our mind*. There is no objective world, only the subjective. When we talk about the physical world, it is not 'out there', but 'in here'.

Poetic Interlude

Lines composed a few miles above Tintern Abbey,
On revisiting the banks of the Wye during a tour.
July 13th 1798.

. . . That blessed mood
In which the burthen of the mystery,
In which the heavy and weary weight
Of all this unintelligible world,
Is lightened: – that serene and blessed mood,
In which the affections gently lead us on, –
Until the breath of this corporeal frame
And even the motion of our human blood
Almost suspended, we are laid asleep
In body and become a living soul:
While with an eye made quiet by the power
Of harmony, and the deep power of joy,
We see into the life of things.

. . . And I have felt
A presence that disturbs me with the joy
Of elevated thoughts; a sense sublime
Of something far more deeply interfused,
Whose dwelling is the light of setting suns,
And the round ocean, and the living air,
And the blue sky, and in the mind of man:
A motion and a spirit, that impels
All thinking things, all objects of thought,
And rolls through all things.

Wordsworth

CHAPTER 4

The Nadis and the Nervous System

Polarity and the Physical Body

In any energy system, it is necessary to first consider the primary, driving polarities. This is as much from without in larger scale polarity, as within the specific functioning of each cell, each molecule, each atom, each subatomic particle, every manifestation of energy. Thus for example, in the larger scale, it is clear that the sensory system being receptive of energy, is negative in polarity or yin. The major sense organs are on the front of the body, while the motor nerves, the active driving, yang or rajas, energy channels underlying the motor power of the muscular structure spread out from within the spinal column, and originate along our back. Indeed the major motor muscles themselves are behind us – the calf muscles, the gluteal thigh muscles and the spinal muscles are all predominantly on the back of the body. So in respect of these two systems, the front of the body is yin, whilst the back is yang.

Within the nervous system itself, overall functional polarity is once again expressed. In the autonomic nervous system, a major component in the controlling mechanism of all unconscious bodily processes, an exquisite balance is maintained through the interaction of opposites. The parasympathetic or cranial and sacral aspects of the autonomic nervous system, including the vagus nerve, with its ramifications to all abdominal organs, is essentially anabolic. Its functions are those of conservation, of indrawing, preservation and accumulation – of yin.

Conversely, the sympathetic nervous system, reaching to the same areas of the body, provides the impetus for catabolic expenditure of body energies and the inhibition of nutrient intake and assimilation – of yang. Between them, a balance is kept and – in the healthy body – the flow of forces and energy remains harmoniously poised.

This balance of forces is *essential* in any energy system. If a function is ascribed to some molecule or molecular interaction whether it is hormonal, enzymatic or whatever, there has to be an equal and opposite balancing force in order to prevent a runaway situation of continuous stimulation or depression of that function. The underlying balance of opposites will always be present.

Similarly, in the endocrine system we can expect to find both the stimulators and the inhibitors. But let us now discuss this in an ordered fashion, and in some detail.

Pranas, Tattwas, Chakras and Nadis

In the yogic tantras, the *pranas*, the vital principle or life energy, are sometimes perceived as a modification or vibration of the antashkarans, whilst in other descriptions they take the place of the tanmantras. But in general, prana is the vitalizing and organizational energy that brings the soul into incarnation. It is, therefore, governed by the karmic record impressed upon the antashkarans which is manifested outwardly as our physical being, both subtle and gross.

Flowing outward and downward as an energy vibration, much as a wave both upon and within water, though in this case with organizational function and intention, the pranas enliven the tattwas, giving rise to the chakras and *nadis* or pranic channels running throughout the body, bringing biological life and coherence to a body composed of otherwise inimical elements. The pranas are thus seen as also five in number or vibrational harmonics, enlivening each of the five tattwas and with functions accordingly. These will be described together with the tattwas and chakras in the ensuing chapters.

Life only exists in a body so long as prana is present and active. While the body itself can be seen as its gross physical parts, prana is fluid and indivisible – inseparable into specific regions. It brings a soul into a body, energizes the growth of the embryo, vitalizes the life span, the metabolic processes, the physiology, biochemistry and anatomy of living tissues; and ultimately it oversees their death.

Prana is known in its universal aspect as *Vayu* which is also translated as 'air' or 'breath', but prana is not the physical breath itself; rather it is the vital energy which manifests in one of its aspects as respiration, the in-breathing and out-breathing of atmospheric air, which gives us life and vitality, through the absorption of oxygen and oxidation of body fuels, releasing usable energy for life's physical processes.

Unobservable, then, by current scientific instrumentation, yet perceivable with the inner eye of consciousness through certain specific yogic practices, lies a series of life-energy plexi, the chakras, distribution points or subtle energy resonance centres, within the etheric body and moulded out of the five subtle tattwas. Each of these chakras or wheels is associated with a particular vibrational state of matter or tattwa and is formed by a pranic vibration, which – travelling throughout the body – transmits its enlivening and organizational nature to every atom, molecule and cell of our physical being. The subtle form of the tattwas woven by the pranic vibration into complex, integrated organizational patterns, therefore becomes the immediate subtle blueprint of the gross physical body, while consciousness, experienced by us at the physical level as our attention, retains its primary human seat, knotted together with the human mind at the eye centre.

From these spinning wheels of blueprint organization arise a matrix of channels, running throughout the body and known in yogic texts as the *nadis*. Literally, 'nadi' means a 'tube'. Like the chakras, they are formed by the interaction of the intelligent, but unconscious, pranic vibration as it weaves the subtle tattwas into the biological tapestry, the morphogenic field, the subtle energy blueprint or etheric body. They thus carry an energetic nature that relates to the chakra and tattvic field in which they have arisen. In the ancient texts, as well as more recently in Dr Stone's Polarity Therapy, the major nadis that relate to the particular tattwas have been mapped out and are therapeutically stimulated or balanced by massage and hand or finger pressure, as in the Chinese art of shiatsu or acupressure.

A Manual Digression

The structure of our entire body – whether seen from the level of subatomic particles, molecules, cells, tissues, organs or the whole body – is a result of the holographic ordering of the tattwas which comprise it. The form which we perceive has not occurred by chance or by random evolution, but is a most wonderful handiwork of the inward Creator. The human physical vehicle, with all its subtle aspects, is a most remarkable microcosm which reflects the full power of the Supreme, and through which He may be realized.

It is no coincidence, for example, that we have five fingers and five toes. The vibrations of each of the five tattwas is matrixed into our hands and feet to permit their integrated functioning in the physical realm of all the five tattwas, with each finger and each toe having a specific tattvic correspondence, (see figure 4-1). The thumb, for instance, carries the tattvic impression of akash, while the sensitive forefinger carries the airy quality of touch, feeling and manipulation.

See how the double-jointed thumb is indicative of will-power – a mental, akashic characteristic – while the forefinger is the primary, manipulative finger on our hand, the air on the air, so to speak, since we use the hand itself as the most common outward manifestation of the airy motor indriya of physical manipulation or grasping. Notice, too, how our beckoning finger is once again this forefinger – a physical link to the mental interaction and manipulation of others, while to have someone 'under one's thumb' means that they are subject to our will-power.

When we hold a pen, it is primarily a combination of the activity of our thumb and forefinger, supported by the other three fingers, that gives rise to written communication. And writing requires the intelligence given by akash and the conceptual ability and fleetness of air, underlain to a lesser degree by the supporting lattice of the other tattwas.

Similarly, with the other three fingers. The middle finger, representing the fiery, expanding principle amongst the tattwas, is the longest, in most of us. Indeed, in palmistry, the length of the middle finger is used as an indication of the drive and outgoing energy of the individual. You can readily check these attributes on yourself and friends and, in fact, many people are already aware of how the structure of a hand, let alone the intricate finger-

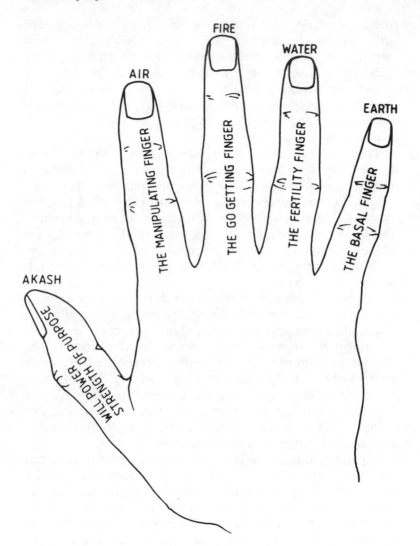

Figure 4-1. Tattvic correspondences in the fingers

prints, accurately mirror the psychological constitution of the individual. And as we have seen, the psychological constitution of the individual arises from the interplay of the mind and the subtle tattvas.

Nothing in nature or in our lives happens by coincidence. Everything has a relevance and a correspondence, is a part of the pattern of the karmic manifestation of our life.

To complete the picture, our little finger represents our earthy nature and the ring finger relates to the watery tattva, the element of procreation and it is no coincidence that we wear a gold ring on this finger to indicate our married status and, according to folklore, to stimulate our fertility. The existence of such practices, as well as the derivation of many words in our language which we take for granted, but which have a direct relationship to our inner human constitution, leaves us with the interesting conclusion that somewhere along the line our ancestors possessed a wisdom which is only rediscovered from time to time, as the ages progress. Technological or 'scientific' superiority does not in any way give us the right to consider ourselves a superior expression of the human race. In fact, the environmental destruction of our planet in the course of a single century, puts us in quite the opposite light and demonstrates how out of tune we have become with both ourselves and with nature.

Return To The Nadis

According to Sanskrit literature, there is a woven tapestry of over 72,000 nadis[5]. Of these, some are primary, (see figures 4-2, 3 & 5), and others increasingly peripheral and minor in function – like the ramifications of the nervous and blood circulatory systems – though the nadis are in no way to be directly equated with them. Of these nadis, three (*Ida*, *Pingala* and *Sushumna*) are primary. Starting at the left and right of the basal centre, Ida and Pingala represent the primary polarized linkage between the chakras. Sushumna passes down the central axis of the spine, through the position held in the gross physical body by the cerebro-spinal fluid. Recent research in cranial osteopathy has shown that there are regular rhythmic and physical pulsations through this fluid, which extends from the fourth ventricle or cavity in the brain, where it washes over the pineal gland, down to the base of the spinal cord.

---

[5] Some texts say the the figure is 720,000. In fact, the number matters little – it simply means: a lot.

The full function of this fluid-filled cavity is not at all understood by modern physiology and certain theories based not only on these rhythmic physical pulsations, but also on proposed electromagnetic or more subtle sub-atomic wave patterns (scalar waves, electron plasma waves and so on), allied to a controlling function of the pineal gland as a determiner of bodily rhythms (which is already known to have an influence on the circadian and other bodily rhythms), sound highly plausible and worthy of greater research.

In this respect, we immediately find correlation between the subtle nature of the pranic energy flowing in the Sushumna and the rhythms of electromagnetic and allied energy fields, products of activity within the subtle state, which may be an integral part of the functioning of cerebro-spinal fluid.

The Sushumna is said to be tamasic or yin in its outer nature and fiery red of colour. Within it, lies the lustrous *Vajra* or *Vajrini* nadi, of yang or rajasic nature and within this lies the sattvic nadi – the *Chitra* or *Chitrini*. Thus, in this central axis, all the three modes or gunas are present in balanced form. Yin is present in the yang and yang within yin. For this reason, Sushumna is also said to be the neutral, zero-balanced or sattvic nadi, from which all others are derived.

At the base of the spine, at the *Muladhara Chakra* lies the *Kundalini*. Kundalini is the quiescent aspect of the manifestation of life energy, quiescent because it has reached the nethermost pole of creation in its association with the *prithvi* or earth tattwa. Said to lie in a coil (which may signify only energy in potential form, ready to 'spring'), kundalini has been the subject of much, often incorrect, western speculation.

In those forms of yoga where the inner attention is directed to and consciousness is awakened in the bodily chakras, the ultimate purpose is the conscious awakening of this potential energy for use in the ascent of the mind and soul to the source of all pranic energy in the sky of the body, in the sub-astral zone. This process requires years of mental and bodily purification and most of those practitioners who claim to have 'awakened' this energy are unaware of the full implications of pranayama and kundalini yoga and have not had conscious contact with the kundalini at all. If they had, they would be able to perform many of the riddhis and siddhis – the miraculous powers that come with the conscious entry of the practitioner's concentrated attention into the realm of the five subtle tattwas.

As described, on either side of the Sushumna lie the nadis of Ida and Pingala connecting between the chakras as they rise from either side of the basal muladhara chakra to the space between and behind the eyes, the seat of the *Ajna Chakra*.

At this point, they enter the Sushumna, making a plaited knot of three, after which they separate once again, continuing upward to the 'sky' within, the source of the pranas.

One must remember to visualize these nadis and chakras, not as fixed objects and tubes, but as vibrating dances of energy enlivened and maintained in existence from within. Indeed, a molecule, comprised of subatomic particles, spinning into observable reality out of the fabric of vacuum should be seen in the same light.

Nadis, Networks and Focal Points

The nadis, then, form a lattice of physiological intelligence within the subtle, tattvic fields or etheric body, weaving the characteristics of the tattwas into a holographic tapestry from which the organs, systems and gross anatomy of the body, as we scientifically perceive it, is fashioned, as their final outward expression.

One can envisage that within this subtle matrix are formed positive, neutral and negative zones or cells, out of which is crystallized the cellular structure of the body with its electrical potentials between the nucleus, the cytoplasm and the cell membrane, reflecting the activity of the more subtle polarization.

The pranic currents of the nadis, imprinted with the tattvic characteristics which they pattern, also flow – according to Dr Stone – in five primary channels throughout the body in a form reminiscent of the lines of force surrounding a magnet, (see figure 4-3). But remember that such drawings are only two-dimensional, linear represen-

Chart of the subtle pana currents in the human body and their chakras as whirling primary *functional* centers of energy.

The six ventricles of the brain – relate to the six spinning chakras

Energy lines on Feet and Hands

These energy lines are purely functional and physiological as longitudinal influence arising from the chakras and forming the five sensory and the five motor currents flowing through the body to each digit of the hands and feet. In the treatment of functional blocks or disturbance of the five senses these areas are useful when the physiology is mostly involved.

(see opposite page)

Psychic phenomena and special sense development is due to the stimulation of a chakra by concentration of mind energy or interest in its function. Animals depend on the keenness of one sense for their direction and safety. The two petaled center in the forehead is the seat of consciousness in the brain. It descends as a dual current in a serpentine twisting motion polarizing and depolarizing in each center of the five etheric fields.

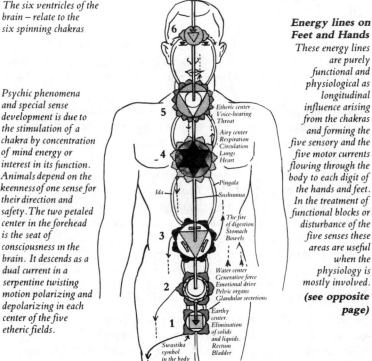

Etheric center
Voice-hearing
Throat

Airy center
Respiration
Circulation
Lungs
Heart

Pingala
Ida
Sushumna

The fire of digestion
Stomach
Bowels

Water center
Generative force
Emotional drive
Pelvic organs
Glandular secretions

Earthy center.
Elimination of solids and liquids.
Rectum
Bladder

Swastika symbol in the body

The center line through the body is the location of the path of the ultra-sonic energy substance as the primary life current and the core of being. It flows through the sixth ventricle of the brain and the spinal cord. It has five stepdown centers below the brain for the specialization of functions which we call the laws of nature for motion, life and the preservation of the species. These centers in the five oval etheric fields are the core of the wireless anatomy of the finest particles of matter known as chakras or lotuses. As they whirl in a right hand direction from the back, each of the five centers gives off one wave of its special quality of vibratory energy flowing as an electro-magnetic circuit to each finger and toe. In this manner the sensory and the five motor senses are created and function in the body.

Figures 4-2 and 4-3 are taken from: Polarity Therapy: The Complete Works of Dr Randolph Stone, D.O., D.C.

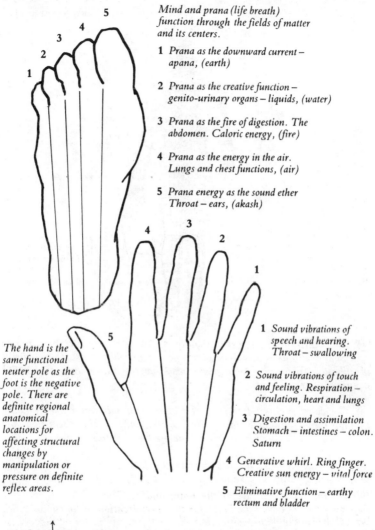

Mind and prana (life breath)
function through the fields of matter
and its centers.

1 *Prana as the downward current –
apana, (earth)*

2 *Prana as the creative function –
genito-urinary organs – liquids, (water)*

3 *Prana as the fire of digestion. The
abdomen. Caloric energy, (fire)*

4 *Prana as the energy in the air.
Lungs and chest functions, (air)*

5 *Prana energy as the sound ether
Throat – ears, (akash)*

The hand is the
same functional
neuter pole as the
foot is the negative
pole. There are
definite regional
anatomical
locations for
affecting structural
changes by
manipulation or
pressure on definite
reflex areas.

1 *Sound vibrations of
speech and hearing.
Throat – swallowing*

2 *Sound vibrations of touch
and feeling. Respiration –
circulation, heart and lungs*

3 *Digestion and assimilation
Stomach – intestines – colon.
Saturn*

4 *Generative whirl. Ring finger.
Creative sun energy – vital force*

5 *Eliminative function – earthy
rectum and bladder*

A spinning center or chakra with a crank inserted
from the back. The wheel gives off shoots of
energy by rotation upward on the left side as a right
hand turn.

*Figure 4-2. Dr Stone's chart of chakras and pranic centres. Note
that in Dr Stone's terminology, 'electromagnetic' sometimes
means what in this book we call 'subtle'.*

Ultrasonic Core

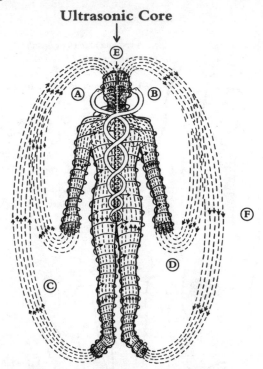

Ⓐ *The polarity of the serpentine brain current is reversed in the center of each oval field where the currents cross over each other, thus stepping down the vibratory intensity of the currents, also changing the nature of its function in every center and field.*

Ⓑ *The dotted vertical lines are electromagnetic wireless waves flowing through the longitudinal muscle fibres of the body, giving them tone and maintaining the body upright against the inertia of earth's gravity.*

Ⓒ *The oval horizontal lines around the body are the electromagnetic wireless currents which give tone to the circular fibres of the muscles. They correspond to the currents from east to west in the atmosphere.*

Ⓓ *The hands should be turned up with the thumbs forward. But for clarity of illustrating the 5 currents going through the 5 fingers, they are shown thus.*

Ⓔ *The ultrasonic energy forms the 6th ventricle of the brain and spinal cord. It becomes the primitive streak and the notochord in the embryo.*

Ⓕ *Electromagnetic energy attracts to its own center of polarity in oval waves. It is prior to the gravity of the earth, because it overcomes it by muscular motion moved by energy impulses. Earth gravity attracts to its center of gravity in straight lines of force by the square of the distance.*

The fine white line in the central core is the ultrasonic energy current of the soul. It is the primary energy which builds and sustains all others. It flows through the 6th ventricle of the brain and spinal cord when these are formed out of its mind pattern energy field. This core is the center of attraction and emanation of all currents from the brain to the extremities. It is the internal gravity of the individual energy and lines of force distinct from the gravity of the earth. This is the true basis for individual therapy.

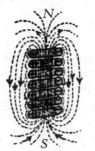

Actual lines of electromagnetic force around a solenoid

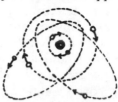

A carbon atom with 6 electrons circling around a heavy nucleus containing 6 elementary units of positive electric charge.

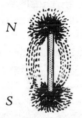

A bar magnet with concentration of iron filings at the poles similar to head & pelvis

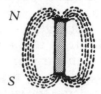

A bar magnet and its field as lines of force

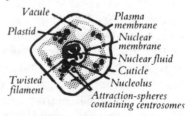

Vacule — *Plasma membrane*
Plastid — *Nuclear membrane*
Nuclear fluid
Cuticle
Twisted filament — *Nucleolus*
Attraction-spheres containing centrosomes

A microscopic cell. The twisted filaments in the center have self inductive electric capacity through oscillation. Chromosomes and tubules are made up of insulating material and filled with mineral salts similar to the ocean, for conduction of energy.

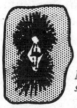

Metakinesis stage

Mitotic cell-division of fertilized whitefish eggs

Figure 4-3. One of Dr Stone's many flow charts, this one representing the primary flow of the pranic currents around the body. Note how the two currents of Ida and Pingala terminate on either side of the brain, thus linking each brain lobe to the opposite side of the body. By 'electromagnetic' and 'wireless' energy, Dr Stone refers to the pranas and subtle tattvic fields. Remember that this is only a two-dimensional, linear drawing in which the relationship of the parts to the whole cannot be adequately conveyed.

tations of energy relationships which are governed by more holographic relationships. The hands and the feet thus become focal points of energy flow, possessing a negative polarity with respect to the shoulders and pelvis. This polarity or potential difference is essential for the movement and flow of energy, as in electricity or any other manifestation of energetic movement. The matrix formed in the hands and feet out of these pranic vibrations with their specific tattvic characteristics, therefore possesses bodily correspondences and relationships through both tattvic resonance, as well as purely mechanical connection at a subtle level.

These energetic factors underlie the practice of foot and hand reflexology, as well as zone therapy, where manipulation and massage of the feet and hands results in a release of energy blockages in the subtle matrix in these extremities and reflexly in the organs and systems that are related to those points through the intricacies of the pattern matrix. Massage of the airy forefinger or second toe, for example, is said to balance the energies of the airy tattwa in respiratory areas of the body, while the thumb and big toe possess akashic correspondences to the brain and neck areas of the body. Energy blockages are normally felt as pain when the reflex area is massaged and may even appear as crystals within tissues. Masseurs of all schools are trained to detect and dissolve these crystals, whether or not they feel that they are working with subtle aspects of body function.

One can visualize that the physical impact of the massage pressure upon the specific point acts perhaps like applied pressure in a plumbing system, creating an energetic wave that travels to the area of correspondence, as well as through reflex resonance. The directed force travels back along the pranic flow-lines to the reflex area of the body, causing the subatomic and molecular patterns at that place to make an automatic adjustment that relates to the change in the subtle substructure. The result is observed in a more balanced physiology and biochemistry and the amelioration or even disappearance of disease and pathology. Perhaps, too, there are other more abstruse mechanisms with which theorization derived from the new physics might provide us. The holographic nature of energy relationships, for example, has been previously discussed.

Physiological Correspondences

Looking from without-in, in western physiological and anatomical terms, on either side of the spinal cord lie the two gangliated chains of nerve fibres constituting the central axis of the sympathetic nervous system, (see figure 4-4), with its links to all the automatically and unconsciously controlled areas of the body – the circulation and heart, the viscera and digestion, the lungs and respiration, and so on. Alongside the spinal column, also run the two major nadis whose function is the conveyance of prana between the chakras, linking them both functionally and energetically with each other and with the source of prana in the higher centres associated with the brain.

In this sense, therefore, there is functional correlation, Ida carrying the moon, feminine, yin or receptive current, associated with the calming qualities of the parasympathetic nervous system, whilst Pingala carries the sun, male, yang or stimulative current associated with the arousing nature of the sympathetic nervous system.

The central axis of the spinal cord contains the motor and some sensory nerve pathways, connected with our experiential and consciousness aspects of physical existence. For while we have the capacity to be aware of our actions and sensory experience, we are unconscious of the physiological and biochemical minutiae of internal body functioning, including that associated with the physiological mechanisms of otherwise voluntary muscular activity and physical sensation.

In all eastern mystic literature, the central path, the Sushumna or Royal Vein is seen as the path of consciousness and it is no coincidence that these aspects of the nervous system which are immediately linked to our awareness, pass along the central spinal axis. It is simply a direct and energetic reflection at the physiological level.

For this reason, too, the Sushumna contains within it a balance of all the three gunas, providing the harmony necessary for the outworking of consciousness in the material world. The autonomic nervous system, on the other hand, is maintained in balance through the Ida and Pingala, the polarized parasympathetic and sympathetic aspects of unconscious, but 'intelligent', pranic activity.

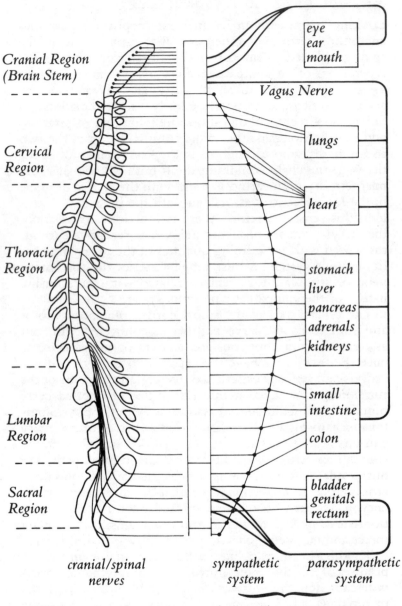

eye
ear
mouth

Cranial Region
(Brain Stem)

Vagus Nerve

Cervical
Region

lungs

heart

Thoracic
Region

stomach
liver
pancreas
adrenals
kidneys

small
intestine

colon

Lumbar
Region

Sacral
Region

bladder
genitals
rectum

cranial/spinal
nerves

sympathetic
system

parasympathetic
system

Voluntary nervous system

Autonomic nervous system

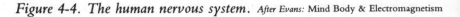

Figure 4-4. The human nervous system. *After Evans:* Mind Body & Electromagnetism

In both eastern and western understanding, therefore, the spinal axis and the central activity of the brain both carry the same functions of informational, organizational and energetic control. And whilst the activities of the spinal column and the associated autonomic nerve tracts lying alongside it are to some degree autonomous in both systems, it is acknowledged that the higher monitoring and control lies in the mental centres or the brain.

Similarly, the endocrine system, linked closely with the nervous system as part of a functional whole, is controlled and administered from above, through the pituitary gland, the hypothalamus and the higher brain centres. Furthermore, just as the nerves ramify throughout the entire body, as do the nadis in their subtle form, recent discoveries using more finely tuned biochemical assays, reveal that the endocrine system, too, has ramifications throughout the body in the sense that many of the major hormones have now been discovered to be produced not only in the major glands, but also in other parts of the body, too, including nerve fibres. *Oestrogen* and *testosterone* (sex hormones), for example, are found in brain cells, while adrenal medullary tissue is found throughout the body in association with the chromaffin tissue of the autonomic nervous system.

We are not, however, seeking parallels that place the subtle elements of human energies directly in exact correspondence with anatomical organs and physiological systems, since this is not the manner by which they come into existence. Rather, the intermerging of the more subtle energies and their interaction results in their precipitation out of the subtle matrix as anatomy and physiology, as atoms and molecules, as bioelectrical and biomagnetic energy domains, with some very obvious overall functional parallels as well as more general controlling mechanisms.

The blood circulatory system with its central cardiac pump and its association with the outside atmospheric world, again uses the central spine of the body as its point of effluence and central traffic control. Blood flows through the aorta and out to the bodily tissues, carrying with it the nutritional and organizational elements required for maintenance of body metabolism. Pranic energy both underlies the organization of this function as well being contained within the oxygen and other molecular substance thus conveyed, and indeed within the vibration of every atom and 'particle' of matter in the body. In fact, it is this intricate and integrated patterning quality of prana, as a stepped-down manifestation of the life force, that I am referring to when I describe the pranic vibration as 'intelligent'.

It is never possible, however, to find the subtle energies of our constitution through objective dissection or examination under the microscope. We will, in this way, only find reflections. There is no physical organ of thought, no place where visual images as we experience them subjectively can be found. These are functions of the antashkarans and the indriyas. We will not discover the pranas, the subtle tattwas or the tanmantras, but only the manifestation of their existence. Indeed we will not find Life or Consciousness by the outward examination of physical matter. We will only find evidence of its mystic presence.

Consciousness is not a development of complex bio-chemistry, as conventional evolutionists would have us believe, (an extraordinary idea, I have always found!). Consciousness is *prior* to the physical and brings it into manifestation. Mechanisms of adaptation are no doubt present and the fittest and most adaptable will always be the survivors, passing on these qualities to their progeny. But pure evolutionary theory, taking – as it does – the premise that life is nothing more than material substance in complex form, seems to me to be remarkably lacking in both common sense and simple observation. It takes no account of the immaterial aspects of being which are the subjective life experience of each one of us. Rigid adherence to outmoded scientific doctrine is very similar in its psychological aspects to human conditioning from religious and social quarters and stems, one imagines, from the same root cause: the inability to accept ignorance as a starting point of our human situation. We would rather bind ourselves to an illusory feeling of the security offered by a leaky boat than realize that we might as well admit to being lost in a vast ocean! And interestingly enough, the root of the word ignorance is to *ignore*, to simply overlook what is present before us, rather than to be lacking in instructed or learnt knowledge.

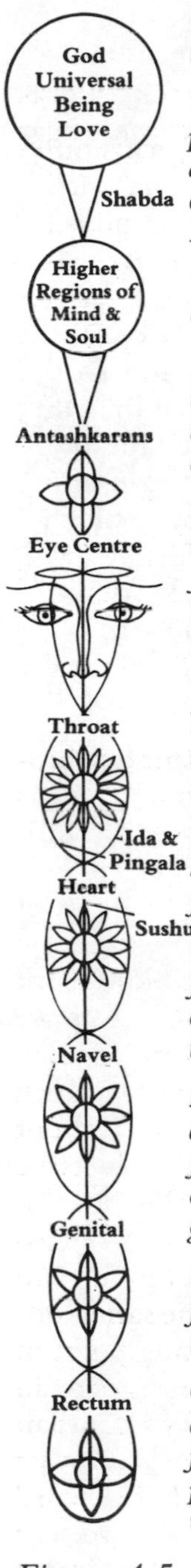

God
Universal
Being
Love

The Source of everything. Known to different cultures by many names.

Shabda

The Shabda or Word is the central creative current or power of life, the primal Life Force emanating from God and sustaining the creation. It is the primary vibration, experienced in mystic transport as Sound. And from this Life Stream, or Sound, also comes Light.

Higher
Regions of
Mind &
Soul

This includes the purely spiritual regions as well as the causal realm of Universal Mind, and the astral region.

Antashkarans

The human mind is comprised of the Antashkarans. This is the 'organ of thought' or the energy field in which thoughts exist. The pattern of destiny is also built into this centre.

Eye Centre

The soul and mind are knotted together at the Eye Centre in the waking condition, but are drawn out into the tattvic fields of the body and inert matter through the medium of the ten indriyas. The area that includes the Eye Centre and the Antashkarans is also known as the 'sky' of the body.

Throat

The pranas flow out from the sky of the body as Ida, Pingala and Sushumna, representing the three primary modes of pranic vibration (positive, neutral, negative) in the central spinal axis.

Ida &
Pingala
Heart

The pranas carry the cohering and patterning power of the Shabda, the life force into the realm of the five subtle and five gross tattwas.

Sushumna

Vibrating with intelligence from above, prana patterns the five subtle tattwas, forming, by its movement, the six chakras and the innumerable nadis. This subtle tattvic tapestry is sometimes known as the etheric body.

Navel

Patterned by prana, the subtle tattwas become the immediate blueprint of the grossly observable physical body. The five subtle tattwas precipitate, condense or dance into observable physical existence, through the medium of the gross akashic or vacuum state.

Genital

Thus are built up the complex patterns of subatomic and fundamental natural forces, forming molecules and the integrated biochemical and bioelectronic tapestry.

Rectum

Contrary to modern scientific opinion, life is not the outcome of a self-determining molecular complexity. In fact, the patterning of physiological and biochemical processes are actually maintained by the life force from within.

Figure 4-5. Schematic representation of the subtle human constitution.

107

Concluding

Up to this point, we have described in general terms only, the human constitution of soul, mind, pranas, tanmantras, tattwas, indriyas, chakras, nadis and their gross physical manifestation. This is summarized in figure 4-5. However, we are now at a point of confluence in our narrative, where the characteristics of the five tattwas, the five pranas, the five indriyas, the six chakras and so on, need to be considered individually, knowing that in reality they are all woven together into one complete tapestry.

Moreover, we are also in a position to begin more specific correlations with modern endocrinology, biochemistry and physiology. From hereon in, therefore, we will consider each centre and bodily region separately, describing the activities of each as we go, and showing – as far as possible – how each plays its part and relates dynamically to the whole.

CHAPTER 5

Down to Earth

The Muladhara Chakra and the Prithvi Tattwa

Starting from the base, the first chakra or centre is the *Muladhara* or rectal centre. The pranic vibration, working within the *prithvi* or earthy tattwa of this level, forms four petals or energy aspects, seen with a reddish or crimson hue when perceived with the subtle sight developed by certain yogic practices. Spinning out from this four-petalled, organizational centre are the extensions of its intelligence network in the form of those nadis constituting that part of the cohering, subtle matrix by means of which the finer details of earthy administration within the body is performed.

As we have described, the chakras and nadis are formed by the life-directed vibrations of prana, as centres of administration and organizational resonance. Thus, when prana is withdrawn at the time of death, the centres cease to exist and, like the pranas themselves, evaporate or disappear, like the ripples from a pond, when the wind or breath of life subsides.

In yogic practice, there are certain mantras or mental repetitions which are made with the attention fixed within at each centre. The thought-shapes of these mantras approximate to harmonics of the energy vibrations of each chakra and, by means of resonance together with persistent and determined practice over the course of many years, they permit the practitioner to focus his attention upon and enter into the consciousness of each centre and effectively become the 'ruler' of the energies administered there. This we all do unconsciously all the time, the pranic intelligence reflecting outwardly as the unconscious bodily control mechanisms. These are the autonomic nervous system, the endocrine system, the biochemical control network whose cellular intelligence stems from the nucleus of each cell, plus other energetic control systems within the body, the bioelectric, biomagnetic and crystalline nature of which modern physiology is only now gaining an awareness.

Through conscious effort and mental exertion, it is possible to gain limited control over some autonomic functions, especially those already closest to our awareness, such as heart rate. In fact, modern understanding and medical research involving simple forms of meditation have actually observed that meditators are able to exercise some degree of conscious control over bodily functions normally considered autonomic or unconscious. From this realization that mental and emotional energy patterns are reflected in the gross physical body, therapeutic techniques involving positive inner visualizations and the use of mental energy to correct energy imbalances and disease within the body are increasingly being added to even conventional medical practice. Biofeedback equipment, for example, trains the user to develop a relaxed state of mind by monitoring brain wave patterns that indicate to him his degree of relaxation.

This process is also the mechanism by which psychosomatic afflictions take root, through the pranic energy imprinted with our mental and emotional patterns, spreading throughout the body via the chakras and nadis and, in a very real sense, placing a harmonic, reflecting the vibrations of our personality, within every atom and cell of our body.

The prithvi tattwa of this first centre, roughly translated as earth, is the lowest and most tamasik of all vibrations within the body, creating coherence and obstruction in energy fields to the degree that we experience its outward manifestations as being solid, despite the fact that modern physics tells us that solids, too, are mostly 'space' and in fact consist of vibrating or oscillating energy patterns. Remember that the tattwa itself, in blueprint form, possesses a subtle aspect to its nature, though also manifesting outwardly as the 'earth' or 'solid' with which we are familiar.

Thus, the solid aspects of the body are maintained by the subtle matrix from the earthy energies distributed through or patterned by this centre. The pranic current at this level is known as *Apana*, the 'downward breath', which governs the excretory and eliminatory processes. Thus the bones, flesh, skin, hair and solid aspects of body tissues take their basal controlling energy and existence from this chakra, tattwa and pranic vibrational administration area.

Our conscious human experience of the prithvi tattwa is manifested through the tanmantra of odour and the earthy sense indriya of smell, its gross physical link being located in the olfactory tissues of the nose. Our sense of smell is thus the outward expression of direct earthy perception and the functions of elimination and excretion, through the rectum and anus in particular are this chakra's most outward site of action. Sluggish activity of the earthy element leads to an unclean colon and constipation, resulting in a spread of uneliminated toxins throughout the body. The breath takes on an odour from within the stomach and intestines, while the sense of smell may itself be dulled.

The body's major outward organs of final elimination and excretion are the colon/rectum, the kidney, the skin and – for airy respiratory waste products – the lungs. Both water and earthy tattwas are fundamentally involved in these former processes, the most earthy being the eliminative functions of the colon and rectum, the skin and kidneys both requiring greater activity of the watery element for the excretion of solids in solution. Dr Stone also comments that overall control of the kidneys is a function of the intricate nature of the airy tattwa. Earth by its solid and dense nature can impede the flow of the other elements and in an unbalanced condition leads to the multitudinous conditions of tissue thickening and loss of mobility – arthritis, tumours, arterio-sclerosis and heart disease.

The interesting book, *Biotypes*, by Joan Arehart-Treichel, which has largely gone unnoticed, documents considerable medical evidence for the psychosomatic energy linkage between personality and health. Thus, for example (and very generally), arthritis is normally traceable to a rigidity, tightness and suppression of emotions at the mental and emotional levels, giving rise to solidification of physical tissues.

Naturally, each part of the physical body contains a mixture of all the tattwas with, frequently, an active preponderance of one or more. Thus there are fluids in bones as well as solids; fiery calorific and nourishing aspects within all cells and tissues; airy constituents transported to every area, and so on. The body is an indivisible functioning energetic whole, a microcosm of the macrocosm, a dynamic vibrating dance of interwoven energies, at whichever level – biochemical, atomic, subtle or any other – you care to make examination.

In Ayurvedic medicine, the essential tattwas active within each part of the body are carefully studied and monitored. For by use of herbs and other natural methods, including yoga, the balance may be restored in these underlying energy fields, thereby permitting any diseased or disharmonized tissues to re-arrange themselves into a harmonious or healthful condition, even resulting in the disappearance of pathological symptoms. This is true of all healing – the higher up within the vertical energy spectrum one can work, then the less energy is required to create a greater effect at the lower, physical (or emotional and mental) ends.

Endocrine Definitions

Although many people will already be aware of the unique nature of the endocrine glands, it may be as well before going any further, to provide some definitions. An endocrine gland is one which secretes chemical substances (hormones) directly into the blood stream. These are then carried to other, often remote, parts of the body where they have powerful controlling effects upon cellular functioning. Each endocrine centre plays a role in body physiology which is directly related to the attributes of the tattwa administered through its corresponding chakra or pranic centre. And we will be discussing these relationships as we proceed.

An *exocrine* gland, on the other hand, is one which secretes a fluid locally. The salivary glands, for example, in the mouth secrete saliva or the glands in the stomach and intestines secrete digestive juices containing enzymes and even hydrochloric acid. There are generally considered to be six major endocrine centres in the body, (tabulated in figure 5-1), just as there are six major physical chakras (see figures 3-2, 4-2 and 4-5).

Endocrine Centre		**Location**

Hypothalamus

Hypothalamus
& Pituitary

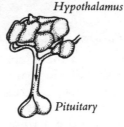

Pituitary

Brain

Thyroid &
Parathyroids

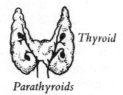

Thyroid

Parathyroids

Throat

Thymus

Thymus

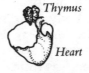

Heart

Heart

Pancreas

Intestine

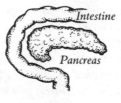

Pancreas

Intestine

Gonads

Ovaries
and uterus

Testes
in scrotum

Sacral area

Adrenals

Adrenals

Kidneys

Lower
abdominal
cavity

Some sketches adapted with permission from Hormones: The Messengers of Life, Lawrence Crapo, W. H. Freeman & Co.

Figure 5-1. The bodily endocrine centres. Compare with figures 3-2, 4-2 and 4-5.

113

Endocrine Aspects – The Adrenal Glands

Associated with the muladhara chakra are the adrenal glands. Earth or prithvi is the base on which the body structure rests. It represents the grossest point of contact with the physical universe. This centre therefore has a primary responsibility for the maintenance of existence on the physical plane. In Sanskrit writings, it is sometimes given the symbolic shape of a square – the solid foundation into which all other structures may be fitted. Similarly, the ruling deity of this centre is said to be Ganesh, seated on the elephant *Airavat*, the symbol of solidity, of being firmly anchored in physical life.

The adrenal glands, too, whose hormones take their biochemical vibration or form from this chakra, are an essential part of the body's life maintenance mechanism, often described as the 'fight or flight' system. It is worth studying these hormones in some little detail because their individual functioning – as much as it is understood – plus their vibrational, energetic (i.e. molecular) shapes present some intriguing analogies and clues as to how the subtle energies manifest themselves and their organizational capacities as gross physical matter.

For the next few pages, therefore, we enter into a more biochemical and physiological discussion of this endocrine centre. If it is beyond your scientific threshold, just read it lightly, picking up any points of general interest, skimming through to the section, Hormones, Molecules & Vibrational Resonance. *You won't miss anything of the general trend by doing this, but it is there for those who have that kind of a mind to be interested in such details.*

The adrenal glands are situated, as the name implies, on top of the kidneys. They consist of a cortex, or outer part, which produces different hormones to those that come into being within the inner medullary tissue.

The adrenal cortex actually synthesizes over forty different *steroid* substances, playing a major role in body metabolism and usually classified into three major groups, according to the manner in which they affect cellular metabolism. These are *gluco-corticoids*, such as *cortisol* and other *catabolic steroids*; *mineral-corticoids* like *aldosterone*; and *anabolic steroids*, which include the *sex hormones*. Their various activities are not, however, sharply delineated.

The adrenal cortex is itself divided into three relatively distinct cellular layers, with aldosterone being produced solely in the outer layer, while cortisol and the catabolic steroids are synthesized in both of the other two layers.

The Adrenal Medulla, Adrenaline and Noradrenaline

Making the fourth category of adrenal hormone, the adrenal medulla produces a group of substances known as *catecholamines*, molecules derived from the amino acid *tyrosine*. In this sense, they are not pure peptide hormones, but are peptide[1] derivatives, the structure being relatively simple, (see figure 5-2).

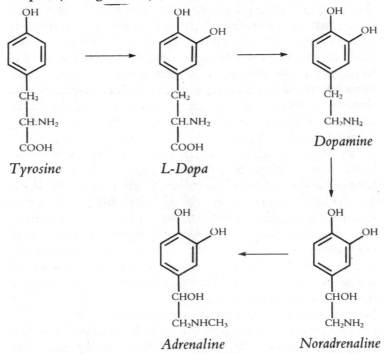

Figure 5-2. Tyrosine, noradrenaline, adrenaline and dopamine

[1] *Peptides, polypeptides* and *proteins* are all characterized by their composition as amino acid strings. The distinction between them is fairly arbitrary, in that polypeptides and proteins simply contain a larger number of these amino acids than peptides.

Three of the principle catecholamines presently known to science are *adrenaline, noradrenaline and dopamine*. Adrenaline, also called *epinephrine*, is synthesized in chromaffin tissue such as that found in the adrenal medullae and elsewhere along the sympathetic nervous system. Noradrenaline and dopamine are more strictly considered as a neurohormones produced, respectively in post-ganglionic, sympathetic nerve endings,[2] and in the brain. They are largely responsible just for local activity at their point of release. While about eighty per cent of the chromaffin cells in the adrenal medulla appear to be given over to the manufacture of adrenaline, the remaining twenty per cent are involved in noradrenaline production.

Adrenaline is the hormone that makes your heart go bang and surge into action when you get a shock or feel tense. It is yang in nature, preparing all parts of the body for action – to flee or to defend, to be alert through all the senses. It gives endurance and staves off tiredness while the work is there to be done. It is the emergency hormone that stimulates rapid deployment of bodily energies for dealing with stressful situations. Physiologically, adrenaline acts on the heart, lungs and blood vessels to increase the circulation of nutrients and oxygen to body tissues and organs. In addition, the production of glucose and fatty acids from body stores is increased, providing greater fuel supply to support any exertion – muscular, cerebral and otherwise.

Adrenaline behaves as the classical hormone, being released into the blood by the chromaffin cells and affecting other tissues and organs at distant bodily sites. Noradrenaline, on the other hand, is more local in its activity being released due to sympathetic nervous stimulation by the nerve endings themselves and therefore only acting on tissues thus innervated.

In most respects, the two hormones have similar, but not identical activity, mirroring the close association between the sympathetic nervous system and the endocrine system. Of the two, adrenaline would appear to have a wider range of effects, befitting its role of being more

[2] Post-ganglionic and pre-ganglionic sympathetic nerve fibres refer to nerve fibres or cells on the through route to an organ or tissue, either *before* (pre-) the ganglion alongside the spinal cord, or *after* (post-) it.

generally circulated in the blood stream, with noradrenaline being generally more specific and less potent.

Interestingly, noradrenaline can be converted to adrenaline by an enzyme which is only found in the adrenal medulla, the organ of Zuckerkandl and, in tiny amounts, in the brain. In addition, an extremely high, local concentration of glucocorticoids from the adrenal cortex must also be present for this transformation to take place.

The chromaffin cells themselves are activated into catecholamine production by pre-ganglionic sympathetic nerve impulses through the intermediary of the ubiquitous neurotransmitter, *acetyl choline*. In this sense, they can be considered as post-ganglionic sympathetic nerve cells, specialized to release their catecholamines directly into the blood stream.

It is also of interest that electrical stimulation of those parts of the hypothalamus that invoke normal sympathetic response, including the release of noradrenaline at post-ganglionic nerve endings, also elicits the release of catecholamines from the adrenal medulla. Furthermore, it has been reported that electrical stimulation of specific parts of the hypothalamus leads to selective release of particular catecholamines from the adrenal medulla.

The hypothalamus has a central function in coordinating endocrine and nervous activity and the electrical link is of some considerable interest in respect of its relationship to patterns within the vacuum and subtle states.

Since this is only likely to occur in times of extreme stress, one can postulate that noradrenaline in the adrenal tissue acts as something of a buffer against emergencies, a storage pool of adrenaline pre-cursor.

The Adrenal Cortex

While the adrenal medulla is linked directly to the sympathetic nervous system and is activated through direct innervation, the adrenal cortex is modulated by endocrine linkage to the anterior pituitary and hypothalamus, in the brain, and thence into the higher brain centres. As mentioned previously, there are three categories of adreno-cortical hormone.

Catabolic steroids are, like adrenaline, released in increased amounts during times of stress, when they temporarily decelerate cell metabolism. In this respect, cortisol works in tandem with adrenaline. For while the latter brings body fuels out of storage for use under stress or in emergency, cortisol prevents the storage of nutrients as fuel by blocking the secretion of the pancreatic hormone *insulin*. Insulin normally triggers the build up of glucose, amino acids and fatty acids into the body storage fuels of carbohydrates, proteins and fats. In addition, cortisol works across the grain, producing fuel for immediate activity by aiding the conversion of amino acids into glucose.

Catabolic hormones also affect cell membranes, superlatively important structures that act as selective gateways to molecular and electrical interchange, increasing their rigidity and making them less permeable to ions, including sodium and potassium.

Since the interchange of ions is essential in all cellular processes and is the mechanism by which nerve impulses are transmitted, treatment with catabolic steroids will upset all body metabolism especially amongst nerve cells. This therefore interrupts the free flow of energy from the more mechanistic aspects of brain function up into higher levels of mind energy, and large doses can cause emotional instability, depression, irritability and even temporarily schizophrenic states.

It has been generally established for some time that the release of both catabolic steroids like cortisol, as well as the adrenal sex hormones, is regulated through the anterior pituitary gland. In fact, its removal results in the gradual atrophy of the two cortical cellular layers responsible for cortisol and sex steroid production. We discuss the mechanism in a little more detail in chapter ten, (there is a schematic diagram on page 255), but basically the anterior pituitary gland produces the *adrenocortico-trophic hormone* (ACTH) which stimulates the various transmutations that are required for the conversion of the steroid pre-cursor, *cholesterol* into cortisol. The hypothalamus is also involved, while rising cortisol concentrations also feed back to inhibit pituitary ACTH production.

In general, therefore, cortisol and catabolic steroids are concerned with body preservation, the being-present-in the-physical-world-ness, the attribute of the earthy tattwa. Blood pressure is maintained and the overall nutritional well-being of the body is fostered and encouraged, with an emphasis on balance being maintained according to the various circumstances of physical origin.

Because of their suppressive action upon cellular metabolism, these hormones or their synthetic similars are used therapeutically to relieve the symptoms and give temporary relief from the inflammatory reactions which are really a part of the body's positive defence to infection, injury or invasion by any foreign substance. Thus, they are widely used for conditions such as arthritis and asthma, but their effects can be disastrous, their prescription being blatantly superficial and symptomatic. Their 'side-effects' are not really side-effects at all, but *direct effects*, including high blood pressure, changes in water and fat metabolism, osteoporosis due to interference in bone metabolism, sticky blood platelets accompanied by myriads of small blood clots, increased susceptibility to infection and a depressed immune response, plus the characteristic moon-like, puffed-up face. *Every cell in the body is in fact affected adversely.* Not really a good advertisment for an intelligent approach to disease.

One is so amazed that modern medicine is often so lacking in any deep, basic understanding and strategy in its approach to health and healing. And while one appreciates that dealing pragmatically with the health problems that beset us every day may lead to unsubtle and symptomatic remedies, the overall conceptual framework and understanding of the human constitution is in drastic need of re-evaluation, in order that better solutions to bodily disharmonies may be found *before* the point of pathological breakdown arrives, requiring the emergency, symptomatic treatment.

The second group of adreno-cortical hormones are the *anabolic steroids* which include the sex hormones of *testosterone* (male hormone), *oestrogen* and *progesterone* (female hormones). The major sites of sex hormone production are the ovaries and testes, but sex hormones control far more than just reproductive physiology. This is why taking the hormone contraceptive pill has such a wide range of dangerous effects. That research, however is beyond the scope of this book and I would direct your attention to Dr Ellen Grant's excellent and detailed survey of the subject, *The Bitter Pill*.

In addition to the gonads, the adrenal cortex of both sexes also produces all three of these major steroid sex hormones and, indeed, after menopause the adrenal gland is a women's major source of oestrogen. Both male and female adrenals manufacture small amounts of oestrogen and progesterone, but while men produce high levels of testosterone from both the testes and the adrenals, women convert only small quantities of the adrenal testosterone pre-cursors (*androgens*) into active testosterone. This admixture of sexual polarity is of considerable interest and is discussed more fully in the next chapter.

The reproductive capability represents a distinct aspect of the preservation and survival role inherent in the activity of the earthy tattwa and its endocrine outworking. Hence its hormonal linkage with the adrenal endocrine centre. This reasoning would also explain why the major part of female oestrogen is produced in the adrenal cortex after menopause, when the powerful reproductive urge and phase of life has subsided. It could also be used to understand why virilism in women is usually due to excess androgen production from the adrenal cortex rather than the ovaries, although the reproductive functioning is normally disturbed by such excess, usually resulting in infertility. The hands-on- hips, domineering archetype of the virile women is clearly an expression of positive earthy rootedness, more akin to the functioning of the rectal chakra, than that of the sex centre.

Additionally, the archetypal, 'aggresive' or outgoing nature of the man, coupled with the more harmonizing and receptive attributes of the woman are both essential aspects of the balanced survival of our human species and hence, once again, we have functional linkages between earthy preservation and sexual polarity. And since every human, man or woman, requires both aspects to be present in their basic make-up, as a reflection of this natural psychology we find both male and female hormones being produced by both sexes and from the earthy gland of the adrenal cortex, too.

Actually, the terms 'preservation' and 'survival' are somewhat basic, and at the emotional level, these qualities appear as one's groundedness or solid presence within the material affairs of life. And a number of excellent books have been written describing a woman's change from the intensely reproductive and motherly phase to the more outgoing and earthily-connected stage of life after the menopause. In the absence of 'wise women' within our modern society, these phases of life are little understood and women, subjected to social pressures, prejudices and taboos, often find themselves floundering in their mid-forties, when the children have left home, and new feelings come upon them but with little or no guidance available from others. Rather than welcome with understanding a shift into a new direction, with new opportunities for fulfilment and growth, some even resort to hormone therapy in an attempt to prolong the earlier phase, while others find themselves emotionally unbalanced for no apparent reason.

Anabolic steroids promote cell growth by stimulation of both metabolism and the production of proteins and sugars within the cells. The polar opposite of catabolic steroids in their effects, the cell membranes become flexible, permitting an easy and flowing transport of substances. The result is an increase in nitrogen retention, a build up of body protein – especially in muscles – and generally vigorous cell growth and activity. They have thus been used by athletes for endurance and body building, especially by boxers, wrestlers and so on, a clear indication of their role as vibrational messengers and lower harmonics of the subtle earthy tattwa.

The effect of anabolic steroids, including that of the various contraceptive hormone pills, has been the subject of much medical observation and explains many of the other effects of the Pill including abnormally high blood glucose levels, (leading in some cases to diabetes), high blood pressure, weight gain, headache, emotional imbalance, nausea and many other problems. This is to be expected, for these steroid substances affect probably every cell in our bodies.

The final group of adreno-cortical steroids are *mineral-corticoids*, which include the major adrenal hormone, *aldosterone*. Aldosterone performs a similar 'solids-preservation' role by acting on the kidneys and other bodily sites to conserve salt, maintaining the essential sodium and potassium balance, as well as blood pressure.

In fact, aldosterone is never administered therapeutically to patients because it can result in a very rapid rise in blood pressure.

Aldosterone release is controlled by a number of factors including the levels of sodium and potassium in the blood, indirectly through pituitary stimulation of cholesterol conversion to a general steroid hormone precursor, *pregnenolone*, but most importantly via feedback from the kidneys. Certain cells in the kidneys are influenced to produce the enzyme, *renin*. Stimulating factors include blood pressure sensors, the anti-diuretic posterior pituitary hormone, *vasopressin*, and stimulation by noradrenaline and the sympathetic nervous system. Renin then enters the blood stream where it catalyzes the formation of the substance, *angiotensin*, via a number of intermediaries. Angiotensin then stimulates the adrenal cortex into aldosterone production, (see figure 5-3).

Dr Grant points out that this is one of the mechanisms by which oral contraceptives increase blood pressure, through an increase in the concentration of blood renin and hence of aldosterone.

Hormones, Molecules and Vibrational Resonance

It is important to appreciate the power that these hormonal molecules or energetic vibrations contain. It is necessary, too, I believe, to maintain a conception of a molecule as an oscillating, vibrating energy complex. Remember the atomic content and the understanding given by modern physics. A molecule consists of electronic, magnetic, gravitational and other forces all vibrating in a complex manner that is not at all comprehended by science. Our analysis of the atomic arrangement of molecular structure is creditable, but should not beguile us into feeling that its more inward energetic nature is of no importance. All molecular interactions take place *because* of this inner nature and structure, which scientifically we do not, as yet, comprehend at all. In fact, in terms of the most recent theories of modern physics, with subatomic particles and the fundamental forces being seen as disturbances or activity on the oceanic face of an energy-rich vacuum, a

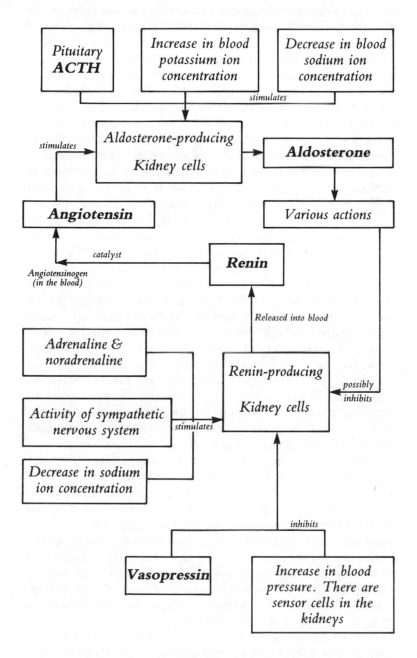

Figure 5-3. Preservation of bodily solids

molecular complex is simply a vibrating pattern that reflects the more inward vacuum and subtle states.

My own intuition, therefore, is that the energetic shape of such highly and universally active hormonal molecules represents in some way an energetic or vibrational harmonic of the more subtle tattvic fields, polarized according to its yin or yang function. This vibration then courses through the body and by vibrational resonance is able to create the purposed effect on the various and multitudinous target sites. This, of course, has an 'observable' molecular aspect which has become the major research emphasis of modern endocrinology, but it does not represent the full story, even if all the biochemical pathways became known to us. And we are far from that state of knowledgeable ignorance, as any biochemist will acknowledge.

Clearly, the individual shape of each molecule must represent its function in energetic terms. Generally speaking, hormones are of two molecular families – *steroids* and *peptides*. The vast majority belong to the latter group and are, like proteins, composed of the basic, life-supporting amino acids, a relatively small group of molecules without which the existence of living organisms is impossible. Steroids are closed ring structures (see figure 5-4) and generally speaking steroid hormones are produced by the adrenal and gonadal centres only. It is therefore tempting to propose that the steroid ring, being of a more complex and dense nature, is appropriately an outward physical manifestation of the denser earthy and watery tattwas.

Indeed, steroids all have one common pre-cursor, cholesterol, (see figure 5-5), which is manufactured in the liver and the adrenal cortex itself, as well as being consumed in the diet. And it is cholesterol which gives us problems of heart and arterial disease by way of blockages, because of its solid nature. In fact, the classic case of heart disease is the personality rooted firmly in the practical earth of life, often running on his nerves and hyperproductive of adrenaline, firmly attached to the possession of things of this world, thereby drawing the solidity into their own body through their own mental and emotional nature.

But in fact, while the fashion has become to avoid foods high in cholesterol, the evidence actually points to the life-style and personality of the individual being the more signi-

Cholesterol
(Full structure)

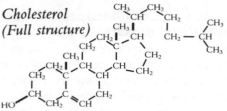

Progesterone

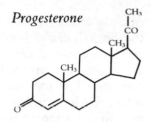

Cortisol

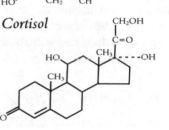

Aldosterone

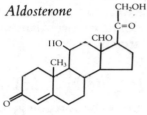

Oestrogen

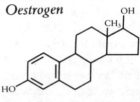

Testosterone

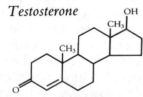

Figure 5-4. Steroid ring structures: cholesterol, cortisol, aldosterone, oestrogen, progesterone, testosterone.

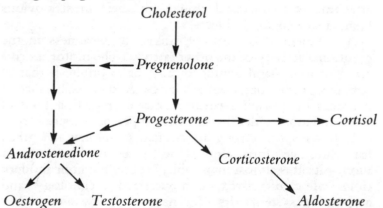

Figure 5-5. Cholesterol and steroid hormone synthesis. Each arrow represents one molecular transformation, catalyzed by a particular enzyme. The names of some of the intermediaries are omitted. In fact, molecular transformation occurs as a continuous and flowing energetic re-shaping of the atomic and probably subatomic structure. Our representation as a series of steps is merely a convenience, but can be misleading.

125

ficantly causative factors than diet. Consider, for example, the Somali camel herdsmen who consume a high cholesterol diet containing over ten pints of camel's milk per day, yet remain relatively free from hardening of the arteries. It is the inner tattvic patterning and imbalance which is the primary, causative factor, causing solidification of areas where the earthy tattwa is not meant to be so active, overrunning and pulling into the lower earthy vibration the balanced activity of the other more subtle tattwas.

Psychological Aspects of the Earthy Tattwa

From the foregoing, it is clear that the human weakness associated with this lower chakra and tattwa is that of attachment to worldly objects and the fear of their loss, including one's body and this makes considerable sense. For it is through the solid property that surrounds us that our attachment goes out. Very few of us lay personal claim of ownership to fluids and atmospheric gases. If we wish to do so, they must first be encased in solid surroundings – bottles, canisters and so on. Generally, therefore, our attachments to physical things, in their most obvious form, relate to solid objects.

Attachment is, of course, linked to weakness in the emotional activity of the other tattwas. The motor indriya and balanced manifestation of air, for example, is that of 'grasping' or 'getting hold of' things. And out of balance, it becomes the grasping nature, avarice or getting hold of more and more under the influence of personal desire or ego.

In this respect, strong attachment to money and greed for more, one of mankind's oldest vices, is of interest, for money itself is almost intangible, especially in our modern times of credit cards, computerized technology and accounting systems. Its very nature of airy intangibility exercises our mind more avidly in its attempts to gain permanent possession. The relentless pursuit of high finance, therefore, becomes the indulgence of the airy intelligent and the mentally adroit, while the accumulation of material possessions is the more outward, physical manifestation of this tendency. The weakness, however, lies in the mind, not in the mere possesion of material

goods, and a man may be quite detached though sur-
rounded by his possessions, whilst another may be deeply
attached to very little or to his inward desire for more and
more.

The human mind, the antashkarans, takes on the shape
of these external objects (including other people) when we
perceive and later recall them to memory or think of them,
usually with personal desire for them or a wish to be rid of
them. These vibrations or waves in the mind are known as
Vrittis or *Chitta Vrittis* and it is the first object of all yoga
and true meditation to still these mental oscillations before
any real inward spiritual progress can be made. Thus the
weaknesses of our human nature, the imbalances in the
various energies of our constitution, need to be overcome
or controlled before we can even think with lucidity, let
alone progress in meditation.

For as the mind moves out from its centre and plays or
reflects against the five subtle tattwas without our fully
conscious control from within, so do the five emotional
weaknesses of all humans come into being. These are earth
with attachment, water with sensory indulgence and lust,
fire with anger, air with greed, and akash with selfishness,
egotism and an unconscious and continuous expression of
self-identification. And just as the lower four tattwas take
their roots from and are created out of akash, so too is the
weakness of akash, that of self-centered awareness, the
mainspring out of which all other weaknesses flow. Take
away one's sense of self and all attachment, lust, anger and
greed disappear automatically.

The ultimate and long-term control of these weaknesses, therefore, lies not so much in 'fighting' them directly,
though of necessity one struggles on a day-to-day basis,
but in attaching the mind to its own inner creative essence,
the Shabda, whereby the over-active ahankar or ego
simply dissolves, as the true identification of our being
with our inner source becomes more deeply established.

Psychologically, the earthy tattwa manifests as a strong
material perception, underlying the astrological signs of
capricorn, *taurus* and *virgo*. Earthy natures readily understand how to work with physical energies. Often people of
their senses, they are governed by pragmatism and practi-
calities, with idealism only being infused into their nature

127

from an admixture of the airy element, in particular. They are people whose material needs are of considerable importance to them and they will hold on with great persistence to their physical possessions.

Convention, habit, ritual and the outer forms of social life are woven into the solid fabric of their lives and in spiritual people of earthy disposition, the tendency towards disciplined and habitual behaviour is a common experience and can be of considerable advantage to them.

Earthy natures are usually efficient, sometimes obsessively so, and whilst they are not necessarily assertive, they will act quite pragmatically to ensure that the fruits of their endeavours are not lost. They are dependable and like time to think before they act, something that an airy, more spontaneous nature might find annoying and difficult to tolerate. Earthy natures, for their part may view the flights of airy personalities with some reserve and even suspicion, being dubious of the lively and the imaginative. Similarly, the drive of fiery natures may be experienced by earthy types as drying or parching, resulting in a feeling of being drained. Watery characteristics on the other hand, with their sensitivity and emotional understanding, give energy to the earth signs, permitting them to flourish within the context of their own nature. For the emotions of water will themselves feel contained by the presence of good and solid earth, without the threat to freedom that such solidity may engender in air or the earthy blocking of expansive energies experienced by fire.

Very few people, however, have the qualities of just one tattwa influencing their nature, and the variable combinations are apparent in the different characteristics we all display. For into our natures, too, worked into the tattvic play, is woven the patterning of our karmas which make us do what we do, make us go where we go and meet the experiences within both the outer and inner fields of the tattwas, that we are predestined to experience.

Overactivity of the earth tattwa can lead to a heavy and overly practical approach to life in which imagination and flair cannot gain expression, while excessive stubbornness, without feeling for the emotions of others, accompanied by a narrowness of outlook, can result in a cynical attitude, in the absence of airy mental ideals.

Earth in combination with air can lead to the inventive and imaginative approach to physical problems, making such people excellent scientists or industrial designers as well as good administrators, where a further admixture of water will infuse into their personality the sensitivity to others that is required for kindly personell management and leadership.

Watery natures in combination with earth alone are, in their most negative aspect, the bearers of burdens, both physical and mental. This is the *kapha* constitution of Ayurveda, characteristically manifesting itself as well-developed, even heavy or overweight individuals, whose skin is oily, but cool and lacking colour, and with thick, soft wavy hair. Kapha people are described as slow, sleeping a lot and possessing plenty of stamina and staying power. Mentally, comprehension may be dull, but their memory is retentive. Without the activity of air and fire, water and earth in combination can become obsessively conscious of their own needs, above all else. Frustrated in their need to fly, to move and to enjoy adventure in their life, they can, at worst, become miserly, manipulative and greedy in an indrawn manner. At their best, they are well-grounded in their perception and understanding of everyday happenings, facing events with great fortitude and strength of purpose.

An understanding of the tattwas predominating in our make-up can be an invaluable aid to improving one's relationships with others and comprehending one's own characteristics. We all have a tendency to mistrust those qualities in others that are alien to us, so an appreciation of the manner in which our different characteristics come into being can be of great help, for we would no more feel intolerant of water for being wet that we should of watery types for being sensitive and emotional. The problem is, of course, that the patterning of our life has devolved upon us according to our karmas and its meaning is only apparent as it relates to our struggle towards spiritual perfection, whilst still encased in the vibrations of the tattvic energy fields. We are thus constrained to act according to our inner nature. So it is not, as they say, what we do – it is the way we do it.

Poetic Interlude

I do not think there is anyone who takes quite such a fierce pleasure in things being themselves as I do. The startling wetness of water excites and intoxicates me: the fieriness of fire, the steeliness of steel, the unutterable muddiness of mud.

G.K. Chesterton

CHAPTER 6

Sex and Water

The Svadhishthana Chakra and the Jala Tattwa

The second centre is that of *Svadhishthana*, situated at the root of the genitalia, with six energy aspects or petals and a colour variously spoken of as vermillion or whitish-black. The Hindu deity is *Brahma*, in his limited procreative aspect, or *Vam*, who is seated symbolically upon a white *Makara*, a mythical creature of the water, similar to an alligator.

The watery tattwa of *Jala* or *Apas* is the dominant facet of the subtle matrix administered through this centre, providing the energetic basis for the procreative aspects of our physical being. Blood, urine, lymph, semen and all the other bodily fluids are also a part of this energy field in its outward physical manifestation. Our bodies are said to be sixty-five per cent water and the embryo itself develops within the fluid-filled, amniotic sac. Water is the basis of all life-forms on this planet, being the medium through which almost all substances may pass, conveying not only solids in solution or suspension, but also electrical and magnetic energies. Water, too, in both its subtle and gross states is said to be a matrix for the conveyance of subtle energies. The pranic energy at the level of the jala tattwa is known as *Vyan* and it is responsible for the circulation of blood, as well as the maintenance of all body fluids in balanced condition.

The Gonads, Sex Hormones and Sexual Polarity

The hormonal or endocrine glands taking their patterning from this centre are the gonads. Here, in humans and in most other species, we have the interesting condition of separately polarized sexes, appearing physiologically and indeed in all other aspects of our being – behavioural, mental and emotional. Since yin and yang attract and interact to make a balanced whole, so man and woman come together, though it would be perverse to maintain that the result was always one of harmony and balance! Ideally, however, this would be the situation and it does indeed occur within the limitations imposed by physical existence, where imbalance and the play of the gunas is of the essence, first one predominating and then another, with – in many instances – only brief periods when the sattvas guna of harmony has the ascendant role.

The gonads, being polarized into male and female, produce hormones with masculinizing and feminizing functions. Interestingly enough, all the sex hormones produced in the ovaries and testes are steroids, capable of being transmuted by the body, one into another. Even the female hormone, oestrogen is very similar in molecular appearance to the male hormone, testosterone, though the polarity of the subtle causative patterning is strong enough to ensure that under normal circumstances female remains female and male remains male.

The phenomenon of very similar molecules having opposite properties is not at all unique to sex hormones but is found throughout all living organisms. While the molecule of haemoglobin, for example, is a carrier of oxygen in the blood of many creatures for the purposes of oxidative energy *release* in metabolic processes, the similar molecule of chlorophyll is universally responsible, almost without exception, for the capture and *storage* of solar energy in the plant kingdom. Energy that is then spread, via food chains, to all other living creatures. Without green plants and trees, the other species would die with great rapidity. Which is why the rape of our planet's forests and vegetation is so monumentally idiotic. But then, nature maintains its own balance and any species that gets out of hand is ultimately curtailed in its devastation. This is also a law of nature. Nature is like a gyroscope, with automatic, self-balancing characteristics. For negative activities are self-limiting, containing within them the seeds of their own destruction.

Back with the molecules of similar structures, we have the remarkable case of stereo-symmetry. Any two or three dimensional shape or form will have a mirror image of itself where the left becomes the right and vise versa. In chemistry, molecules, too, exhibit this feature and are found in both forms, known as *stereo-isomers* of each other. They are distinguished according to their property of being able to rotate the axis of polarized light – itself an interesting energetic phenomenon – either to the right (*dextrorotatory* – *D*) or to the left (*laevorotatory* – *L*).

In nature, a substance is normally found in one form or another. All the 'main' amino acids for example, exist only in their L-isomer whilst DNA is found only as a right-handed helix. In the laboratory however, a prepared substance will normally be a mixture of the two forms.

It is as if, as we suggested earlier, that the motion, spin and spatial arrangement of molecular and atomic constituents can be yin or yang in their characteristics at a biological level, according to the polarities within the subtle formative matrix. Thus the L and D forms of molecules, which not only affect the senses as sweet and bitter or pleasant and malodorous, also appear from modern immunological studies, to be treated as friendly or hostile by the body's biochemical and physiological defence system, according to whether they are of L or D isometric form.

This kind of evidence and thinking also places some considerable rationale behind the point of view which feels that naturally prepared substances and food supplements are superior to those of artificial manufacture, due to the quality of their vibration or energetic constituents, because stereo-isometry is unlikely to be the only difference between natural and laboratory synthesis. In fact, according to certain theories in modern physics, there can be many virtual or subtle energy substructures which all manifest as apparently identical molecules at the physical level while containing quite different vibrational aspects in their hidden dimensions. Similarly, it sounds a note of warning to those wishing to irradiate our foods with gamma and X-rays. We just do not understand enough about the physics, and especially the subtle physics, of food biochemistry to take such risks.

But returning once again to our theme, the male and female sex hormones are responsible, together with the genetic constitution, for the determination and maintenance of primary and secondary sexual differentiation. The designation of male or female is determined, from a physiological point of view, at the moment of fertilization. Each normal human cellular nucleus contains 46 chromosomes (23 sets of pairs) or strands of DNA. Each spermatazoon and each ovum contain just 23, exactly one half of each original chromosomal pair. It is the arrangement or patterning of the nucleotides comprising these ultra-long DNA molecules that provides the biochemical template from which the elements of our body are constructed – both our individual characteristics, as well as our basic cellular mechanisms and molecular interactions.

One of these pairs holds the biochemical key to sexual polarity and are designated as the sex chromosomes, X and Y. *X is female and Y is male.* Thus XX leads to typical female development, while XY gives rise to normal male development. Since the female (XX) can only supply an X in the ovum, it is the male spermatazoon, which can provide an X or a Y, that holds the key to the sex of the forthcoming child.

It is the yang, male or Y chromosome which directs the synthesis of proteins responsible for male development, one of the key substances being the *H-Y antigen*, the presence of which determines whether the generalized, embryonic gonadal tissue will develop into ovaries or testes.

Within these gonads are manufactured the male or the female hormones, whose vibrational existence oversees the remainder of the differentiation into yin or yang sexuality.

This description is of necessity a simplification of a process which is only partially understood by those involved in embryology and genetics. Many fundamental questions remain unanswered, not the least of which are – where does the life come from in the first place, is there a morphogenic patterning determining embrylogical development, of which DNA is just a hologram, and – given an ordered and structured universe (which surely is apparent to observation) – how is it that apparent chance is the determining factor as to which spermatazoon unites with which ovum?

According to yogic philosophy and the mechanisms inherent in the laws of karma and reincarnation, the soul takes a birth with those parents where its previous actions, desires and inclinations lead it. The parents and the child are inextricably bound together and each unwittingly have already penned the invitation to each other for the conception and birth to take place. The sex, characteristics, innate strengths and weaknesses both mental/emotional and biological, are already written.

The embryo therefore develops and – say the mystics – the soul, which is designated to that embryo, 'wakes up' after three months, when a consciousness of its situation first arises. By this time, all the major organs and systems are laid down within the embryo. All that is required then, is organized growth.

From the moment of conception, the karmically encoded pranic vibrations begin to operate upon the differentiating cellular patterning of the embryo, according to the destiny already laid down for the life of that soul in incarnate form and partially expressed as the DNA within the nucleus of each and every cell. By the time the child is born, it already has the means for expressing its individual personality and its life's course is already set.

Any defect at any point in the sexual designation mechanism can result in impaired sexual determination. This defect can be in the chromosomal arrangement, in the production of H–Y antigen or its precursors, in the gonads and their role in hormone manufacture, or in the target sites upon which the sex hormones operate.

Thus it is possible to have children and adults with multiple X chromosomes (XXY, XXXY, XXXXY) who develop as normal males or with a missing Y chromosome (X). It is thought that about one in 125 conceptions are X in nature, since there are many defective spermatozoons, but only about three per cent survive as far as childbirth. This condition is known as Turner's syndrome and the children – who develop as females with non-functional fibrous ovaries – are short in stature and have skeletal and other anomalies.

Again, there are rare cases of XX, genetically normal females, but with well developed testes. In these cases, the

H-Y antigen is present. Geneticists assume that this indicates that the region of the Y (male) chromosome that regulates the formation of H-Y antigen has been translocated into another chromosome, from where it is still active. Though this presumes that the DNA is the only mechanism that results in the formation of the H-Y antigen. A presumption that may be misguided, when looked at from the point of view of a 'whole integrated system' of which DNA is only one aspect. Most true hermaphrodites are 46 XX (genetic female) in their chromosomal distribution, yet the testicular tissue has developed in response to the presence of the H-Y antigen. Under these circumstances the genitalia and secondary sexual characteristics (hair patterns, breast tissue, body shape etc.), are likely to be sexually ambiguous and most so called sex-change operations which so tickle the public imagination are usually on those unfortunate people whose genetics and physiology are in a muddle, the operation being an attempt to reinstate a determined sexual polarity, one way or the other.

Research scientists, however, are well aware that there are more aspects to this than just Y chromosomes and H-Y antigens. Very rarely, for example, it is possible to get 46 XY *females* with either normal or abnormal H-Y antigen activity.

Similarly, it is clear from observation that within a range of variety, all physical aspects of a normal man have male characteristics, while the same is true for women and female attributes – from the size of the feet to the way the hair grows, to the texture of the skin. That all bodily processes are related to sexual polarity is born out from the evidence of 'side' effects in women taking contraceptive hormone tablets where almost every part of the body can be affected in some way. Indeed, the nucleus of every cell carries an imprint of the sexual polarity in its DNA patterning, a factor which must have meaning in the overall bodily economy.

So it means that there could be a sympathetic resonant connection and response between the energy patterning of molecules that originate under the direct control of the highly polarized gonadal chakra and the polarization of the sex-determination section of each cell-nucleus. Indeed, it would seem certain that just as all our personality and karmic record are encoded into the subtle vibrations of our physical being and thence into each atom, molecule and cell, that the sexual polarization of our nature is likewise vibrationally programmed into every part of our body. No wonder the aura or atmosphere of some folk seems to breath sensuality and sexuality.

Sex Hormones and Germ Cells

The ovaries and testes both possess two functional aspects. Firstly, the production of the germ cells – the ova and spermatazoa – and secondly, synthesis of the sex hormones, which are responsible at a biochemical level for the development, functioning and maintenance of both the reproductive organs, as well as the secondary sexual characteristics. These include the breasts, general body shape, patterns of body hair, and so on. They are also involved with the development and maintenance of libido, behavioural patterns and general emotional condition, though to what degree is very much a matter of medical debate, since social and environmental conditioning clearly has a strong role to play.

The Testes and Male Polarity

At this point, we again become technical and you may, if you wish, prefer to skim through this and the following section, The Ovaries and Female Polarity, *to the more general section,* Men and Women, *picking up on only the more non-specific comments scattered throughout.*

The *testes* produce spermatozoa continuously from puberty to old age, within coiled *seminiferous tubules* and under the intimate nutritional, mechanical and endocrine guidance of the *Sertoli cells.* The male steroid hormones or *androgens* are synthesized in the interstitial *cells of Leydig,* situated between the seminiferous tubules, (see figure 6-1). Of these androgens, the principle hormone is *testosterone,* ninety-five per cent of which is manufactured by the Leydig cells with the source of the remainder being the adrenal cortex, as we have described in the previous chapter.

137

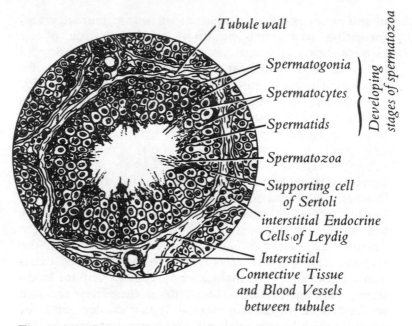

Tubule wall

Spermatogonia

Spermatocytes

Spermatids

Developing stages of spermatozoa

Spermatozoa

Supporting cell
of Sertoli

interstitial Endocrine
Cells of Leydig

Interstitial
Connective Tissue
and Blood Vessels
between tubules

Figure 6-1. Cross section of a seminiferous tubule in the testes (of a cat). Redrawn from A Histology of Body Tissues, M. Gillison.

As with all steroids the common pre-cursor is cholesterol, which itself can be manufactured from *acetate.* Testosterone, however, can be converted into a hormone with even greater androgenic effects by an enzyme found in certain target cells, including the seminiferous tubules, the prostate gland, the skin and perhaps the brain, as well as the cells of Leydig themselves.

Furthermore, a small quantity of testosterone is itself converted into one of the most important of the *oestrogens* or female hormones, in both the Leydig cells and some peripheral tissues. Its role in the physiology of reproduction is not understood, but as a reflection or lower harmonic of the presence of the yin within the yang, or the combined presence of male and female polarity for balanced overall energetic functioning, its existence can be understood, as discussed in the last chapter.

The characteristic of steroid hormones, including testosterone, of being carried in the blood by a protein carrier, is quite common, in which case the hormone itself is largely deactivated until it reaches its target organ. Further transformation of a hormone into a more active form within target cells is also of frequent occurrence. These two factors can be perceived as a biological way of putting a sword into a scabbard until required for use.

Androgen production in the testicular Leydig cells is controlled from above, through the pituitary gland and the hypothalamus, in a feedback system similar to the one described for adrenal cortisol, though somewhat more complex and with a number of factors remaining little understood (see figure 6-2).

Briefly, the hypothalamus, under neuronal or electrobiological control, is stimulated to produce the decapeptide (ten amino acids), *gonadotrophin releasing hormone* (GnRH). GnRH then stimulates the anterior pituitary to produce the two hormones, *LH* and *FSH*, which act on the Leydig cells and seminiferous tubules respectively, to synthesize testosterone and spermatazoa. The testosterone is then thought to feed back negatively to the hypothalamus and the pituitary, inhibiting further GnRH and LH production. Additionally, the seminiferous tubules are also a source of the hormone *inhibin*, which is thought to feed back in a similar fashion, inhibiting GnRH and FSH synthesis.

This linkage of the lower endocrine glands to the pituitary and hypothalamus would seem to be a direct reflection of the three major spinal nadis energetically linking the chakric centres of organization with the two petals of the ajna chakra. For at a lower harmonic, these petals reflect a facet of their functioning in the anterior pituitary and the hypothalamus. We discuss this in greater detail in chapter ten, but note how the law of polarity is similarly applied in both the endocrinological as well as the yogic descriptions.

For on the one hand we have a positive stimulation resulting in a negative feedback and thence a reduction in stimulation, which of itself again leads to an increase in the positive. And on the yogic side, we have the positive and negative energetic patterning and polarized subtle currents underlying their manifestation as the biochemical pathway. The creative patterning within the locked-in potential of the gross akashic or vacuum state is also involved, being the point of origin and formation of the four lower

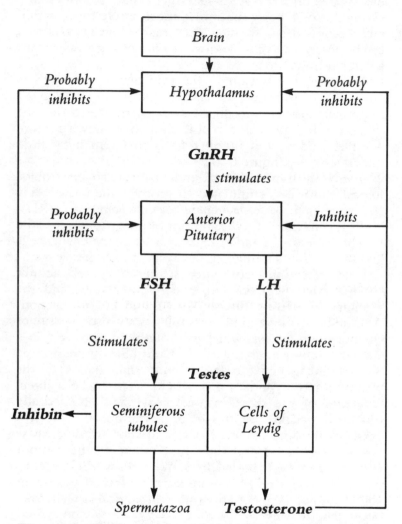

Figure 6-2. The hormonal regulation of testicular function

tattwas as subatomic particles, a theme that was introduced in chapter three and is discussed more fully in chapters nine and twelve.

Furthermore, the hypothalamus is linked directly into the brain by neurological pathways and in our thinking, this also means a direct linking into the vacuum state control centre that underlies the brain as its subtley energetic blueprint. Because, although the pattern of hormonal and physiological pathways is partially understood, even if all the biochemical processes were open to observation, it would still not provide us with the answer to how the parts are put together and integrated into one whole, living human being.

The Ovaries and Female Polarity

The *ovaries* and the associated reproductive organs present a considerably more complicated picture than the testes because the amazing process of pregnancy, embryological development, birth, breast-feeding and care of the infant are all involved. Men may sometimes complain of a woman's complex nature and at least in this respect, they would seem to be quite correct! Though it is hardly a matter for complaint.

The ovaries differ from the testes in that the *germ cells are produced before birth*. In fact, initially, about four million develop, of which around two million are still present when the child is born. Further regression continues during childhood, so that by puberty only a few hundred thousand remain. It is the development of just one of these immature ova and the preparation for its possible fertilization, implantation and pregnancy that underlies the *cyclic* menstrual or oestrous cycle with which women are familiar.

Furthermore, because of the rigours of pregnancy, childbirth and rearing a child, nature has set up a pattern whereby a woman becomes increasingly less fertile after the age of 40–45 and by the age of 55 or earlier has usually ceased the process of ovulation, altogether. While a man can usually father a child until the day he dies, there would be little point in a woman being able to give birth shortly before her death, because the natural processes of aging would ultimately leave the child without a mother, even supposing that she could physically cope with a demanding infant in her later life.

Menopause, therefore, has a practical aspect to it and, as with all of biochemistry, though some of the molecular and biological changes and pathways are understood, a comprehension of the basic patterning mechanisms underlying how, why and when it should occur, are totally lacking.

Within the ovaries, each ovum is contained inside an envelope or *follicle* of cells. The outer, *thecal* layer (see figure 6-3) consists of an external fibrous capsule and an inner, vascular layer of tissue. Then, within that, and immediately surrounding the ovum, lie the *granulosa* cells.

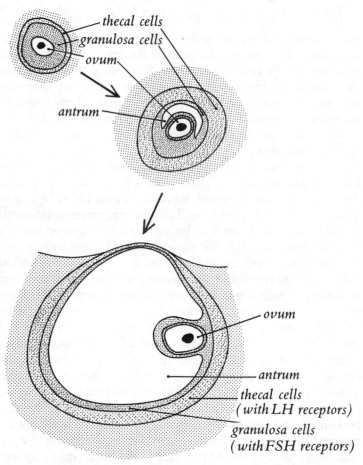

Redrawn from Essential Endocrinology, *Laycock and Wise.*

Figure 6-3. The development of the ovum and ovarian follicle during the pre-ovulatory phase of the menstrual cycle.

As each menstrual cycle 'commences', taken by convention to be the end of menstruation, a few of these ovarian follicles begin to develop under the influence of, once again, hypothalamic and anterior pituitary control and subsequent ovarian feedback. Interestingly, the process is very similar to that found in the man. In fact, the two identical pituitary hormones of LH and FSH take their names from their role in the woman. In simplified form, the cycle goes like this:

Firstly, the inner layer of thecal cells synthesize receptors to LH. LH subsequently binds to these receptors stimulating them to produce *androgens*. At the same time, the granulosa cells form FSH receptors and under its influence produce an enzyme which catalyzes the conversion of the thecal androgens into a limited quantity of oestrogen, (see figure 6-4). The thecal cells themselves produce only a small quantity of oestrogen.

The granulosa cells, in the maintained presence of FSH and the increasing level of oestrogen, begin to synthesize LH receptors, becoming self-supporting. Any antral follicles which have not reached this level, now fall back as the rising oestrogen level inhibits pituitary FSH production. Usually, only one follicle remains to respond to the final LH surge, also accompanied by a smaller surge in FSH.

Oestrogen then further stimulates proliferation of the granulosa cells which by this time are secreting a fluid that fills a cavity, the *antrum*, which forms around the ovum. When the follicle is fully matured, the ovum is separated from the antrum, by only a thin layer of granulosa cells on the inside, which are connected to the outer layers by just a narrow stalk. As these granulosa cells develop, and with the synthesis of specific LH receptors in their outer layers, they produce their own oestrogens, the follicle thus maturing under its own local biochemical feedback, with the regression of thecal cell activity. The individual follicles thus become 'self-supporting' and in any follicles that have not reached this stage, there is regression as the rising level of oestrogen production negatively feeds back onto pituitary FSH production and its associated hypothalamic GnRH synthesis.

Under normal circumstances, usually only one follicle is left and as the oestrogen level rises higher, the pituitary is further stimulated to produce a marked surge in LH production, accompanied by a smaller surge in FSH.

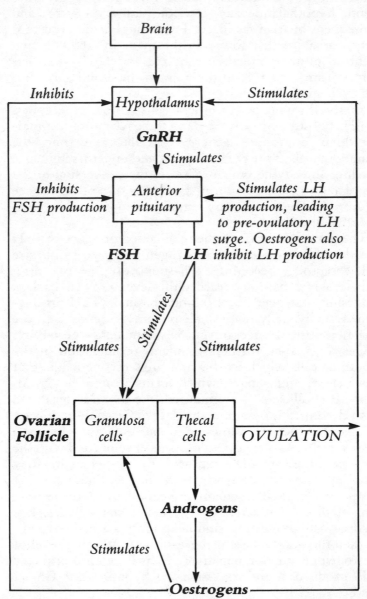

Note that oestrogens both stimulate & inhibit GnRH & LH production – a toning effect. The mechanisms are little understood.

Figure 6-4. Pre-ovulatory hormonal control of ovarian function

This LH surge stimulates the final follicular maturation and within twenty-four to thiry-six hours, the follicle ruptures, releasing a mature ovum. The ovum, finding its way into the enveloping tendrils comprising the opening to the *fallopian tube* which leads down into the uterus, then awaits fertilization by a male spermatazoon. This may indeed be already waiting at the door, or be on its way up the vagina, through the uterine opening, along its endometrial lining and up the fallopian tube, in the upper part of which the all-important meeting takes place and fertilization occurs.

The biochemical ramifications of this process have been studied in detail and yet the real formative patterning underlying it is far from understood. Why only one follicle usually reaches maturity ahead of the others, for instance, is not really comprehended. Nor is there any single and universally accepted hypothesis that accounts for the endocrine changes which surround puberty, nor for the cyclic effects of oestrogen on pituitary and hypothalamic function.

Indeed, as I have previously pointed out, biochemistry is itself only a convenient language for describing observable cause and effect, knock-on-knock molecular processes. Even the micromechanisms of molecular interaction at an energetic level, are little understood, let alone the interactions at an atomic, subatomic or vacuum state level. And just as it is possible to macroscopically build houses and monuments without a knowledge of molecular structure, so too do observations of molecular and physiological pathways allow us to perform even genetic engineering without understanding the underlying formative and subtle blueprint, or even suspecting its existence.

Once understood, however, it immediately throws light on the integration of all the molecular processes and makes an even deeper investigation possible.

Just as a knowledge of chemistry has helped preservationists understand the processes of decay in old and weathered buildings; or an appreciation of materials science and atomic structure gives engineers a deeper knowledge of the stresses and strains within metallic and engineering materials, so too does a perception of finer, morphogenic energies present a beautiful and aesthetic picture of mechanisms inherent in the outworking of life energies.

Returning, however, to our ovarian theme, whether or not fertilization takes place, the follicular granulosa cells, incorporating some of the thecal cells, now reform into a highly significant body known as the *corpus luteum*. The corpus luteum synthesizes not only oestrogens, but in place of converting androgens to oestrogen also produces a new and allied steroid hormone, *progesterone*, still under the support of pituitary FSH and a low level of LH, (see figure 6-5).

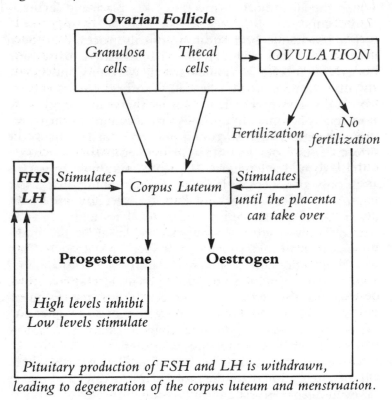

Figure 6-5. Post-ovulatory hormonal control of ovarian function

If pregnancy occurs, the corpus luteum continues its steroid support until the foeto-placental bridge takes over, usually by the twelfth week. If pregnancy does not take place, the pituitary withdraws its support due to feedback information received from the endometrial layers of the uterine wall. The result is that the *endometrium* which has

been prepared for a possible implantation under the stimulation of oestrogen and later progesterone, now breaks
down and is eliminated in the processes of menstruation.

Parallel with the activity of testosterone in men, oestrogen is also responsible for the development, maintenance
and functioning of both the female reproductive systems, as
well the secondary sexual characteristics. Actually, there
are a number of similar steroid oestrogens, of which
the major one found in free circulation is known as
17β-*oestradiol*.

Oestrogens, in the absence of androgens, are responsible
for such characteristics as the accumulation of fatty tissues
in the breasts and buttocks, broad hips and the patterns of
body hair. It is also considered likely that both androgens
and oestrogens are involved in processes within the central
nervous system, as well as with libido and various other
aspects of feminine behaviour. But although exposure of
the brain to sex hormones is known to affect the early
develpment of rats in respect of both genital and behavioural factors in adults, their involvement in human brain
and behavioural development is only speculative, the
required experiments being, fortunately, impossible to
perform.

However, with the structure of molecules being able to
modify, as well as be created out of, the subtle substructure
of the vacuum state, it would seem probable that an
arrangement of subatomic particles forming a molecule (ie.
oestrogens, testosterone etc.) possessed of sexual energetic
polarity – male or female – would also be present in the
brain. For it is there that the consciousness-mind-physical
matter linkages have their primary activity and where
mental characteristics of male and female are similarly
expressed.

Graphically, if one visualises the vacuum state as a three-
dimensional sheet out of which subatomic particles spin and
dance into existence from formative patterns on the 'other
side', then it is the nature and polarity of these subtle
patterns which is manifested as molecules of a certain shape
and function. And these molecules likewise affect the nature
of energetic movement in the more subtle state.

The molecules of oestrogen and testosterone therefore
represent male and female vibration and polarity, and one

would expect to find them active in every cell of the body as well as in the brain-mind interface. And this is indeed the case.

The corpus luteum, then, synthesizes the hormone progesterone, one of the most potent of the naturally occurring *progestogens*, which – as the name implies – are progestational or promote pregnancy in their general effect. Progesterone is of particular interest in that not only is it a major sex hormone, but it is also a precursor to all the other major steroid hormones, (see figure 6-6), and is therefore produced in all cells that manufacture steroids from cholesterol. And as we have said, both progesterone, oestrogens and testosterone are also synthesized in small quantities by the adrenal cortex.

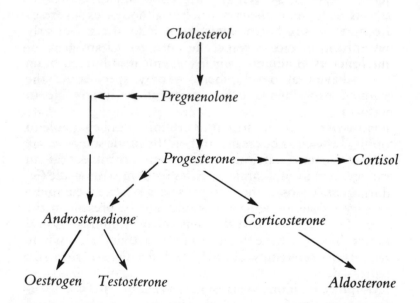

Figure 6-6. Cholesterol and steroid hormone synthesis. Each arrow represents one molecular transformation, catalyzed by a particular enzyme. The names of some of the intermediaries are omitted. In fact, molecular transformation occurs as a continuous and flowing energetic re-shaping of the atomic and probably subatomic structure. Our representation as a series of steps is merely a convenience, but can be misleading.

Progesterone acts in some respects as a polar opposite to oestrogenic activity, for while oestrogens prepare the way for fertilization to take place, progesterone is concerned with preparations for, and the maintenance of, pregnancy. There are many internal changes that take place, but the most commonly known of the outer effects is the wet, slippery, alkaline and fertile cervical mucus produced under oestrogenic influence. As oestrogen levels decline after ovulation, this then changes to thick, dry and acid mucus which is inimical to spermatazoa. Furthermore, while oestrogen stimulates pituitary and hypothalamic gonadotrophin release (i.e. LH and FSH), high concentrations of progesterone inhibit their release.

And there are other opposing functions too. Progesterone, for example, binds to renal aldosterone receptors, preventing aldosterone from enacting its normal role as a stimulator of sodium absorption. The *decreasing sodium ion concentration* thus motivates an increase in aldosterone production, to restore the sodium balance. Oestrogens, on the other hand, *directly stimulate salt retention.*

In Chinese thinking, one could describe oestrogenic activity as the receptive yin aspect of the feminine, yin, biological system. Conversely, progesterone, with its stimulation of endometrical proliferation and the promotion of the intensely active period of gestation and embryological growth, is clearly an outgoing yang or rajas aspect of this yin, procreative, female function. Endocrine activity during both pregnancy and breast-feeding also follows some interesting pathways, as far as they are understood, and many patterns emerge upon examination in the light of the thesis of this book. A deeper analysis may be attempted at another time, but I am attempting to present here only enough of the biochemical complexities to show how they are understandable in terms of a more fundamental energetic paradigm. Too much physiological detail may prove of little interest to many readers, who nevertheless are interested in the general theme.

Actually, lactation and breast physiology are a superb example of endocrine linkages. Without going into the ramification of details, oestrogen and progesterone, the anterior pituitary hormones of *prolactin* and *somatotrophin* or *Growth Hormone*, the adreno-cortical hormones such as cortisol, certain placental hormones, insulin – the pancreatic hormone, thyroid hormones and finally the posterior pituitary hormone *oxytocin*, which provides the neuroendocrine linkage between suckling or nipple stimulation and the ejection of milk – all these are involved in the processes involved with the development of breast tissue, milk production and ejection.

Moreover, the pituitary hormone prolactin seems to be responsible for the suppression of the normal oestrous or menstrual cycle and thus the protracted period of infertility during lactation. And the duration of this period has strong emotional linkages, since it normally continues for as long as there is a close relationship of mother and child with complete dependency upon breast milk as a source of nutrition. In fact, if the signs of a return to fertility are observed, such as the presence of fertile, cervical mucus, then a mother can often reverse the process, by taking the baby to bed with her and generally deepening the close physical ties.

Such emotional–endocrine linkages would appear to be mediated via the hypothalamic-pituitary connection, the hypothalamus receiving neurological and electrical messages from the brain, which is itself connected into the subtle states moving towards the mental and thought levels.

Similarly, the effects of emotion and stress on the menstrual cycle have been well-documented, though the *pathway of feeling to biochemistry* is not understood by conventional science. Stress in the early part of a cycle can delay ovulation while nature awaits a better opportunity for the potential start to a pregnancy. Continuous and severe stress can even result in *amenorrhea*, the complete loss of menstrual cycles, as was experienced, for example, by women in concentration camps during the last world war. After the lifting of the stressful circumstances, cycles slowly return to normal, depending upon the individual.

Disorders of the reproductive system are many and various, since any part of physiological, genetic or biochemical pathways can be prone to malfunction. The primary causative patterning will lie further within the subtle fields out of which subatomic matter is derived, and although many gonadal dysfunctions can be viewed in terms of biochemistry, there are some interesting anomalies which give us a few clues as to the activity of the higher formative matrix. Most cases of precocious puberty, for example, appear to have no immediately obvious endocrine cause. In a large number of patients, however, there is an abnormal electroencephalogram (EEG, electrical brain wave pattern) and a tendency towards epilepsy. With our understanding of electrical brain waves as a reflection of subtle state activity, an abnormal EEG would suggest abnormality in the subtle morphogenic energy fields. And precocious puberty is clearly an example of formative, bodily patterns being disturbed.

Similarly, amongst mentally subnormal or otherwise disturbed people, there is a higher incidence of chromosomal disorders such as *Klinefelter's syndrome* where testicular failure occurs due to a mixed chromosomal content (XXY instead of XY for a normal male). One assumes that the genetic malformation indicates a distorted or disharmonized subtle energy matrix showing itself as both mental disturbances, upset genetic patterning and gonadal or endocrine disorders. In fact, endocrine disorders, being functionally closer to the inner energy patterning, have far higher incidences of associated emotional and mental disharmonies than any other physiological disorders, with the exception of those related to the central nervous system.

Finally, the question has to be asked as to *why* oestrogens and androgens are so similar in molecular structure or energetic shape? If men and women are reproductively so different, then why are their hormones so similar? The answer has to lie in the fact that we are dealing with a polarization of energy. And just as positive and negative *charges* in electricity, or north and south *poles* in magnetism are opposite, but of the same *nature*, so the male and female hormones must represent a real, energetic polarization, first expressed in the subtle state and then reflected in the molecular patterns formed out of the spinning and charged subatomic particles that constitute all physically observable matter. The exact nature of this polarity, from a scientific point of view, is clearly a matter for deeper research.

Men and Women

The entire mental-emotional-physical energies of men and women would appear, then, to have male and female, yang

151

and yin characteristics expressed throughout. As we described, the sex hormones themselves affect not only the sexual functionality of the physical system, but also almost all aspects of physiology, as well as the emotional life. Generally speaking, women express yin and receptive characteristics in both their psychology as well as their physical sexual structure. Conversely, men, archetypally, are yang and outgoing. One is on shaky ground here, especially in these modern times, and these are, of course, very broad generalizations, especially at the psychological level! But without the softer, yielding, receptive, more adapatable and giving warmth of a woman, the child cannot receive the early affection that helps to mould these human qualities into his own personality.

Similarly, the firmer role of the father or man adds tone and (again, very generally speaking) the qualities of rationality and determination in outward expression. Although these qualities may be mixed, psychologically, between and within individual parents, the polarity of both characteristics is required for the balanced raising of any child.

So women generally, have a warmer heart and a more emotional approach, while men are more determined and rational. And the question is: how, therefore, does their subtle energetic constitution differ, giving rise to these differences?

Some clue to this lies in the psychological qualities of the watery tattwa, those of sensitivity and feeling. And the primary division of sexual polarity lies in this procreational tattwa and organizing chakra. Within the confines of the extremes, all polarity can be relative. Thus, while water is yin in respect to the drive of fire or the lightness of air, within water itself or any of the other tattwas, there is also a polarization. The yin of water is its flowingness, its warming qualities and its non-confrontational approach, its yang is the restless and surging drive of emotional force, the raging torrent or the cold, storm-tossed ocean.

Female sexual polarity, therefore, expresses the yin aspect of a yin tattwa, while the male takes on the yang characteristics. And the primary patterning for this lies in the antashkarans or human mind. These yin and yang attributes are present within each tattwa and depending, therefore, upon the individual mental patterning, each person's personality will contain a preponderance or a balance of these possibilities within the emotional or subtle tattvic spectrum.

And just as the inner or superior energy, in this case the mind pattern, rules the outer or inferior – the emotional and physical – so too does the inferior rule the superior through the flow of the return current required to complete the circuit. This polarity, therefore, expressed at the outer biochemical level of endocrine activity, can therefore affect the inner level of emotional functioning, as we observe with the other effects of the contraceptive Pill. In fact, there are emotional changes associated with all endocrine activity in particular, and more generally with the ingestion of many, if not all substances at a molecular level, whether they be drugs or food.

Cellular and Biochemical Intelligence – The Cell Mind and DNA

The DNA, nuclear biochemical intelligence present in each cell of the body is something which has intrigued me as to the mechanism by which it is specifically related, (which it must be), to overall body patterning and organization from a subtle energy point of view. And it seems to me that it must once again be one of holographic resonance and coherence, based upon the fact that the DNA, just like the first nucleus in the fertilized ovum, contains the biochemical blueprint for the entire body.

Whilst this patterning is essential in the embryo, it is not at all clear, using allopathic or linear paradigms, why it necessary for the cells in the tip of the nose, for example, to have the intelligence required to pattern the growth of finger nails, or the size of the feet or to create certain enzymes required by the digestive system. And neither do cells attempt, under normal circumstances, to function in any way other than in their appointed modality, though the health and smooth functioning in these cells can and does vary radically from individual to individual according to innumerable factors both from within and without.

Suppose, however, that the real blueprint for body function and format is located in a higher, more subtle area of energy. This, indeed, is part of the thesis of this book.

This morphogenic field therefore (which is none other than the pranas, tattwas and other subtle forces we have been discussing) has its own structure, oscillatory patterns and laws of energy relationship. It is a formative matrix that relates directly, specifically and in complete detail[1] to the manifestation and functioning of the gross physical body. Note, however, that this field is not something separate or away from the biochemical energy level, but is *within it* in a creative sense, not just a *part* of it. It is more intermerged than a dye in water, more primary, essential and fundamental.

As described in the section, *The Body as a Tattvic Hologram*, (chapter three), the bodily cellular structure that we perceive outwardly is underlain by a subtle organizational matrix within the vacuum and subtle tattvic fields. It is patterned by mind and pranas. This holographically integrated matrix thus provides each cell with its own 'cell mind' or administrative centre. DNA and the cellular nucleus are simply a reflection of this subtle holographic structuring. *The discovery that every bodily cell contains a reflection of the whole has given us a tremendous clue to the way in which this mysterious, multi-level body machine is constructed.* A clue which has been largely neglected by believers in the conventional, materialistic paradigms.

The biochemical interchanges, therefore, in particular tissues of the body, and which are 'controlled' by the DNA and cell nuclei, are actually stimulated into specific activity by the patterning in the subtle morphogenic field. In other parts of the body where this activity is not required, the cellular DNA and corresponding subtle intelligence remains quiescent for lack of a particular resonance to activate it. But, as in any intelligent system, when *the parts – like soldiers – are aware of the whole, though still restricting their activities to performing only their alloted task*, the whole benefits greatly from this background knowledge within each individual soldier. Or put more simply, when the soldiers know what the overall plan is, they can fight more effectively and more intelligently as

---

[1] cf. "Even the hairs of your head are all numbered" – *St Matthew*, Ch. 10, v. 30.

one integrated army. Thus the knowledge of the part concerning the whole is by no means wasted. Rather it is essential for the coherent functioning of the whole.

In fact, it is yet another manifestation of the microcosm containing within it the image of the entire macrocosm. We are back with the Hermetic axiom, "As above, so below." Man himself contains the ability to reach out (or rather *in*) within himself and contact the source, as well as all the parts of creation. And this mechanism is reflected within each and every cell in our body.

DNA – An Indication of the Subtle State Hologram

In chapter three, it was described how a hologram is a method of storing an image, just like a photographic slide or print. The difference, however, is two-fold. Firstly, it requires special projection equipment for the image to become apparent. Looked at with our normal eyes it does not look much like anything. Secondly, every part of the hologram can be used to project an image of the whole. Some of the detail will be missing, but essentially the complete character of the whole is reflected in the part.

The comparison to DNA and the cellular nucleus should be clear, for the cellular nucleus is a part that represents or could be projected as the whole. The analogy does not, however, stop here. The mechanism by which a hologram is formed is one of *interference* or admixture of energetic waveforms in the electromagnetic frequencies of visible light. Similarly, with our model of the molecule as the effect of intermingling vibrational patterns within the vacuum and subtle state, we can visualize how the complex molecular structures of the body can be formed. They are the result of interference patterns in morphogenic or formative pranic vibration in the subtle realms of energy.

DNA and no doubt the cell nucleus itself can therefore be seen as a necessary part of the process by which the vibrant, energetic and continuously maintained, subtle state hologram can project itself as the ordered biochemical patterns and pathways with which we are familiar.

The Cell, The Soldier and Subtle Organization

The image of each cell possessing its own 'cell mind' or organizational structure within the subtle physical realm leads us to a new understanding of disease and ill-health. We have already suggested that good health and a feeling of well being arise from harmonious energy patterns at the subtle level and conversely, dis-harmony or dis-ease leads to the experience of poor health, tiredness, mental-emotional unrest and so on. To really make use of this generality, however, for the re-creation and maintenance of health we need to understand the specifics of how this subtle matrix is ordered. That is, the mechanics and interrelationships of this subtle energy system – how, in detail, it actually operates; how the weaving of the tapestry takes place. When we understand a machine, then we can begin to repair and maintain it in a truly knowledgable fashion.

Because of its all-pervasive, ubiquitous and outwardly featureless nature, there can be a tendency to think of the vacuum state as being simply a bland and unstructured sea of energy at high potential. This is actually not the case, for the structure we perceive on the outward physical side of things (subatomic particles, atoms, molecules etc.) arises because of structure within the vacuum matrix.

So it must possess as highly ordered, structured and organized a matrix as the outward physical reality it gives rise to. This being the case, the primary area of vacuum state research – both theoretical and practical – must be directed towards understanding the details of how this fine tapestry is woven.

And this is required firstly for the bodies of living creatures where the life force is more directly involved in the vastly more intricate patterns, interrelationships and connections than we find in the second case of so-called 'inert' matter, which is held in structured form by a more diffuse vibration of the Primal Energy Source, or Shabda.

It is clear that, in living creatures, each cell, like a soldier, has a certain degree of individuality, of autonomy, and is yet held firmly within the organizational structure of the whole. Just as we have nerves, blood vessels, hormones and a multitude of connectors at the gross physical level, so too – though governed by different laws of relatedness – must there be a pattern of organizational interchange at the subtle level, between and within the individual cell minds, or focuses of subtle energy administration. This we see reflected in cell structure, the DNA, as well as the nervous system, hormonal messengers and so on. These are all parts of the whole picture.

Much of this subtle patterning, however, will remain at the subtle level, within the vacuum and more subtle states, without specific external manifestation. We do not, after all, physically perceive the thoughts that make us move about and do things. Even at the manifested physical level, however, there must be an energy network that is more refined than the neuroendocrine system. For each cell soldier needs to be in instant physical communication, at least with his immediately adjacent fellows.

Such an organizational communications network does exist and some of the evidence of this was presented in *Subtle Energy*. I am referring to the bodily electronic and magnetic aspects and will not go into all the details again here. But recent research by two Americans, Dr James Said and Philip Callahan, has added an even greater dimension to this thinking.

Philip Callahan is the scientist who discovered that the antennae of insects are actually highly tuned receivers for the laser-like, infrared emissions of molecules used by insects as communicators of food, location, sex, territory and so on. These infrared laser emissions (masers) are highly individual and specific, reflecting the nature and condition of the emitter molecule itself. Similarly, the antennae of insects are tuned specifically for the reception of these emissions.

This is a fascinating discovery in itself and I will be discussing some of its other implications in a future book, but it means that molecules emit infrared patterns that reflect their condition, structure and position. This is just what we need for intercellular and indeed intermolecular communication. It is, in fact, radar and radio communication at the cellular and molecular level. Once again, man makes a 'discovery' only to find that living creatures have been at it all along!

Now, infrared electromagnetic emission and absorption takes place continually in all substances above the temperature of absolute zero. Infrared is what we experience as radiated heat. It is emitted due to the fiery excitability and motion at the molecular and atomic levels. Emission and absorption go on simultaneously all the time.

Scientists, of course, know about infrared emission and absorption because it is a continuous aspect of all matter at temperatures above absolute zero. But it has largely been ignored as a medium for potential bodily organization because it is so ubiquitous, difficult to experimentally monitor at a detailed level, and because the discovery of such a system of bodily integration would considerably upset conventional models in the life sciences, demonstrating them to be hopelessly lacking.

It would also be yet another nail in the coffin of Darwinian theories concerning the origin of life from dust and water. For such interwoven and whole complexity within living organisms could never have evolved in a linear, piecemeal and random fashion. It is our minds which are fragmented, not nature.

So Said and Callahan have suggested, as I did in *Subtle Energy*, that electromagnetic cellular and molecular emissions are an integral part of bodily organization, at the manifested level. And they suggest that the primary level is at that of the infrared, because energy at that level is being continuously emitted and absorbed – transmitted and received by every molecule and atom within the body.[1]

Ultraviolet and other cellular emissions and communications are produced due to *stimulation* or as a reaction. They are hence a secondary system of intricate flags and semaphores.

So far, so good – but do not forget that all gross physical manifestation, including this infrared activity, is due to movement and patterning within the vacuum and subtle states. In other words, just like the energy pattern we call DNA, the entire physical network is also a reflection of the subtle organizational structure.

In fact, it would make an interesting project to determine the infrared and general electromagnetic emission characteristics of the beautifully structured double helix of the DNA molecule itself. It looks remarkably like a tuned

[1] The emissions actually cover both infrared and microwave, at millimetre to centimetre wavelengths.

emitter-receiver for electromagnetic wavelengths, perhaps at multiple, yet ordered, frequencies. Indeed, this would be the case with all molecular structures.

Actually, molecules do not exist as little blobs, but as vibrating energy mosaics which includes what we call their electromagnetic 'emissions', and the study of biochemistry needs to be enlivened by this understanding. For it is only *our* human conception that makes us think of tiny molecules moving along in the cellular system of the body as minature sealed envelopes until they reach their destination. This is quite simply untrue. The situation is continuously dynamic, and highly ordered. It has to be so, for with all the vast intricate sea of energy moving, vibrating, emitting, receiving, if there is order at any level, it has to be total. There cannot be any allowance for randomness.

Now once again, you can see why I insist that the life force is primary in the organization of living bodies. Such a wholeness cannot be the chance juxtaposition and evolution of subatomic energies and forces. For they are themselves only effects upon the energetic vacuum sea.

The intricacies and implications of this paradigm in the study of the human energetic constitution and hence of health and disease, are immense. Consider, for example, cancer. Cancer is a disruption to the normal functioning of cell-life. It may be caused by ionizing radiation which breaks up molecules, by chemicals which perform a similar role, by non-ionizing radiation which disrupt the energetic harmony of molecular structures, and so on. Anything that can cause cellular disharmony at an organizational level will result in cancer.

Is this then, the common denominator amongst all the causes of cancer? If so, it would certainly explain why no 'cure' for cancer has been forthcoming, since the primary problem has rarely, if ever, been addressed. It would also explain why and how the exposure to cancer-inducing agents may not manifest for upwards of twenty years. For if the disruption is actually at the subtle level, causing a disturbance to the subtle matrix, *to the cell minds themselves*, then, naturally, it may take some while before such a disturbance can no longer be held in check by the organization of the surrounding or related subtle tapestry.

In addition, our own mind and karmas pattern and are

responsible for the inward structuring of this mosaic. Hence the observation that cancer patients have certain characteristic personality traits. For energetically, these traits or patterns are reflected in the subtle, cell mind matrix as cancer-inducing cellular disruptions.

Furthermore, cancer – as well as AIDS and heart disease – are a direct reflection of the degenerative conditions prevalent in our modern lifestyles. All lifestyle and activity arise from our minds. The nature of our mind is reflected both in our body as well as in our outer life. The indiscriminate pollution and rape of our planet for personal, financial profit and the pursuit of material possessions indicates the degree of spritual consciousness – or rather the *lack* of it – amongst us humans at this time. We are all responsible for the planetary destruction, to one degree or another.

The degenerative condition of our mind and our environment are thus automatically reflected in the diseases to which we are prone.

The 'cure' for cancer, therefore, and other disease can be approached at both a planetary, as well as an individual level. If all humans worked together to make the planet a pleasant place, the more wholesome mental attitude and planetary conditions would automatically result in greater health and a diminution of all such bodily reflections of inward and outward disharmony.

However, for the individual, caught up in the present world conditions, the 'cure' for cancer or any disease, becomes individual, because we are each energetically different and because health and disease are essentially a personal concern. And these differences in individual energetic constitution can only be comprehended within the context of the holographic and holistic energy model.

Fortunately, this kind of energy medicine *is* being developed in many parts of the world at this very time. But considerable research remains to be done before we can understand specifically and rigorously the way energy is integrated and related at the subtle level and how physical manifestation of subatomic particles and forces actually takes place.

But this research is going on, often in private laboratories, because it is outside the presently accepted paradigms of conventional research. Dr Said, who wrote the foreword, is one such pioneer, working with Philip Callahan and others.

There is also the French scientist who has been able to cure cancers in other species by using modulated magnetic fields to disrupt certain electromagnetic energy patterns that he has discovered are characteristic only of cancer cells. But he has not been permitted to try it on humans. Radiation therapy, chemotherapy and surgery rule the day in conventional practice. Rather gross approaches, lacking in energetic finesse, you will perhaps agree.

Dr James Said's Holographic Model

Dr Said has used an essentially holographic model of the human energetic structure. Starting from first principles, he has employed a form of sacred geometry concerning the inward structure of creation and the first manifestation of the tattvic essences in the causal realm. From this he has been able to demonstrate, exactly, the manner by which the chakras, nadis and the entire acupuncture system of meridians and acupoints comes into being. This is a very great achievement. The acupuncture system, he has shown, is actually derived entirely from the fiery tattwa and represents the involvement of this fiery tattwa in all parts of the body.

This is interesting for it also provides the rationale behind the experience that the acupoints have differing electrical potentials to the surrounding body surface and can be stimulated by electromagnetic excitation, as well as by the more conventional use of needles. I am referring here to electro-acupuncture, magnets and the use of lasers and monochromatic light, which are all used to stimulate the acupoints.

Electromagnetism, which includes light, is a physical expression of the expanding fiery tattwa and hence couples readily to the acupuncture system, being of the same nature, though at a lower vibrational harmonic. It also demonstrates quite neatly why acupuncture bears a relationship to the nervous system, for the electromagnetic aspects of the nervous system are woven from the fiery tattwa.

Remember that the key to understanding this is that what appears on the outside is woven from within, out of energies that are closely interrelated to each other in a holographic and non-linear fashion. This is contrary to the linear models of energy relationship which we are presently taught in our schools and universities, and to which we are unconsciously conditioned. We are dealing with energy systems where the parts all relate to each other, whatever their physical location, and which make up one indivisible whole.

Dr Said is presently engaged in preparing his first book. His work represents a tremendous breakthrough in the science and modelling of the energy tapestry, both subtle and gross. He has also produced some prototype equipment that is able to test the condition of all physical energy levels, gross or subtle, without the linkage to the human mind which we find in dowsing, radiesthesia and radionics. This makes it more reliable. It is based upon the continuous infrared and microwave emissions and absorption associated with every atom and molecule of the body.

His model is also capable of defining experimental procedures for the extraction of usable clean energy from the vacuum state. Something with which our planet is in great need. Greater and more urgently by far than most of us realize, actually, if our civilization is to survive nature's whiplash response to our unconsidered activities over the last few centuries.

Understanding the Tattwas and Indriyas

The watery, jal tattwa has the sense or indriya of taste as the primary means of its direct perception with the tongue its organ of perception and the underlying experiential aspect or tanmantra being that of flavour.

Water is essential for the sensation of taste, as you can readily observe by drying your tongue with a cloth or tissue and then placing some substance upon it.

The indriya of procreation is the action or activity most associated with that of the water tattwa, the external genitalia being the organs of this activity, in addition to their association with the kidneys, bladder and excretory system of the body.

With our western background of scientific thinking, it requires some vigorous and perceptive thinking to understand the simple depth in this eastern manner of perception. As I have often said, it does not in any way invalidate western methodology and conceptualization, but it does provide a deeper level of understanding. The complex, western mind is often so habituated to conceptual entanglement that the the power of the simple is judged as naive and a great potential for advancement is lost.

If, for example you have difficulty experiencing, from without, what is meant by the tattwas even at a gross physical level, try sitting alone, when you get a chance, on some cliff-top overlooking the sea, when the sun shines clear and strong out of a bright, blue sky.

I well remember many years ago, sitting on Beachy Head, feeling so clearly and subjectively, *through experience, not intellect*, the distinction between and the qualities of these elements. The great mound of solid rock and earth beneath; the liquid ocean rolling powerfully, waves breaking on the shore-line; the sun – radiant and scorching, a plasmic fire too bright to contemplate directly though 93 million miles away; the air scintillating and sparkling with freedom and vibrancy. And interpenetrating all, a finer integrating fabric or power of akash; a web of energy not lost even in the spaces between the stars where the other four elements hardly penetrate, a creative lattice out of which the subatomic particles of the grosser tattwas dance into being.

So, sitting free amongst the elemental forces, become aware of your own body and those of other living creatures. Still, for a while, if you can, the continual bombardment of your own thoughts and see directly how all these elements are woven most mysteriously into life forms. Imagine the tensions that must be inherent at the subtle and grosser levels for these otherwise inimical elements to be in such close and complex association with each other.

Put your attention on each of the five senses. Imagine yourself with only that one sense in operation and see how it is directly related to the tattwa of which it is the perceptive mechanism – the tongue with water, for example, or the eye with light and fire, electromagnetic vibration being the radiant and expansive aspect of the fiery tattwa's manifestation. Fire is a poor translation with a restricted meaning inapplicable to the wider activity of tejas.

Then consider the ear and hearing, faculties so closely associated with intelligence and rational thought, the quality brought to the human species by the activity of the subtle form of the akashic tattwa. In no other sense does there appear such appreciation through thought and intelligence, of the external world. We hear words and interpret them as *language*. Through words and sound come our major mode of communication with each other. Speech is articulated in the throat, where the chakra of the akashic tattwa is manifested, under the inner guidance of buddhi, the discriminatory, akashic quality found only in full development in humans. Air may be required for the transmission of sound in the physical world, but the subtlety of akash is required for its inner, intelligent appreciation.

In fact, akashic activity underlies our mental interpretation of all the five senses, and is present in the intelligent integration of all our actions through the medium of buddhi, our discriminatory faculty, which sorts out the impressions gained through the sensory indriyas and manas, formulating any executive action to be taken by our ego, ahankar, as necessary. Speech requires the greatest degree of intelligence for both its understanding and expression; sight following second with its ability to read and write, as well as discriminate intelligently amongst the wealth of visual input we receive. But though we may use our intelligence or akash in the perception or even further enjoyment of touch, taste and smell, it is not so essential for our basic experience of these senses.

Air is manifested within us as the indriya of touch or feeling, whose major sense organ is that of the skin, especially the hands with their fine ribbing of fingerprints providing a greater surface area for intricate sensation. The delicacy of air is manifested in the actions of holding, grasping and sensing with the hands. How sensitive are our fingers and how clever their manipulations. Rational thinking might have unthinkingly placed earth as the tattwa of touch and sensation, but a moment's reflection provides us with an understanding of the greater subtlety required by this sense and its associated actions. Air and fire are also the major tattwas of the nervous system – electricity and subtle sensitivity. See, too, how this indriya of 'grasping' is manifested not just through the hands but through other parts of the body – the feet and head of football players, for example. Actually, the word manipulation itself comes from the latin *manus* or hand, so manipulation means 'formed by hand'. And of all the astrological signs, it is the airy natured who are always said to be the most unconsciously manipulative. Astrologers speak of the 'fiendishly clever fingers' and mercurial quality of geminis, for example, often full of ideas and getting themselves into the position that suits them, changing constantly, regardless of its effect upon others; intolerant, in fact, of them for being unwilling to immediately change plans or even personality.

Associated with earth we have the sense of smell, a gross and earthy connection with the world, a direct perception of molecular structure, closely associated with the sensation of taste, that of the watery tattwa next above it, in which the molecules dissolve for their finer sensory appreciation. The olfactory cells within the nose are the earthy organ of perception, while its active principle is expressed through the eliminative function of the anus, via the rectum. Some schools of psychology have unwittingly found within the human personality these energetic associations between the nose and the anus, as well as the tongue with the genitalia. This we also experience in the act of kissing – a kiss on the lips is more sensual than a peck on the cheek, while an open-mouthed kiss with the tongue in action is immediately sensual in a sexual sense.

The association of the eyes with the feet and their action of walking is quite clear, for we need our sight to see where we are going, as indeed we do for our hands to function successfully, but while we can learn to use our hands without sight – as does the musician who cannot watch both hands simultaneously and may even shut his eyes, watching neither – we cannot easily walk or move about without our sight. Calorific energy is required, too, for movement – a clear manifestation of the fiery tattwa. And walking, or going places, is certainly the most physically expansive form of human activity, the mode in which the fiery drive is most eloquently expressed. See, for example, how the unrelenting, subtle, emotional drive of fire, as well as its physical manifestation, is required in the athletic prowess of an Olympic runner. Or how these same fiery qualities are combined with the dexterity of air in the incredibly fast and accurate teamwork of international basketball players.

Looked at in a more holistic way, we can say that the tattwas are an energetic essence which we *experience* in a variety of ways. Their subtle aspects give us our sensory and motor indriyas, as well as our human psychology and the substructure or subtle vibrations which give rise to our physical forms. We also experience these tattwas, through our indriyas, as the material substance of this world which therefore appears to us as solid, liquid, gaseous and so on.

But to appreciate this, it is necessary for us to relax our grip on the feeling that the world of our senses is outside of ourselves.

The point is that although we might describe the world of gross physical substance as the 'primary objective reality', this perception is actually incorrect. The external reality of the fiery state of substance, for instance, the sensation of sight, the ability to move about, the emotional desire and drive to do so, the experience of frustrated or unbalanced drive (anger), the fiery qualities within body function – all these are a part of the way that the fiery tattwa is built into our being, into our human stucture. No one aspect of it is more real than another. It is only the focus of our attention that may make it seem so. And similarly with the other tattwas.

So we are 'floating' – lost – in the ocean of these five tattwas, these five essences. We are led through the nose by our mind which is itself tightly gripped by the things we perceive through our five senses – so much so that we consider them to be the only 'reality'. And *this* is Maya or illusion.

However, we digress, but not unwittingly, for rather than put all the comparative thinking concerning the tattwas into one section of the book, I have interspaced it throughout to add variety and allow time to mature for what may be new thoughts to many readers. Sleeping on an idea, I have always found, is an excellent way of letting new concepts infiltrate one's thinking processes and gain maturity. And as the months and years go by, the understanding deepens and experience grows. This is a factor of inner growth and seems to be a univeral principle, regardless of whatever tattwas are particularly active in one's make-up.

The Sensitive, Psychological Characteristics of Water

Psychologically, water is the tattwa of sensitivity and emotion, in the more restricted sense. The primary response from one whose dominant keynote is that of water is emotional and receptive. Experiences great or small are taken into themselves and *felt*. Their nature is truly of the fluid element. Water will permeate with enveloping sympathy, perceiving subtleties and nuances left unobserved by others. To one with little active water in their constitution, the reactions and mode of being of watery types is an enigma. The dryness of the other tattwas finds comprehension of the sometimes surging emotions of the watery types, a subjective exercise of considerable difficulty. In fact, we instinctively call a callous or hard, insensitive individual, a 'dry-fish' – an interesting expression, since a fish is essentially of the water element. Fire will scorch water by sheer insensitive drive, while air will loftily overlook water's quiet sensitivity in its airy conceptualizations and ideals. Earth may feel at home with water, if the need for sympathy is felt, but the solidity of earth may injure the water's feelings on the one hand or provide a welcome containment and relief from emotionality on the other.

Water is not assertive, seeking more to flow around obstructions than to knock them aside. Watery personalities are intuitive and often psychic, sensitive of vibrations and influences. In their most positive state, they are warm and sympathetic lovers of creation, the solace of many weary hearts, receptive and good listeners, able to understand the feelings of others empathetically rather than rationally, comforting to the dryness of the other tattwas.

Those whose watery nature is overactive and imbalanced find themselves awash with emotion and feeling, full of reactions and undercurrents which confuse the minds of other types, who may have no personal experience of that degree or depth of feeling. They can become highly impressionable, seeking continually for signs and portents, apprehensive and self-protective. Water-logged by emotion, uncertainty, paradoxical feelings and absorption in how they feel about themselves and their life experiences, misery and depression can become their day-to-day companions from which they can see no way out.

The great founder of homoeopathy, Hahnemann, appreciated the effect of the subtle, psychological constitution of human inner life upon the outward manifestation of disease, and many of the homoeopathic remedies are prescribed for the mental and emotional patterns rather than for the more outward actualizations of these inner energies in the physical symptoms of ill-health and disease.

So self-absorption, dwelling in one's own emotional ocean, is the major source of the difficulties faced by this personality type. If this can be turned to positive advantage, then the inner well-springs of love will give rise to feelings of compassion and understanding.

The tendency to become overly introverted also means that such people readily run away from difficulties rather than face them. Easily worn out and devitalized by their worries and concerns, they can become fearful of the events of life, being under the sway of their negative reaction patterns.

In association with air, considerable inner conflict can arise as the light and fast moving, conceptual idealist is brought into contact with the grossness of life, experienced and felt deeply through the watery tattwa. The result can be swings of mood and activity, at one time rushing about under the sway of air with the latest new idea seeking expression, and at the next moment cut to the quick, stopping dead in their tracks as some event, seen as a source of difficulty to the airy nature and associated with the manifestation of their airy concept or ideal, grips their emotional reaction. Resentment and hurt may then set in as the mode of expression, until the next cycle of new thought rises to the surface.

The imaginative capacity of air combined with the introvert tendency of water towards feeling hurt, can lead such a person to be a dreamer, an escapist and a spinner of fantasy – even around their mundane outer life.

Air and water, at their best and most integrated, combine intellect with emotional sensitivity: the grasp of the abstract with an intuitive feel for life's inner processes. The result is that there is a depth, humanity, and a synthesis of many points of view expressed in their ideas, through the watery appreciation of others' manner of thinking, combined with the fleetness of conceptual linking derived from air. These kind of people have fertile and active imaginations and are creative in whatever their sphere of life. Their ability to tune in to others and to readily verbalize their perceptions makes them excellent in the healing and counselling professions or in any activity involving both people and creative thought.

Life is a struggle and a superficial approach might lead one to believe that the combination of opposites or extremes, whether within oneself or in relationships, is a recipe for disaster. However, a mastery of these apparent opposites within oneself and a bringing together of these facets under the eye of greater consciousness, gives one a broadened perspective and a far higher outlook and understanding. To bring the effect of all these tattwas into integrated harmony within one's being is to move towards the ideal of the perfect man, one who can function well in all spheres of life and with all manner of people. For all of us, however, hemmed in by the karmic patterning from our past, such an ideal can only be realized within, by rising above the tattvic energy fields into higher realms of inner consciousness, love and bliss. And this does not happen so much spontaneously, as by many years of sincere meditative practice of a high order.

The Central Fire

Spinal Correspondences

It is an interesting exercise at this point to once again look at the spine as a whole, according to classical western physiology and anatomy, comparing its divisions with those of yogic philosophy, (see figure 7-1).

At the base we have the coccyx, a section of fused vertebrae. It is our tail, situated at the most earthy part of our body, upon which we sit. Here we find the earthy tattwa and the muladhara chakra governing the organization of solids within the body.

Next, we have the sacral area from which flow the nerves to control the rectum, bladder and genitalia. These lower areas correspond to the earthy and watery centres from which sexual polarity, procreative function and bodily fluids are administered. So far, we would seem to be in correspondence with the classical view of the nervous system and spinal divisions, though clearly there is an admixture of function as the subtle centres exercise their control over the gross physical, through the mechanisms of causative formation.

Third is the fiery or navel, *manipuraka* centre governing the food factories of the body – the intestines, the liver, pancreas and so on. Here our classical distinction begins to break down because the nerves to these systems are associated not only with the third, lumbar section of the spine, but also with the lower thoracic area below the diaphragm. These western spinal divisions are, however, somewhat arbitrary and the diaphragm – which separates the operations of the three lower centres from the three higher – is in many respects a better division, since it relates to a specific functional aspect of human anatomy. It is also interesting to note that the nerve supply to the pancreas comes from *higher up* in the spine than the area of

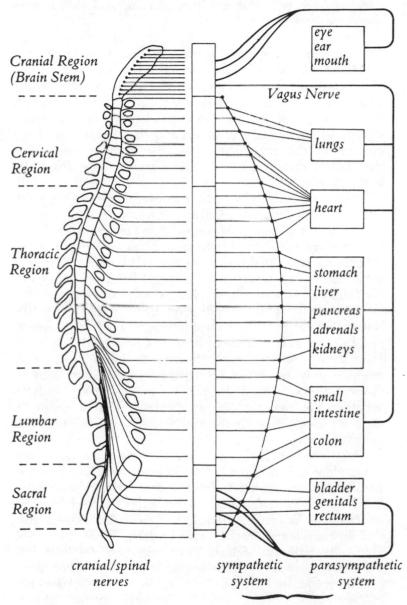

Cranial Region
(Brain Stem)

Cervical
Region

Thoracic
Region

Lumbar
Region

Sacral
Region

eye
ear
mouth

Vagus Nerve

lungs

heart

stomach
liver
pancreas
adrenals
kidneys

small
intestine

colon

bladder
genitals
rectum

*cranial/spinal
nerves*

*sympathetic
system*

*parasympathetic
system*

Voluntary nervous system   *Autonomic nervous system*

After Evans: Mind, Body and Electromagnetism.

Figure 7-1. *Spinal correspondences.*

the gut over which it has jurisdiction, and this link is discussed later in the chapter.

Above the diaphragm, we have the upper thoracic and the cervical sections of the spine with their nerve supply to the heart and lungs. Here we have the heart or *hridaya* chakra with its tattwa of air, which correlates well, whilst above that is the throat chakra with its faculty – through the mouth – of making intelligent speech, related very closely to the element of akash and the expression of the content of the antashkarans or the human mind. The throat and mouth receive their nerve supply from the lower cranial nerves.

This is of interest for the motor functions of speech require a high degree of intelligence found only in man and related to the presence of the subtle akashic tattwa. This, like the zero point of the physical vacuum, behaves as an interface and control point for the subtle tattvic energies from below and the mental functions from above. Hence we find the nerve supply reaching the throat area from the lower cranial region, a reflection, most probably of the linkage upwards of the subtle aspect of akash into mental and thought energies. In addition, of course, the throat is intimately connected with the mouth and an integrated nerve supply from the higher brain centres, related to consciousness, would appear to be essential. Though whether the majority of us operate from a point of consciousness when we use our throat and mouth is open to debate!

The *ajna* chakra, being above the spine and holding a controlling function over the lower centres has an exact parallel in the pituitary gland and the hypothalamus, a topic we will be discussing at some length in the appropriate chapter. The hypothalamus provides the neuroendocrine linkage between the brain and the other endocrine glands, partially through the intermediary of the pituitary.

Finally, it is worth pointing out that the major sense organs are located with a direct neuronal integration and linkage into the brain and higher mental faculties, including the indriyas or 'mental sense organs'. The senses, being our normal means of experiencing physical reality and in many people, *the only channel for experiencing life*, are hence very close, experientially and anatomically, to our centre of mental attention. In fact, we feel our thinking centre to be right behind our eyes, the sense organs which we take as our primary means of perception of the world and through which the major part of our attention flows out into physical 'reality'.

We put our hand to our forehead, for example, when we wish to remember something or when thinking deeply. We do not strike our knees or any other part of our anatomy!

Biogravitational Coherence and the Life Force

That the brain and spine are the staff of physical existence is not in dispute. Even embryologically, the development of the child starts with the growth of the notochord, the primary pattern for the spine, embryonic development taking place from the central axis outward. Firstly, the morphogenic patterning of the pranas weaves the subtle tattvic blueprint into embryonic existence. Once the subtle chakric centres of subtle energy administration are established in simple form, then the ramifications and complexities can commence with material substance drawn in from the mother and fitted into the the pattern through the formative power of the subtle and vacuum matrix.

But the central administration lies in the brain and spine, expressed outwardly as the central nervous system.

This cohering and attractive blueprint is sometimes called the *biogravitational field* of the body, because the spinning together of material, tattvic substance through the inner power of the life force is an attractive and organizational power above that of the simple gravity of material attraction, particle for particle, upon the creative web of vacuum or akash. And the essential focus of this life-giving force is located in the brain and spine.

The understanding, therefore, of physiotherapy, osteopathy and chiropractic, as well as many other forms of therapy that the health of the body lies primarily in the condition of the cranial vault, the spine and the central nervous system, is entirely justified. All the major organs hang from the spine and have a relationship to it, both structurally, as well as in their nervous and blood supply, through the spinal cord, the autonomic nervous system and the central artery, the aorta.

The limbs themselves are simply a leverage system, attached to the spine, in order to overcome the forces of physical gravity. In terms of polarity, the shifting flow of electrical impulse results in muscular contraction and expansion in order that we may move our otherwise inert torso and head around the world of our karmas.

Note, too, how the soft, sensory and yin parts of our body and limbs are on the front, with the yang, motor aspects at our back. Even the blood vessels and nerves that supply the muscles of our arms and legs with warmth, nutrition and organizing coherence run along the frontal, protected area of our body before passing to the muscles at the rear.

With our back, we present our musculature to the world, harder and more tolerant of physical abuse and injury than our soft 'underbelly'. With eyes and sense organs only in the front of our head, we keep our senses where our heart is and maintain a protective physical configuration against danger and the rigours of life. And when we wish no longer to have association with something, we simply 'turn our back' on it, for the life connection to be broken.

The cohering and organizational power of the life force from within is a law of nature that is not recognized by conventional medical science. However, it is a very real force, with a multitude of ramifications and expressions at the physiological and biochemical level. It is the presence of this force which keeps living forms alive. The intensely complex tapestry of biological activity ceases, almost immediately, as soon as it is withdrawn, matter reverting to the relatively still and simple structure inherent in dead objects and which are maintained in manifested existence by only a highly diffuse form of the Shabda or primal Creative Word.

How it is that scientific paradigms fail to take account of the significance of the difference between dead matter and living organisms is a subject for some consideration. For the assumption that life is caused by biochemical complexity rather than biochemical complexity being due to the energy of life, is surely both naive and superficial.

We should, however, return from our digression to the subject of fire.

The Fire Centre – East and West

Fire is the nearest translation available for the *tejas* tattwa, whose control point is situated in the *manipuraka* or *nabhipadma* chakra, so called – according to the the Gautamiya Tantra – because the fiery tattwa makes it as lustrous and sparkling as a gem *(mani)*, the colour being a dark red, and the number of petals, eight. *Nabhi* means navel, which tells us the level at which this chakra is located. The pranic vibration here is known as *Samana* and is concerned with the distribution of nourishment throughout the body.

By tejas or 'fire' is meant the quality of energetic expansion and activity, giving rise to exertion and movement. In outward expression, it can be *experienced* as calorific in nature and hot, heat being directly related to the rate of molecular or atomic movement. Thus we find that tejas governs the kitchen and larder of our body, where food is digested and stored, being made available for later use as required. Intestinal function and assimilation is given energy from this point, as well as the control of nutritional metabolism. Under the influence of the fiery tattwa and its associated pranic patterning, the basic nutritional constituents of carbohydrates, triglycerides (fats) and proteins are broken down by the digestive system into sugars, fatty acids and amino acids and then reassembled as storage and structural tissue in the liver, adipose and muscle tissue, respectively. As demand requires, the reverse or yang energy route is later followed as sugars, fatty acids and amino acids are again made available to active body metabolism.

The associated gland is very clearly the pancreas, which has both exocrine and endocrine functions. In its exocrine aspect, enzymes are secreted directly into the gut for the digestion of food, while the endocrine cells (*Islets of Langerhans*) within the pancreatic tissue, are responsible for hormonal secretions.

The Islets of Langerhans, first described by Langerhans in 1869, represent less than two per cent of total pancreatic tissue, indicating that it is not the *size* of a key that is important, but its *structure*. Three types of cell have been observed in human pancreatic endocrine tissue, designated the α, β and γ cells, (see figure 7-2). While the α and β cells are responsible for the production of the hormones *glucagon* and *insulin*, respectively, the γ cells are associated with the presence of *somatostatin* and *gastrin*. A further pancreatic polypeptide (*PP*) has also been recently demonstrated, though at present, its function appears obscure.

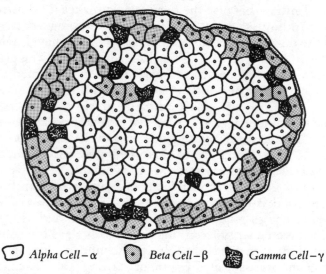

◻ *Alpha Cell* – α   ◼ *Beta Cell* – β   ▨ *Gamma Cell* – γ

Redrawn, with permission, from Hormones: The Messengers, of Life, *Lawrence Crapo*, W. H. Freeman & Co.

Figure 7-2. The Islets of Langerhans, within the pancreas

Though the roles of somatostatin, gastrin and PP are little understood, insulin and glucagon activity have been well documented as major factors in the biochemical regulation of carbohydrate, fat and protein metabolism. Unlike the thyroid gland, however, whose role in body metabolism is more of a controlling nature, insulin and glucagon are a duo whose role lies in the storage and availability of body fuels, a part of the administration of bodily fire.

Imagine the power of these two hormones, these two energy patterns, lower harmonics with relationship to the subtle aspect of the tejas tattwa. Their influence is felt within practically every cell of the body. Insulin is the yin, storage hormone. Under its prompting, glucose is converted into glycogen and stored mostly in the liver and muscle tissue. Amino acids are converted into proteins in muscle tissue, while fatty acids are amalgamated into triglycerides in adipose (fatty) tissue.

If insulin is pre-eminently the 'storage of nutrition', the yin hormone, the keeper of the larder, the prompt that directs nutritional energy into stored, potential form, then glucagon is the opener of the larder door, the opposite polarity (yang). While insulin secretion seems to be stimulated by a post-prandial increase in blood levels of glucose, amino acids and fatty acid concentrations, glucagon is brought into action when we miss a meal or two, in order to maintain an adequate supply of fuel for the brain (especially) as well as the other bodily tissues. The brain uses up a prodigious amount of glucose in proportion to its size, compared with other body tissue. An interesting fact that no doubt relates to the its role in the translation of subtle energies into the physical and vice versa.

Physiologists are well aware that the metabolic rates and the usage of body energies are only incompletely understood. Why some of us are lean, whilst others run to plumpness is still quite a mystery and it seems probable that the equations of bodily energy will balance more readily if one considers that the body has the means for the transformation of energies in and out of the subtle state. 'Food for thought' may indeed be just that and can explain why mental activity can make us so hungry.

Insulin

We now embark upon a short section concerning scientific aspects of insulin, which may be lightly skimmed over if you are not of a mind to follow the biochemical details and diversity.

Insulin is actually the only hormone known to lower the level of blood glucose, while glucagon, adrenaline, cortisol and others have the converse effect. Insulin appears to act in two separate, though interconnected, fashions. Firstly, it facilitates the transport of glucose across cell membranes. For most cells cannot take up glucose even in the presence of a favourable glucose gradient across the membrane. Very little simple diffusion takes place.

Notable exceptions to this general principle are cells of the liver and central nervous system which do appear to rely upon diffusion and a favourable glucose gradient, and erythrocytes (red blood cells), gastrointestinal and renal cells which rely on a glucose-sodium ion liason and an ion pump mechanism which operates independently of insulin.

Secondly, insulin directly affects intracellular metabolic pathways in a variety of ways. Glycogen synthesis, for example, is mediated by the insulin-sensitive stimulation of a glycogen-building enzyme or catalyst, whilst simultaneously inhibiting the effect of an enzyme involved in the breakdown of glycogen to glucose. Similarly, amino acid and fatty acid transport across cell membranes and into cells is facilitated by insulin and their subsequent anabolism into structural and storage tissue as proteins and fats. Insulin is thus involved in the process of bodily growth and development. And interestingly enough, insulin also facilitates the formation of cholesterol, the steroid hormone precursor. The activity of this chakra is thus linked downwards to the function of the two lower centres, helping to provide the substrate for their outward endocrine encoding.

A low level of insulin synthesis would appear to be continuous even in the absence of other stimuli, but apart from an increase in blood glucose and certain amino acids, there are a number of other factors which influence its secretion (see figure 7-3).

The Islets of Langerhans receive innervation from the autonomic nervous system providing the other principal regulating input, the dominant effect of sympathetic stimulus being inhibitory, while the parasympathetic promotes insulin output. This is of interest and fits the general pattern of autonomic control, for while the sympathetic nervous system has general functionality as the stimulator of autonomic body function, in this case insulin production is actually diminished or inhibited. Insulin, however, is pro-yin in its general metabolic role and hence the net effect of insulin inhibition is stimulation of metabolic activity. And the converse is true for the parasympathetic promotion of insulin synthesis and body metabolism. This is yet another example of the complex patternings of the

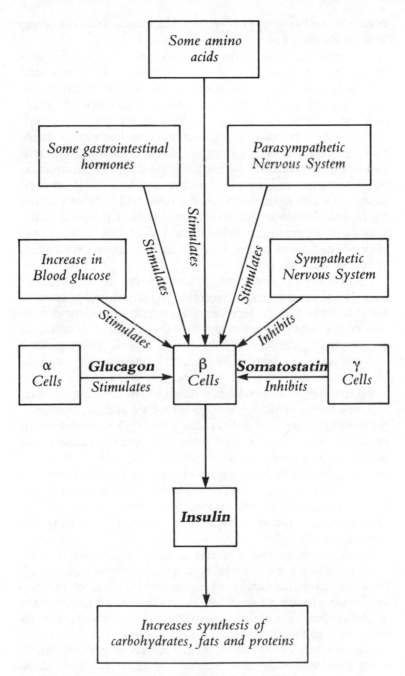

Figure 7-3. Factors influencing insulin synthesis

cosmic duality, the yin within the yang and the yang within the yin.

Amongst other substances which influence insulin production are all those hormones, enzymes and so on which increase the level of blood glucose and certain amino acids, such as pituitary growth hormone and adrenocorticoids, thereby indirectly stimulating insulin release. Catecholamines like adrenaline, will have complex effects since their stimulation of the sympathetic nervous system will depress insulin output, while their general role in increasing blood glucose levels will increase it. In a situation such as this, we can again perceive the tone and balance created by harmonious interaction of opposites, the yin and the yang. For adrenaline is essentially a yang hormone, but it is prevented from going too far by the counterbalancing effects of insulin.

Any complex energetic system such as our human mental–subtle–gross constitution will naturally contain these bio-gyro, self-correcting facets and in any investigation of the subtle state energy fields, one can also expect to find such an interwoven lattice of energetic interactions.

Amongst the stimulators of insulin production we also have the anabolic steroids, the body builders, including the sex hormones, though the full mechanism remains unclear.

The general principle would therefore appear to be that those interactions and substances which are essentially yin, or take body energies into potential form, stimulate the production of insulin, either directly or indirectly. Conversely, those which consume energy and are intrinsically yang in nature, will primarily depress insulin production. But then the counterbalancing effect comes into play as glucose and amino acid levels rise, thus adding tone to the general energetic balance.

Finally, the gastrointestinal hormones of *secretin* and *gastrin* and the pancreatic enzyme, *pancreozymin-cholecysto-kinin* all stimulate insulin manufacture. These, of course, are involved with good digestion, an aspect of fiery tattvic activity, facilitating the assimilation of a wide range of nutrients, and are simply providing advance warning of a meal about to be digested, with the concomitant rise in body nutrients ready for both storage as well as immediate utilization.

Glucagon

The interplay of glucagon and insulin presents a beautiful example of energetic polarity at work for the maintenance of a total, harmonious system. For in almost every way, glucagon and its control factors are diametrically opposed to insulin. Glucagon release, for example, is stimulated by sympathetic nervous messages and inhibited by the parasympathetic.

There is no need, therefore, to go into the details, as we did with insulin. The nature of the energy balance is clearly expressed, an excellent and simple example of the opposing pranic polarities flowing between the chakras as Ida, Pingala and within Sushumna, and appearing outwardly as biochemistry and bioelectrical nervous system activity.

Somatostatin

Also produced in the pancreas is the hormone *somatostatin*, found, too, in the hypothalamus, where it is an inhibitor of the pituitary production of growth hormone, as well as in the stomach, large and small intestines, the salivary and thyroid glands. Its pancreatic function, however, can only be surmised, perhaps as a part of the regulatory function over the growth and maintenance of the cells that produce insulin and glucagon. For its general function appears to be that of inhibition of further growth, maintenance of the status quo, a kind of sattvas guna thread running throughout the body at a molecular level.

It is noteworthy that within the Islets of Langerhans where these three hormones are all produced, a positional polarity is adhered to, the glucagon-producing cells being on the periphery, around the centrally positioned insulin-manufacturing cells. The somatostatin-producing cells are found intermingled here and there throughout, (see figure 7-2).

New Paradigms in the Life Sciences

The role of somatostatin in both pituitary and pancreatic function is an interesting factor and leads one into some intriguing speculation, because the presence, production and activity of hormones away from their traditionally understood manufacturing and target sites is becoming a matter of frequent discovery as biochemical assays become more accurate and more able to detect smaller quantities of substance. Somatostatin, for example, could be considered to possess an energetic 'frequency' at the molecular level that is resonant with growth factors, both central – as displayed in the link with the pituitary growth hormone – as well as peripheral via its association with insulin and glucagon and other bodily physiological processes. Energetically, one could perceive it as a homoeostatic keynote or vibration.

This line of thinking leads one into an interesting area of biological theory, where all biochemistry is reunderstood more accurately, according to the understanding of modern physics, not as the interaction of 'solid molecules' as we are shown in classical biochemical texts, but as interplay of the intensely energetic subatomic particles and forces by which each molecule is more accurately described. That is, even within the understanding of mainstream modern physics, biochemistry presently employs a paradigm or conceptual framework which is a considerable simplification of the energies which are actually known to be at work.

If we add to this the subtle, inner, substructural aspects of those theories or models of modern physics which acknowledge the existence of a hidden and deeper reality, then biochemistry, as a study of energy interactions at the molecular level, seems superficial and lacking in finer detail. Its paradigms appear unable to accommodate even the subatomic, the bioelectronic and biomagnetic, let alone the other more subtle aspects, known by biophysicists and others to be active within the human constitution.

Such an approach would probably require the formation of a mathematical model of human energy interactions, based upon a fusion of biochemistry with such concepts in modern physics as scalar electromagnetic theory and vacuum state understanding, discussed in later chapters. Such a model would of course be highly complex, requiring many years of research, with the use of advanced computing facilities. The practical advantages, however, would be an understanding of the body and mind as an integrated energy complex and from it would automatically emerge advanced therapeutic techniques for both physical, emotional and mental imbalances. It would also advance the study of robotics, making the existing electronic approaches seem like Victorian steam engines by comparison. Such is the nature of all scientific progress.

The Fiery Tattwa

The fastest moving of all physical, expanding and radiating energies is that of electromagnetism. Also a manifestation of the fiery tattwa, it is perceived by the eye, where subtle tejas energy activates the retina to be responsive to the very small section of electromagnetic vibration we perceive as light. Electromagnetic radiation moves directly and in straight lines (more or less), interacting with the solid, watery and airy substance through which it passes. This, for instance, underlies the phenomenon of rainbows, as well as why sticks and straight objects appear to bend when entering water.

The incessant, background buzz of electromagnetic radiation, excitable fiery energy from electrical and TV broadcasting, from microwave radar cloud mapping and communications, from electrical appliances and cabling, plus the interruption to the earth's natural electromagnetic properties by modern buildings, equipment and lifestyle, all have their effect on all living organisms, as modern research is now discovering. This subject is discussed in some depth in my previous book, *Subtle Energy*, and from a practical point of view I will only comment here that it is best to sit at a good distance away from your TV set, do not live under or near electricity pylons, avoid underfloor electrical heating systems, do not sleep on or under electric blankets unless they are switched off, do not have electrical cabling in your bedhead or trailing under the bed, and treat your microwave cooker and home computer or VDU with considerable distance and respect.

As we discussed, the agni or tejas energy domain directs digestion and is involved in the metabolic process of storing and releasing energy for bodily action. Air fans the flames of fire, so to say, providing the oxidative fuel through which the fire can manifest, while water is the carrier of heat and fuel throughout the body. Whenever there is an imbalance in this energy system, stagnation can be the end result, but the primary cause may lie in imbalance in either of the air, fire or watery tattvic fields.

Those forms of energy medicine, such as Dr Stone's Polarity Therapy, which comprehend the manner in which the tattwas operate in the body have a supreme advantage, therefore, in that they can more readily move directly to the heart of a problem and find release of energy tensions both emotionally and mentally, as well as physically, before disharmony can appear outwardly as pathological symptoms of tissue degeneration.

Dr Vincent Lad, in his book, *Ayurveda*, comments that repressed emotion of the fiery type, such as anger, leads to toxic conditions, also changing the flora of the small intestines, the bile duct and the gall bladder, aggravating the watery, mucous membranes of the stomach and the intestines, large and small. Frequently, the resultant symptoms become those of allergy to pollen and dust, flower scent, certain foods, and so on.

A hyperactive fiery tattwa, by drawing energy from air, depletes the protective airy function of its immune system regulation, resulting in lowered immune and protective response and in symptoms of allergy to substances with which the body should, under balanced circumstances, be able to cope. The link between allergy and emotion is clearly drawn and the apparently neurotic behaviour and emotionality often associated to a greater or lesser degree with allergy, can thus be readily understood.

Psychosomatic and Placebo Effects

The tendency amongst some members of the healing professions to dismiss physical symptoms, once they have been traced to psychosomatic origins is a reflection of poor understanding of the human energy complex, for we are just one complex in which all outward expression, whether of outward physical action or within our bodily processes, reflects what lies within. Indeed, the appreciation of psychosomatic effects needs to be expanded to understand the total energy picture and to permit the physician to help the patient to an even greater extent.

The most consistent finding in trials of drugs and therapies is that in an appreciable percentage of cases, an administered placebo effects a cure. This is normally dismissed by thinking, "There was nothing wrong with the person, anyway. It was just psychological." In fact, more research and thinking needs to go into *how a placebo works. I would go as far as to say that the placebo effect is arguably the most important discovery of all modern medicine and pharmacology,* (and the most overlooked), because it points to a real energetic pathway linking mind, emotion and body. And it is an understanding of this linkage that will form the basis for twenty-first centry healing techniques.

The ability to mobilize the patient's own inner energies is of great importance to any physician, whatever his calling, for this in itself can effect a real cure, as is evidenced by the use of placebos. And it is a real *energetic* effect, calling upon the higher mental energies to repattern themselves, and thence the manifested energies that underlie the symptoms. Indeed, if this mobilization is not engendered, then a patient's subconscious can equally well work *against* any applied treatment. As any doctor or therapist knows, when the patient *really* wants to get well, then more than half the battle is won. But the subconscious contains many unhealthy mental and emotional patterns that bring about disease, and are more than difficult to shift.

Asthmatic patients, for example, have frequently been observed to come from backgrounds where they have been taught in early life to repress anger and other negative emotions. The 'cough and splutter' of repressed feelings is the beginning of this kind of manifestation and the observation that the asthmatic tendency is considerably curtailed when patients are taught in psychotherapy or through bioenergetic techniques to release their pent up repressions and emotions, shows the power of these inner causative energies. Any therapeutic technique that does not consider the emotional and inner life of the individual is so superficial as to be genuinely considered naive, however much energy and resources have been channelled into its development. Symptomatic relief is fine for emergency use, but long-term improvement in well-being is quite another matter and requires a far deeper approach.

Three Aspects of the Healing Process

Actually, one can also expand this concept and understanding of the placebo effect *to the therapist or physician*. For just as the attitude of mind and human intention of a cook becomes encoded into the food, affecting those who eat it; or the care of a craftsman is woven vibrationally into his creation at the vacuum state level, so too is the intention and understanding of the healer an integral part of the patient-therapist dynamics involved in any healing process, even regardless of the efficacy of the remedy applied.

And this, like the placebo effect, is an energetic phenomenon involving real energies at subtle levels.

In general, therefore, one can say that any healing process involves three integrated aspects:

1. The patient – his attitudes and belief systems.
2. The physician – his skill, attitudes and belief systems.
3. The therapeutic technique itself.

With any therapeutic technique, whether drug-orientated or more natural, we know from the placebo effect, that results can be obtained purely by going through the motions of applying the technique – by administering a placebo pill, for example. This mobilizes the mental energies of the patient and effects a healing even at the biochemical and physiological levels.

I have not seen the results of any placebo trials where the physician also thought that the pill was a real medicine, but depending upon the charisma and depth of rapport between the patient and the healer, I would imagine there to be a greater or lesser enhancement of the effect. This will be partially because the patient's desire to be healed is reinforced by the healthful, positive, understanding and confident air of the doctor, but will also be due to a subtle encoding of the physician's expectations and concern *into the subtle substructure of the medicine itself*, which is then ingested by the patient and integrated into their own energetic complex.

Secondly, any applied therapy requires a *belief system* or

a conceptual framework in which it is to be understood and administered. If a doctor or therapist loses faith in his system, his efficacy automatically declines because the inner empathetic rapport between himself, patient and technique is lost and the dynamics of his situation loses tone and balance. For his own happiness and well-being, he needs at this point to reconsider his options and his modus operandi.

Skill, training, attitude, experience, intuition and a penetrating understanding of the underlying belief system or science can all contribute to a caring and healing approach to any therapy, much as an Olympic athlete is at one in mind and body, so that there is no blockage in the free expression of energy from within-out.

Actually, this energy of the athlete is often so mentally and hence physically funnelled and concentrated that Michael Murphy and Rhea White have written a lengthy book, *The Psychic Side of Sport*, which relates innumerable instances of how this concentration can unconsciously result in mind–over–matter 'miracles'. The intense desire for achievement coupled with the unblocked channelling of energy from within moves the player faster than ever before, psychokinetically moves objects such as golf balls and footballs, opens up a spontaneous mental glimpse of inner cellular and physiological processes and so on. In fact, it even provides the inner impetus for lucid or mystic moments, or spiritual experiences. In the eastern martial arts and wrestling, the development of their Ch'i or subtle energy is an intrinsic part of the training, its mastery leading to the legendary and miraculous anecdotes sur-rounding the great practitioners.

So the quality of mind and energy in the physician is of considerable importance in the healing process because it is not only transmitted directly to the patient, but also becomes manifest in the doctor's own skill and presenta-tion of himself.

Finally, the therapeutic technique itself must be valid, for the third aspect of the healing process to play its central part. This is not a book in which we discuss the available options, but as we have previously said, the essential function of any therapy is to balance and harmonize the energy network of our human constitution. Therefore, the deeper the conceptual framework of any applied therapy in terms of its perception of human life energies, then the more effective will be the results obtained.

In the light of the foregoing, it is clear that the tendency amongst some proponents of modern drug-orientated medicine to criticize alternative therapies on the one hand, and to miss the crucial relevance of the placebo effect, on the other, stems from a lack of appreciation of the existence of the patient as a living, vibrant human being – an integral part of the healing process. Furthermore, the mental attitude and personality of the physician, as an intrinsic aspect of this process is also often overlooked or considered as being of no importance. And yet it is the kind and understanding, as well as the skilful, doctor who receives the gifts from grateful patients. Kindness and a caring approach must work hand in hand with scientific method.

So while modern medicine purports to effect healing primarily through only the third aspect of the three defined, many alternative therapies are active in all three, and hence their popularity. Some may even be deficient in the third aspect of therapeutic technique, but the belief system of the healer and patient and the dynamics generated by the relationship are themselves of a real and valid healing quality and require the existence of the belief system for their efficacy to become apparent.

In this sense, therefore, not every therapist can help every patient, because the energetic dynamics need to be right before the magic can be woven at a real and subtle level.

I am purposely not attempting to delineate which therapies fall into which categories, for in practical terms it may not matter. But the point is that the pragmatic and down-to-earth approach of the third aspect alone – a characteristic of modern science, generally – while apparently 'safe' from a conceptual point of view, is actually the most severly limited of all. And since, as humans, we are limited in our perceptions, it has become the conventional approach to healing. But it is not the most comprehensive and powerful. The scientific knowledge encapsulated within it is of tremendous value, but its conceptual horizons need greatly expanding for it to give rise to truly great methodology. A new healing paradigm could then emerge in which all aspects and approaches to well-being are harmoniously integrated. And this would be of great benefit to humanity, surely the primary objective of all medicine?

The Tattvic Fabric – Subtle and Gross

It maybe useful at this point to reconsider one's under-standing of the tattwas.

For convenience of expression, I talk in this book as if they were both subtle and gross. In fact, the tattvic fabric is just one, linked through our experience, though our mind – itself enlivened by consciousness. It is one whole which we experience at subtle and gross levels as our mind's attention moves inward and outward. This, in-deed, is true of our experience of the entire creation as we ascend and descend in meditation. So the tattwas are a subtle essence which manifests to our experience in a variety of ways – sensory, motor, emotional, as well as in body structure and function etc. They are not simple, disassociated and unconnected to each other, but are a tightly woven fabric of integral, interconnected-ness.

In inert matter, this tattvic fabric is only loosely inter-woven, with boundaries developing between the observed states of solid, liquid and gaseous. But in living organisms, this fabric is so complexly integrated by the inward life force that these otherwise inimical states of matter are combined into an intricate tapestry.

Actually, if there were no tattvic boundaries in inert matter, life as we know it would be intolerable, for we would exist in a homogenous goo – a sort of tattvic porridge.

Conversely, if there were more than five tattvic condi-tions, the number of boundaries would make living on this physical plane far too complex. Boundaries between solids, liquids and gases are quite enough for us to handle. With only one or two more possibilities thrown in, we would not know where to put our head or our feet! Think about that for a while, it is quite mind boggling! Yet still some modern thinkers do not acknowledge the relevance of the five elements or tattwas to present-day thought and science. It is no more than man's primordial condition of being unable to see the wood for the trees!

Acid and Alkali, Yin and Yang

Back with our fiery theme, acidity, being yang in nature, is associated with the outgoing rajas quality of the fiery tattwa and thus excess fire energy in the body is also observable as a more acid urine and a more acid system generally. Conversely, a lack of body fire can also be countered by a choice of foods or herbs, high in fire energy. These include both carbohydrates and acidic foods. The range of Chinese tonic herbs, administered for their yin and yang characteristics and their effects upon the different bodily organs, systems and energies are well worth studying in this respect. The popular tonic herb, ginseng, for example, has strong yang characteristics and while useful to those with low fire energy, it may be too powerful for those in an already overly-yang condition.

On the other hand, a person who is low in yang energy, demonstrating itself as an active, nervous disposition lacking in the true and sustained directive power of fiery energy, can benefit from a boost to their inner yang. This would balance out these fibrillations of nervous energy that stem from the attempt to move outward, but are stifled by lack of real energy and a conflict with the yin condition.

The discussion of these topics in their specific relationship to particular disorders and bodily conditions is of great interest, but is beyond the scope of this book. What I am attempting to do here is simply to present a conceptual framework, illustrated by a few simple examples, from which the reader may extrapolate and understand many of his or her own experiences of both themselves and others.

Fire and Emotion

Psychologically, the same characteristics are manifested out of fire as are seen at the physical level. The fire signs of astrology (*aries*, *leo* and *sagittarius*) are known for their relentless drive and active, excitable natures. Fire is the tattwa demanding direct and speedy action, just as light is the fastest moving energy of the physical universe. Fire signs, when unmodified by the effect of other tattwas pour themselves forth in an exuberance of inspiration, aspiration and creative expression of their inner life force. They are enthusiastic and self-motivated, often feeling pride in their super-abundance of life energy, quite unaware that others may be overwhelmed by their drive. Direct, self-willed seeking of their goals characterizes the fiery nature, often revealing a lack of tact in their open honesty. "I say what I think", says fire, "I call a spade a spade" – quite unaware that others may be hurt or consumed by what to them is the best and only way to proceed.

Fire requires space and freedom to express itself and such people ensure it by the insistent pressure of their point of view until others give way. They rush into things, always looking ahead, rather than behind, displaying a quality of childishness in the display of force that they feel is required to accomplish their aims. They may even belittle the sensitivity and emotionality of the watery types, who quietly move aside and hope to be overlooked by the onrush of the fiery nature.

Fire in combination with earth is observed as the overpowering drive of the steam-roller, one who reaches the top of his profession regardless of who is trampled under foot in the process. Fire lends spontaneity to earth, while earth gives direction, perseverence and discipline to fire, plus a grounding which gives such people the ability to test their inspirations. These people can have an influence on world affairs within their own sphere of activity. They are the builders of empires, who spring from nowhere, taking their particular world by storm; the creators of family fortunes, international businesses and global networks. They make their own rules, relying on themselves rather than conventional social patterns, and yet their earthy nature provides a conservatism that relates their ambition to a pride in being seen to achieve what they do.

Water in combination with fire is of interest, providing the framework from which great drama can be created. For while water allows a depth of emotional feeling and instinct, fire gives the ability to express it dynamically in convincing outward manifestation – just the qualities required for the stage actor and entertainer. Personalities of this type do the whole thing and go the whole way. Typified by a lack of self-restraint, they see everything in terms of their own reaction to it and can be highly emotional, excitable and explosively unpredictable. Water and fire make steam and these personality types certainly get 'steamed up' pretty readily. Indeed, even under quiet domestic circumstances, they will find occasion for drama whenever life becomes, by their standards, dull and uninteresting.

Imbalance in the fire energy leads on the one hand to a crude, destructive and restless pattern of behaviour – wild, turbulent, self-centred, reckless of consequences and of the feelings of others – while too little activity in the fiery domain leads to digestive disorders, low metabolic rate and lack of vitality, enthusiasm, confidence and optimism.

The relationship of diet to unsocial behaviour patterns is slowly being recognized by the more modern social workers and a rationale behind such thinking can be readily observed in the interplay of the five elements. Dietary plans, worked out from skilfull observation and a true knowledge of nutrition could work wonders, especially for young and disturbed offenders, before their life patterns have become too habitual to change. The 'short, sharp, shock' to young offenders of our recent British government is so superficial and naive that almost any caring human being could have predicted its failure, before the government wasted millions on the attempt to repress emotional energy that needed balancing out in other more wholesome ways.

Fire in combination with air provides fire with airy conceptual characteristics, which at their best furnishes an idealistic basis for the drive of fiery natures, infusing high and positive intentions and motivations. Out of balance, such folk can neglect their own physical needs, due to a lack of the grounding supplied by earth, burning themselves out through an over-abundance of energy poured forth continuously until breaking point is reached. Without water, they will lack the inner emotional strength they need to develop a deep inner life.

In Chinese thinking, the yin phases of metal and water are thus never entered, so like plants kept in a state of perpetual growth and expansion, their centre is lost and potential, inner energy is never concentrated or restored. The phases of growth, storage and regeneration are necessary in any energy system if its constant integrity is to be maintained.

CHAPTER 8

Air and The Protective Heart

Modern Research in the Life Sciences

The full story of the endocrine system, or more correctly, the neuro-endocrine system is really quite little understood by modern medical science, even at the molecular level, as most researchers will readily acknowledge. New and more sensitive assays have brought the realization that tiny amounts of specific substances – just a few molecules even – can trigger off major events within the body. Modern techniques have identified a host of active peptides, for instance, within the brain, nerve and other bodily tissues with powerful functional activity.

There is also a range of recently discovered natural opioid substances, some with up to one thousand times the potency of morphine. The role of these neurohormones is only very sketchily comprehended, but it is clear that the bioelectrical transmission of nerve signals and the endocrine system of chemical messengers are more closely related than was previously thought, and that they cannot be considered as two separate systems. The body, of course, is one functional, integrated whole energy complex and though for the purposes of modern methods of scientific analysis it is necessary to consider just parts of it, each 'piece' must then be considered in the light of the whole. The fact that the human mind is probably incapable of holding all the scientifically 'discovered' facets of biological functioning in mind in a 'simultaneous' manner is quite clear. However, without the inside-out or top-down approach of eastern thinking, the western scientist is left with this analytical outside-in approach, where he analyses the extraordinary ramification of bubbles on the surface without ever coming to an understanding of the great and causative ocean lying beneath, and which gives so much more meaning to the apparently multitudinous surface patterns, often of seemingly random or chance nature.

A directly logical outcome of a view of causation that is supposed to exist at a purely horizontal level, within grossly observable material substance, is an automatic gravitation towards a Darwinian style of evolutionary theory and bootstrap theories of physical existence. In the context of these theories, life and matter are supposed to have spontaneously appeared out of 'nowhere'. However, with an understanding of causative patterns operating from within-out and without-in, in a vertical energy spectrum that takes in mind and even consciousness, the range of possibilities that can be drawn on to explain our physical experiences and observations of life is enormously increased. And interestingly, it also leads us to an understanding that ultimately the universe cannot be comprehended intellectually, for the intellect and thought are themselves realized to be but one energy field within the whole. And how can a part comprehend the whole?

It is difficult, of course, for any of us to admit that our approach to life is shallow, but as human beings in the physical plane of existence this is the name of the game given to us to play. To find the depth in our own lives is of the greatest importance, for without this, everything else becomes meaningless, just an 'ego-trip', as the popular saying is, but in a far deeper manner than is usually meant.

There can be no end to the unravelling of energy interactions. Currently, biochemistry is holding largely to its molecular level of enquiry. But this, as we have seen, is only an arbitrary staging post, a convenient level at which laboratory and research procedures have ramified and become established, so that biochemical research becomes a discipline for which one can train and hold down a good job with which to support a wife, mortgage and kids. Little funding is available for radically new approaches to the life sciences, but even now the understandings of modern physics and subatomic matter can be brought to bear on the grosser level of molecular thinking in biochemistry.

The result is a vista of complex energy interactions in which the forces of electricity, magnetism, electron plasma waves, scalar waves and a host of other possibilities must all be accounted for. Moreover, the preventive health implications are immense, since disease can be determined as imbalance long before its pathological manifestation. In terms of therapeutic practice, all such research is likely to have value, in that disease is immediately recognized as energy disharmonies and imbalance. Healing therefore 'simply' becomes a matter of how to rebalance the energy patterns.

Some people say that energy medicine is the medicine of the future. It would be more correct to say that conscious application of the understanding that everything *is* energy (as well as consciousness) is the way forward. For even now, even the grosser forms of drug-oriented and surgical medicine are seeking to do no more than rearrange the energy patterns. It is just that the full implications of this approach are not normally appreciated. In this sense, there is no barrier between the conventional medical approach and the so-called alternative or complementary practitioner. They are all doing the same thing. The difference lies in the subtlety of their methodology, from an energetic point of view.

It is necessary to realize, too, the great power of the profit incentive inherent in the structure of the major drug companies and its influence on medical research. The primary motive underlying the research of pharmaceutical companies is the production of biochemically active products for financial profit and for marketing to closely identified markets – either the medical profession themselves or over-the-counter sales to the general public. Company directors are not usually seekers of life's mysteries, they are seekers of financial profit. They are not usually scientists or great thinkers either, but hard-driving, go-getting business folk. So the major source of new treatments for man's ills lies with organizations who are committed to just one approach. And conceptually, it is a gross, highly limited and unimaginative approach.

Research performed by the medical fraternity is often funded by the pharmaceutical companies and naturally – to justify the expenditure from a business point of view – before the finance is forthcoming, there must be hope of new drugs, (not new methodologies or paradigms), integral with the stated research goals.

Independent medical research is largely conducted from within regular medical institutions and broadly speaking follows along strictly conventional tracks. The facilities for new directions are strictly limited by the competition for available funding, the fear of professional ostracism and the possible loss of job or career possibilites, as well as the close and creatively confining atmosphere of such institutions. Within such places, it can become very difficult to step outside the established manner of procedure, even in one's own thoughts, let alone in practice or research. This I have personally experienced while at Cambridge University's famous Department of Applied Mathematics and Theoretical Physics.

I do not intend to be negatively critical in this thinking, but the way forward has to be considered within the context of what is happening and is available right now. Many alternative therapists whose healing follows the basic principles of energy harmonization, could be of great help in establishing new techniques and paradigms, but professional jealousies, differing belief systems, or simply lack of time or opportunity – and certainly understanding – prevents this cross-fertilization from taking place.

The Thymus Gland and the Intricate Mechanisms of Immune Defence

We are, however, digressing from our theme, but perhaps not too wildly, because the next centre or chakra under discussion is that of the heart. And in a very real sense, we need to open the energies of our heart area to permit ourselves to venture into new territory as members of one human family, striving to make life better for *all* its members not just for ourselves, our family or our country.

In the heart area, too, we find the thymus endocrine gland. An organ that until recent years (until the early 1960's) was considered as vestigial and of no importance, without function, but is now known to be at the centre of the body's protective, immunological network. I am reluctant to use the word 'system' because it implies a closed operation with boundaries. In life, this is never the case and the body is one integrated whole – a part of the cosmos, inner and outer, a greater whole in which all life is encompassed.

Specifically, then, the heart, *hridaya* or *anahat* chakra is situated at the level of the heart, horizontally speaking, though within the spinal area. Its function is described in the yogic texts as those of protection, destruction and dissolution of the physical body. Considering that these texts were written some hundreds and others thousands of years ago, while modern medical research has only discovered the protective role of the thymus gland in the last few years, these designated functions, as well as the whole of Indian Ayurvedic and yogic medical understanding, deserve to be taken far more seriously than hitherto by western medical practice.

The destruction and dissolution aspects relate in some degree to the end of bodily life, when the pranas are withdrawn and the five tattwas comprising the body each return to their source in the absence of the life-giving organizational role of the pranas emanating from above the ajna chakra and modulated under the influence of our pralabdh karmas. "Ashes to ashes, dust to dust."

Within the living body, however, the protection conferred by the immunological network of lymphocytes, hormones and other biochemical interactions requires the destruction and dissolution of bacteria, viruses and parasites as well as other toxic and invading substances which disturb bodily function. The power to protect requires the selective power to destroy, as the balancer of polarities. And this is born out by observation of the *continuous* operation of the immunological system. The turnover of lymphocytes or white blood cells is itself prodigious – there are something like a trillion of them in a normal healthy body, about two pounds by weight, sustained, owing to their short life cycle, by the manufacture of about ten million per minute.

The orchestrator of this immune system would seem to be the thymus gland. Not a bad rise to fame for an organ once thought to be useless. Endocrine research into the functioning of the thymus gland is still very much in its infancy. The human thymus, lying underneath the rib cage and close to the heart is really inaccessible to biopsy and only observable during heart operations or in postmortems, both of which imply some degree of illness. Much of the research has therefore, been conducted on lower species and while that gives us an idea of what to expect in humans, it by no means allows us to make any specific assumptions.

In general, however, the thymus is now known to produce a number of hormones that are involved with the maturation of T-cell lymphocytes. Lymphocytes, leuocytes or white blood cells are produced in different stages of maturation in various sites around the body, especially the spleen and bone marrow. Whether there is just one *stem cell* or *progenitor* which later differentiates into both erythrocytes (red blood cells) and lymphocytes, is still very much a matter of medical debate. There are, however, a number of different kinds of lymphocyte that populate the blood stream, the loosely woven network of lymph passages between cells and body, and in most of the interstitial spaces and places of our body. These have been called *granulocytes*, *macrophages*, *monocytes*, *megakaryocytes* and T-cell lymphocytes, amongst others.

Between them, and involving some pretty tidy biochemical and physiological processes, the lymphocytes are responsible for directly combating the effects of invading or even home-grown bacteria, microbes, toxins, allergens and anything else that causes problems at the biochemical level. This is why the lymphocyte population rises in response to any kind of physiological stress – the invasion of microbes or the presence of toxic metabolites produced by internal bodily processes of disease or health, or ingested or absorbed from without. But even in a normally healthy body there is plenty for them to do, to preserve the status quo, to provide the intricate, complex and nifty network of balance between requiring nourishment from without, yet not being disturbed by it. The normal human body quite naturally produces its own toxic waste materials, as well as maintaining a healthy relationship with a host of symbiotic bacteria both in the gut, in the blood and elsewhere, and the maintenance of ordered balance is of course absolutely essential.

Some of these blood bacteria are of particular interest, because they are responsive to the changes in electrical potential that arise when you cut yourself or are otherwise injured. Migrating to that spot, they are then involved in the process of stemming the bleeding by the formation of a blood clot.

So just as the airy tattwa expresses itself in nimble and complex manual dexterity, or in the innovative and multi-faceted mind of the airy nature, so too at the biochemical level does it produce one of the most intricate and delicately balanced of all essential bodily activities. The complexity and universality of this immune system is only surpassed in innate and structured 'intelligence' by that of the central nervous system whose use of the akashic medium as the energy out of which the other tattwas are derived, automatically places it at a higher level of control within bodily mechanisms.

The thymus gland, then, is intricately involved in this process, though a fuller story of the mechanisms involved has yet to be elucidated. It is known, however, that T-cell lymphocyte progenitors migrate to and colonize the thymus gland, where under the influence of thymic hormones, known collectively as *thymosin*, they mature into a number of different, though related, T-lymphocytic types. There is also a strong suggestion that thymic hormones circulating in the blood predispose developing and generalized lymphocytic cells to become T-cell types, thus effectively marking them for thymic migration.

It is also speculated that other thymic hormones stimulate and regulate the production of the other varieties of lymphocyte, outside the thymus gland itself. Certainly, the thymus gland increases considerably in size during the course of any disease, reflecting both its greater activity and its colonization by progenitor lymphocytes.

At least three active, thymic peptide hormones have so far been identified. Firstly, a 49-amino acid, polypeptide or protein, *thymopoietin*, which induces the differentiation of immature lymphocytes into T-cell types and generally promotes their functioning when they are working in the ouside world, away from the thymus itself. It also seems to have other metabolic effects such as those on neuromuscular transmission, though these are not at all understood.

Secondly, there is a small thymic peptide, *Thymic Humoral Factor (THF)*, which is known to help restore human immuno-deficiency, killing cancer cells, returning the functionality of lymphocytes and generally overseeing at least some of the complex, immunological pathways at the biochemical level.

And finally, there is a 9-amino acid peptide, designated *Facteur Thymique Serique* (*FTS* or *Serum Thymic Factor*), by its French discoverer. Its functions, however, are hardly elucidated.

All the endocrine glands are linked into the higher control systems of the body either by endocrine feedback through the pituitary and hypothalamus and hence to the brain via neurological linkage – or directly, by autonomic innervation. In some cases, by both.

Thymic control, however, and its linkage to the central intelligence of the body is little understood at the present time. The thymus does receive innervation from the autonomic nervous system, but so far, no direct biochemical linkage with the pituitary and hypothalamus has been demonstrated. Theoretically and within the general pattern of endocrine activity as well as a result of the pranic linkages between all the chakras in the subtle fields, this would seem a likely possibility.

There is evidence, however of biochemical feedback to thymic activity from the bone marrow, where most of the T-lymphocyte progenitor cells are currently thought to arise. No bone marrow substance, however, has yet been isolated which demonstrates this conclusively.

In many lower species there is clear evidence of linkage to gonadal and adrenal activity. All in all, therefore, thymic activity and the functioning of our immune defence system is receiving considerable attention, especially with the advent of the AIDS virus, which infects lymphocytes and also human brain cells, causing an increasing lack of immuno-capabililty, dementia and other neurological disorders. Since a percentage of people do not actually develop AIDS or show only mild symptoms, it means that the body does have a natural protective mechanism which in some instances breaks down, allowing the virus a foothold.

Recent research (in 1986) by a team of Californian scientists in San Francisco has shown that harnessing the body's own immuno-defence system may prove a better approach to the disease. Essentially, what they have observed is that certain T-suppressor cells, whose normal function is to regulate the total number of blood T-cells after a defence has been mounted by the immune system against an invader, are also capable of countering proliferation of the AIDS virus.

Anything therefore, which stimulates our immune defence system is likely to be of either general or specific help in combating AIDS. This is not the subject of this book, but I have previously compiled a list of such known substances, known scientifically as *adaptogens*, and which are discussed in some detail in my book, *Radiation*.

One should note that the lack of general knowledge or medical recommendation of these substances, many of which have been uncovered as a result of medical research in various countries, but never clinically followed up on any wide scale basis, is not indicative of their lack of efficacy, but rather a reflection on human behaviour.

Remember that the definitive research on the use of citrus fruit to combat scurvy was performed by a Royal Navy surgeon *fifty years* before it was taken seriously and adopted by the admiralty as official policy. During this unnecessary delay thousands of soldiers and sailors died. The reason was that of currently extant paradigms. That is, it was not *believed* at that time that diet could affect health. Therefore, a solution which ran contrary to the current belief system, the idiom or fashion of the time, was immediately discounted as impossible, despite the evidence of hard and clear observation.

Remember too, that scientists are just human beings with emotions, like the rest of us, reacting and thinking according to their education and preconditioned points of view. Science is not truly objective, as we would be led to believe, but is simply a reflection of the attitudes, prejudices, personal philosophies and current idiom or fashion of the scientists involved.

This is why, even in science, there are millions of plodders and so few path forgers, millions of designers and only the occasional real inventor.

Returning, however, to our theme, and just to give you a very broad idea of biochemical compexities, let us follow a part of this immunological trail in simplistic and brief outline. T-lymphocytes produce hormone-like molecules known as *lymphokines* which biochemically attack all invaders. One of these molecules, for example, is known as *interferon*, a compound being used with some success in combating the proliferation of cancer cells. T-cells also stimulate another variety of lymph cells, *macrophages*, which function as biological scavengers, ingesting and swallowing up whatever nasties they can find.

B-lymphocytes, produced in the spleen and lymph nodes, locate foreign organisms and make specific antibodies – biochemical destruction and deactivation agents – against them. This antibody system is a part of the body's protection against bacteria, viruses and potential allergens, and is the basis of the science of immunology. B-lymphocytes are a remarkably adaptive and creative munitions factory with the ability, within limits, to create new biochemical weapons as new invaders are encountered. And once created, these weapons normally stay with you. This is intelligence at the biochemical level and explains why you only get certain diseases once in a lifetime. After that you have the right antibody to fight the virus, bacteria or allergen should it attempt a second landing.

In fact, the thymus generally posseses its greatest weight, in relation to body size, at puberty and it is certainly during youth that much of our basic antibody system to local bugs and toxins is laid down. This for instance, is why we pick up local viruses so readily when we go abroad – because we have never previously been exposed to them and had a chance to build antibodies against them.

Interestingly, amongst the substances with antibody activity, are a group of proteins known as immunoglobulins. Medical research into the herb, pokeroot (*Phytolacca americana*) has demonstrated that it contains further compounds which are directly involved in immunoglobulin synthesis. And pokeroot has been used by generations of American Indian, and now American and international herbalists, to combat illness and infection, including cancer.

Nature has many secrets to reveal to those who trust and are in tune with her, something that many of the best laboratory scientists would probably agree with, especially when one adds up how many earth-changing discoveries have been made by apparent accident or coincidence. Revelation can sometimes come as a 'gift' and is not always the result of effort.

The Airy Tattwa and the Respiratory Process

The tattwa of the heart centre is that of *Vayu* or air, while the pranic current is itself called *prana*, which also means 'breath' or 'life-breath', in the general sense that it is the energy which breathes life into inert material substance for the creation of a living body. In the particular meaning, the heart centre is the organization and energy networker for the incorporation of atmospheric oxygen into physical life processes. Air is breathed into the lungs and distributed throughout the body as the fuel for the lower fiery tattwa to accomplish its task.

One can, in fact, evolve this idea further. For, within a watery matrix, earthy solids are consumed by fire through the oxidative admixture of air for the production of energy by which the body continues in existence. And this inter-action between the tattvic states does not stop there, for the heightened activity and motion at the subatomic level, on the surface of the vacuum or akashic state, automatically reflects inwards, carrying energy from our metabolic processes up into our mental and emotional energy fields. And hence food and all substances can affect our inner sense of well-being, if they become involved in these metabolic pathways. This indeed is our experience. If we miss a meal, we can become irritable, to give just one simple example.

Oxygen is also said to be a 'conveyor' of prana which makes the lungs, the heart and the circulatory system a further method by which subtle energies are distributed throughout the body.

The close functionality of the heart, lungs and airy tattwa will probably be known to most readers but just to refresh your memory, oxygen is breathed into the lungs where it is absorbed by the blood capilliaries. Returning via the pulmonary blood vessels to the heart, this refreshed blood is pumped out through the efferent arterial system to all parts of the body, where the oxygen and nutrients are consumed and replaced by carbon dioxide and other waste substances of the metabolic process. This blood is then returned via the afferent venous system to the heart, whence it is pumped out into the lungs once again, (see figures 8-1 and 8-2), for elimination of the carbon dioxide and re-intake of oxygen.

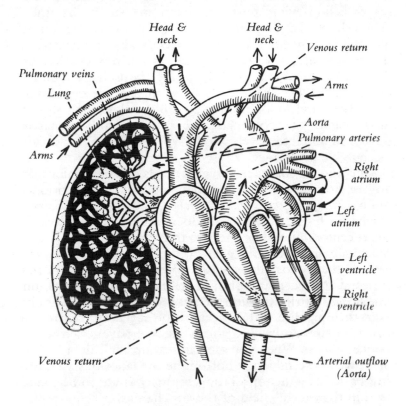

Figure 8-1. Heart and lung anatomy. The direction of blood circulation is shown below in figure 8-2.

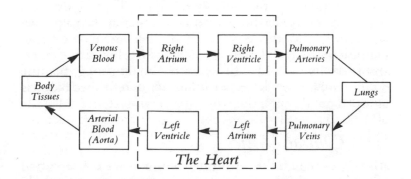

Figure 8-2. The direction of blood circulation

The blood circulatory system is hence the body's conveyor belt carrying substances from one part to the other. The cells of the different bodily organs and tissues under normal healthy circumstances correctly absorb or respond to the nutrients and messengers (e.g. hormones) that are carried by the blood, while ignoring those that are meant for other tissues. The fine tuning of this energy network is incredible and only seems possible to me when one understands the power of the guiding and formative blueprint at subtle levels, underlying its more outwardly observable mechanics.

The hridaya chakra has twelve petals of a blue colour. In mystic literature, it is sometimes said that the practitioner should manifest the *Anahad Shabda*, the *Aum* or *Unstruck Sound*, in his heart. But this does not mean the physical heart centre, but rather refers to the centre of being, which spiritually lies above the *ajna* chakra. The true Shabda, the Word, the Logos, the creative power of God does not descend in direct manifestation below the eye centre or ajna chakra and it is for this reason that the higher forms of yoga start their practice with concentration at this eye centre and do not come down into the physical body as centres of concentration. When you are halfway up a hill already, it is said, why descend to the bottom before laboriously climbing back up to the top? True simplicity is not to be found within the psychic field of the six chakras.

Each petal of each lotus or chakra in the body is, however, appreciable through the inner indriya of hearing, as a sound – just as the chakras are also visible through inner concentration and the indriya of sight. These individual sounds are said to be those from which the Sanskrit alphabet is derived and the Sanskrit tantras contain the exact definition of which letters are derived from which chakra. But I have not included those in this book, simply because they would have little meaning to one who reads no Sanskrit.

Airy Characteristics

Air carries with it the sensitivity required for the sensation of touch and physical feeling, manifesting most particularly in the hands as its organ of action as well as that of exquisite and fine sensation. Imagine the skill of the artist or musician whose deft and nimble fingers spin out the image or sound of their own or another's creative imagination. One would expect many of the great artists and musicians to possess a high degree of air in their make up. The sculptor will be combined perhaps with earth or the painter with fire, while an addition of water can provide the passionate intensity to be woven into their creation, binding the hearts of the rest of us with a spell that is difficult to comprehend, but can uplift and inspire in a most remarkable fashion.

Hands are amazing structures. How much more meaning there is in the touch of hands than of any other part of the body? All cultures use their hands in greeting and in conscious expression as a powerful means of communication, in gesture. No person's hand-shake is quite the same as another's. The feeling and energetic quality reflects the individual as uniquely as the individual markings on the fingers themselves. Palmistry is more than the simple study of just the lines on the hand. Like astrology, it is a reflection of patterns from which, in skilled readers, much information can be drawn – but from the whole hand and fingers, not just the lines on the palm.

Like an image stored in a hologram where the whole can be reproduced from just a part, so too do certain parts of the body contain a reflective map of the condition of the whole energy complex of the body, mind, emotions and karmic patterning. The hands and feet are two of these, while the iris of the eye and the lobes of the ears and the tongue are others. These are focal points for external manifestation of the five tattwas, where the energy of these subtle fields finds a focus of expression, uniquely patterning what is within into external manifestation.

In the mind and emotions, air is the light, conceptual and intellectual principle. Airy natures are usually fast thinkers and may be particularly clever with their hands, also, while concepts can be almost as real to them as things are to the survival needs of earth, or as emotions and instinct are to water. By its very swiftness and clarity, air brings things into actualization by sheer concentration upon the concept, while earth works hard physically to create the same effect and fire drives forward, willing things into actualization. Astrologically, the airy signs are *libra* – the impartial balancer and harmonizer; *aquarius* – the detached, individualistic co-ordinator of events, people and concepts, sometimes given to extremes; and the mutable *gemini* whose outgoing friendliness, curiosity and talkativeness, backed by a rapid perception and synthetic verbalization, make them fascinating companions, always full of new ideas and with a ready charm and turn of phrase.

Whilst fire moves faster than air and may be frustrated by even air's desire to conceptualize before action, water and earth can threaten air's need for freedom of expression. For while earth insists on examining the practicality of ideas, refusing to be rushed into anything, water is suspicious of air's lack of emotional depth and threatens to swamp air's fleetness with what (to air) is unnecessary emotion.

Many of the combinations of air with the other tattwas have already been covered, but in general, air is a good synthesizer of the individual's characteristics and is able to integrate the various aspects of his personality. Air can temper fire's on-rush, adding direction and ability to communicate; while water will provide an emotional base to an otherwise light and dry nature, with earth able to supply the grounding in 'good old common sense' so much needed by the air signs.

Airy natures generally exhibit ease and sociability, mixing well with all kinds of people, for they feel little need to truly empathize or get involved with the problems and feelings of others. Their weakness lies in over-airy-ness and a lack of appreciation of physical limitations, easily over-extending themselves with commitments. An airy nature in a relationship with an earthy one may drive the latter to distraction as he tries to keep pace with his (or her) mercurial partner. Or he may find that the demands made of his practical skills are over-worked by the impatient demands of air as it fails to perceive the gap between the mental concept and the physical reality, expecting earth to be the instant manifester of its physical desires and dreams.

Thought and concept are of such importance to airy natures that mentally and emotionally they are closely identified with them, feeling challenged and insecure if their opinions are ignored or if the quality of their work is criticized. Without the stability of water or earth, airy natures can float from one thing to another without any deep involvement or real knowledge of any one thing. Airy natures tend towards sensitive and active nervous systems, and without the balancing yin of earth or water, they are easily exhausted, needing to give themselves times for rest and recuperation, perhaps entailing a change of scenery to free their minds from the habitual ruts of worries, thoughts, endless plans and mental gyrations. With their agile minds, airy natures are, of course, the innovators. Stephen Arroyo comments that more Nobel prize winners have had a dominant air sign than any other element.

Underactivity of the air tattwa can result in a poor ability to stand back from life's problems, to see them in lighter vein. Detachment from material preoccupations becomes difficult and 'lightness of touch' is missing in both physical as well as social life. Air is the bringer of lightness and sparkle, and without it, humour and finesse are frequently lacking. Those deficient in air, distrust the airy qualities of conceptualization and the love of ideas. Without the gift of verbalization, they can burst out emotionally and irrationally, even violently, when faced with beliefs contrary to their own.

Human Weakness

The true source of our being lies deep within us, beyond the physical, astral and causal realms, beyond even the spiritual regions of manifestation, in the complete unity and oneness of God, Universal Being or whatever name you care to call it. As human beings we are locked into the physical realm of our karmas, and while the universal problem is one of duality, of separation from our Source, in the physical form this separation takes on particular definable aspects.

Under the influence of our karmas, we take birth, and our mind, conditioned by the habits of innumerable past lives, moves out from its inner centre of the antashkarans, putting its attention on the physical world through the intermediary of the five indriyas of perception (yin) and the five of motor action response (yang). The mind thus comes into contact with the five tattwas in its outward movement, giving rise to five major modalities of human weakness. Weakness or 'sin' is thus understood as a movement of our inner attention away from the inner source of our being and into physical reality. In the perfect man, the mind should keep its focus of attention within, using the senses and working through the tattwas, while itself remaining in fully consious control. For most of us, however, our mind plays in the world of the tattwas in the vain search for the peace, unity and wholeness it would experience if it sought those realities within and which it once knew in the realm of the Universal Mind.

The mind, moving outward, thus manifests as emotion and human weakness of five major flavours according to the indriyas which are drawing it and the tattwas with which it is interacting. Starting from below, association with the earthy tattwa gives rise in us to feelings of attachment to the world about us. Most of our attachments and desires for things of the world are for its solid aspects. Our sense of possesion rarely extends to the air or watery aspects of our environment, as discussed in chapter five.

In association with the watery tattwa, we are deeply bound up with sex lust. Indulgence in sex draws our attention down to the lower part of our body with a tremendous wastage of pranic energy or life force. Celibacy, however, can only be successfully managed by a few because of the unbalanced reaction caused by suppression of this immensely powerful urge and natural human inclination. Mystics, therefore, advise a controlled married life, keeping in mind the higher ideal of celibacy. Then, with the practice of meditation and the rise of the attention, the mind, finding far higher enjoyment in the bliss within, naturally discovers an aversion to what it once considered an essential pleasure.

The sensation of taste is also an aspect of lust, an indulgence in an apparently enjoyable bodily sensation which again draws the mind away from its inner centre.

The next higher tattwa is that of fire and the mind in contact with the subtle aspect of this energy field takes on its characteristics of expansion and heat in the emotion of anger. Note how anger can suddenly kindle, like fire in dry timber, and how explosively violent and irrational this emotion can be when running completely out of control. Thus, while attachment binds us solidly to the things of the world and lust drags our attention to lower centres, anger scatters our mind and blows apart our focus of concentration, as we have all experienced.

Next is the airy tattwa with its motor indriya of grasping or getting hold of physical possessions. Its emotion is that of greed or avarice, an imbalance under the influence of ego, in the use of the airy aspect of the human constitution. Essentially, greed leads us into the attempt to get hold of more than we need and a hoarding possessiveness regarding those things that we feel belong to us.

Man unconsciously realizes the airy and intangible quality of ownership. But rather than relax into this reality, he attempts to stem these feelings of insecurity by greedily getting hold of more and more, in compensation for his usually unconscious realization that he can never permanently fix his possessions into orbit around himself.

The weakness of akash is inextricably bound up with the operations of the antashkarans. Essentially, imbalance in our use of akash leads us to a self-centred use of our intelligence through the inner activity of our ego or ahankar. It leads, therefore, to our sense of personal identity, the thought of 'I' and 'mine', with which we have become obsessed.

Just as akash is the 'sky' out of which the other tattwas take their being, just so is its weakness of ego, the source of the other four imbalances.

Man's attention is thus brought into contact with the objects of this world by being drawn out through the five senses, both the mental indriyas and the physical organs themselves. Through these, his attention plays in the tattvic fields and becomes liable to the emotions and weaknesses of attachment, lust, anger, greed and egotism.

His involvement is further complicated by the response he makes through the five mental indriyas of action, manifesting as his activities in physical life. His senses and his actions lead him into 'sin' in its widest sense, and for each action – whether mentally inward in desire form, or outwardly expressed in physical activity – a groove is impressed upon his antashkarans. A karmic seed has thus been sown which must bear fruit in some future birth, unless erased by the practice of deep meditation.

Human Expression and the Perfect Man

One more aspect of human expression needs to be covered. When a master or perfect mystic adept takes birth, he manages the formation of his own karmas. In life, he is always above their limitations in his inward being and always in fully conscious control. He can be in his body whenever he wants to and he can leave his body whenever he so desires.

But in order to express himself as a human being, he is able to do what none of us can manage and that is to use the physical vehicle purely as a means of expression at the human level, *but always under fully conscious control.*

A master therefore will, in a most beautifully perfect manner, display human emotion and activity, whilst being perfectly human. He uses his senses and acts, but is not a slave to them. He will laugh and behave as a perfect father, mother, son, daughter, employee or employer or in any other role. In all situations, there will be a quality about him that is intangibly unique. He will possess things necessary for his physical existence, according to his 'position' in the normal social structure, but he is not a slave to them. He may be married and have children but without our human indulgence. He can be stern, too, as occasion demands, like a mother with her child, but he is never inwardly carried away in anger. He has no greed, but uses things as occasion demands. Above all, although he has the human characteristics of being separate, his ahankar is under full control and is merely a part of his expression as a human being. He is not a victim of ego and self-identification.

In this way, therefore, the perfect mystic is always full of grace, charm and warm, well-balanced humanity

Poetic Interlude

MY GARDEN

A garden is a lovesome thing, God wot!
Rose plot,
Fringed pool,
Ferned grot –
The veriest school
Of peace; and yet the fool
Contends that God is not –
Not God! in gardens! when the eve is cool!
Nay, but I have a sign;
'Tis very sure God walks in mine.

T.E. Brown

CHAPTER 9

Akash – A Matter of Creation

Man, Tattwas, the Lower Species and Evolution

As we have described, the entire physical universe, both gross and subtle is comprised of the five tattwas. In living forms, these tattwas are held together by the patterning of the pranas or life force from within, under the overall imprint of the pralabdh or destiny karmas programmed into the antashkarans, thus completely influencing both our human mind and body for the duration of our physical life.

Just as in the gross physical condition there is a specific phase jump when substances *suddenly* move from solid to liquid and from liquid to gaseous, so too is the spectrum of species inhabiting this planet observed to be non-homogeneous. That is, there are distinct classes of creatures without gradations in between. There are plants, for example, but no creatures that are half-plants and half-insects. There are no species that are part-insect, part-reptile; no part-bird, part-mammal, and so on. In fact, not only is there a 'missing link' between apes and man, but between all the major and most of the minor classes of creature, there are missing links.

Indeed, there are no creatures between inert matter and living organisms, no 'half-dead' creatures, though facetious observations may suggest otherwise! Even viruses are complexly organized and can be killed. But you cannot kill a stone or a dead person! Dead is dead. There is no such thing as half-dead.

The fact that there are a very few species which do possess some of the characteristics of two major classes of species, the duck-billed platypus, for example, or the lungfish, does not provide evidence of evolution, because there are so few of such creatures both living and in the fossil record. And even with these species, it is clear that they are indeed a *mammal* which lays eggs or a *fish* which is adapted to breath atmospheric oxygen. They are, in fact, highly specialized anomalies, not genuine missing links.

For if evolution had progressed by chance along purely Darwinian lines, then surely there would be no definable classes, but only a smooth gradient of creatures from dust to man, with no stepping stones between?

The instrinsic reason for the definition of classes as well as the specific identity of species is determined by the number of subtle tattwas which are active in their make up. Plants, for example, have only the tattwa of water active in them, insects have earth and fire, birds have air, fire and water, while mammals possess earth, water, fire and air. Man alone has all five subtle tattwas active within him.

Note that the operative word is *active*, not *absent*. This means that the degree of tattvic activity can vary within a class and that plants, for example, are not to be considered as totally lacking in earth; just that water is the most active tattwa present in their constitution.

I am aware that this description requires greater elaboration and discussion before such a concept could be made acceptable to our educated western minds, but this would require a full survey of the lower species and the fossil record, plus some detailed discussion of both mystic and modern cosmologies and their relationships. This may be attempted in a later book, but the main point to consider at this stage is that man's physical and subtle physical being is comprised of all the five basic conditions or states of material substance. And it is the subtle tattwa of akash, the inner sky out of which the other subtle tattwas are created or derived, that provides us with our capacity for rational thought, intelligence, discrimination and considered, rather than instinctive, behaviour.

All of life and nature represents an economy and a total, ecologically balanced whole. There is a part to play for every living creature and a role for every human being. The patterning of our karmas is not random, but is set within the context of a grander design. In their inner essence, all souls are of the same source, all are drops of the same ocean. But in outer manifestation, each is placed at a different position and with a different role to play within the tattvic energy fields of the physical universe.

The essence of this system is management and enlivenment of the tattvic domains, for the meaning of creation is represented in the play of life. On our planet, all five tattwas are actively present. Therefore, there are creatures and species formed out of the subtle aspects of these energy domains. Man is constituted of all five tattwas and automatically becomes the king of all species, though whether he is a good or a bad monarch is quite another matter. Higher animals come next, with the subtle element of akash missing. Though possessed of obvious feeling and limited cognitive processes, they lack the human faculty of rational thought and discrimination. They are largely creatures of the here and now, of instinct. Akash being the energy which gives us the faculty of speech and intelligence, they do not have the powers of communication of which man is capable. The human ability to speak and possess a varied vocabulary is unique to him. Other species do communicate in varying degrees – one thinks of the haunting vocalizations of the great whales and dolphins or the capabilities of the apes – but without the same degree of complexity and intelligence.

Actually, their communication is to a large degree by body language – posture, gesture and movement – a direct reflection of their inward state. Just observe any creature closely and for a while, and you will see how it is informing you, mostly unconsciously, of the patterns in its inward and 'instinctive' mind. A dog wagging its tail and even its whole body in greeting; a slinky cat hunting; a chirping, hopping, contented group of sparrows or their sudden rush into flight upon the hint of danger; mating and territorial displays amongst many, if not all, species. Every action is a communication, just as it is with humans, if we are observant enough – if our own mind is not so active as to obscure the messages we could and should be receiving from our fellow creatures and humans.

Species, of course, vary within any class, just as humans vary from each other, in the relative activity of each tattwa active within them. Those who work with animals know that their individual degree of intelligence as well as their 'personalities' or natures vary quite widely, even amongst brothers and sisters of the same parents, just as with humans. And this is because all souls, whether trapped in human or other bodies, bring with them the karmic patterning of impressions or sanskaras from their past lives.

Birds have the subtle tattwas of air, fire and water in their active constitution, those of earth and akash being dormant. They thus have less intelligence than even the mammals but do possess an airy ingenuity, as is evidenced by their nest-building capabilities, their vocal mimicry, their complex social behaviour and their ability to learn and even use implements, such as the cactus thorn used by one species of Darwin's famous Galapagos finches. These qualities are largely lacking in reptiles, fishes and lower species. Birds are highly active or fiery (most of them!) and creatures of the air, while their earthy solidity is penetrated by air spaces, and the subtlety of akash is altogether inactive.

Note, too, how the fiery element manifesting in the electromagnetic sense organ of sight and the activity of going places is superbly concentrated in birds. Their lofty airiness combining with their fiery nature gives them a prodigous line of sight – up to thirty miles, for example, with homing pigeons on a clear day – as well as the ability to travel under their own steam, and with an airy fleetness, for far greater distances than any other class of species on our planet.

Kestrels, for example, that these days we see hovering alongside motorways, are looking as much for tiny beetles and insects, as for small mammals. And I have many times watched the network of vultures that fly high above the city of Delhi. Each one surveys his own patch of ground below, while keeping his eye on the other fellow members of the lookout team, in the search for offal. As soon as one drops to a source of food, the others begin to congregate, the entire event taking place through the murky visibility of Delhi's atmospheric pollution.

Similarly, fish have the elements of water and fire active in them while reptiles have earth and fire. Insects are generally dry and active, also possessing the tattwas of earth and fire.

Finally, plants are of the watery element, with even earth practically dormant and with the other tattwas in quiescent condition. Most soft-growthed plants are at least ninety per

217

cent water, and some fruits – especially in dry, hot climates – are even more. One thinks of citrus fruits and melons, for example, which produce water within themselves by physiological processes (as do all creatures, to some degree).

Note that while we are more specifically talking here about the subtle tattwas, the inner constitution automatically reflects in the gross state. Thus fish, for example, which lack activity in the airy tattwa, derive oxygen for their metabolism directly from the watery condition, through the gills.

Note, too, how the fewer the tattwas, the lower the degree of intelligence. Not only that, but the sudden change from warm-blooded to cold-blooded is indicative of the number of active tattwas present within a creature. The increased complexity of managing a warm-blooded or endothermic body and metabolism, which generates and accurately maintains itself at a more or less specific temperature, seems to require a subtle matrix of three or more tattwas in which fire and probably water, too, are both essential as active constituents. Without this complexity, fire manifests itself as an active and expansive principle, as we find in most insects, but without endothermic characteristics.

One can get some understanding of the manner of tattvic manifestation in lower species from the senses and activities by which they are characterized. Plants have no fire, and as a result they possess no sight, neither do they have the drive to go anywhere. It might be a question asked by an 'enfant terrible' – "why can't plants walk?" But it is a valid question.

Why *can't* they move about, even just a little bit? Plants are creatures geared almost entirely to growth and reproduction, the qualities of the water element. Their appreciation of the external environment is largely of chemicals in solution, a form of taste, through the roots and via the cells of their leaves. Even their dedication to sunlight is photochemical in nature.

Similarly, amongst the other species, insects (fire and earth) are creatures of sight and chemical sensation, through their antennae, for example. Their fire enables them to go places, often at high speed, while their earthy tattwa keeps them in close association with the surface of the planet.

In similar vein, one can analyze the other species, although the skein requires some considerable disentangling, beyond the scope of this book. For the correspondences are not always simply drawn in naive one to one relationships.

Moreover, what we perceive with one sense organ may be perceived by a different sense in other species. Recent research, for example, has shown that insects are aware of smells and fragrances at least partially by the infrared emanations and characteristics of these gaseous molecules picked up by their finely-tuned antennae. Their antennae are actually constructed like the highly complex, precise and mathematically designed antennae used in science for picking up microwave frequencies. So if you want to know how to build an ultra-sensitive microwave and infrared detector, ask the insects.

What this means is: *they SEE what we SMELL*. This is an interesting area of thought, for it leaves one open to considerations of 'reality' and sensory experience. At the very least, it seems that what we experience through our senses is not the 'true and only reality'. How can it be if other species experience it in quite a different fashion? It seems probable that each species perceives the world in its own, quite unique manner. Will the 'real reality' please stand up?

Evolution, Darwinism and Natural Balance

Man has always been a man, throughout the course of our planetary history and Darwinism in its fullest sense is considered incorrect by mystical philosophy. This is because it sees only a section or a window on life's processes at a horizontal level, taking no account of consciousness and the inner causative, creation of energies and life from within.

The limited expression of Darwinian theory, in terms of adaptability of the species, is certainly a mechanism which one sees in operation. When an environment changes, the fittest of any species to live in the new environment automatically gain precedence and greater success. The tree that bends will not be broken by the wind. And this essential adaptability and variety is built into the mechanisms of genetic coding and transmission.

But the same basic species will always be present, filling their niche in nature according to the fine tuning of tattvic activity within them and the continued existence of that niche. We have a tendency to portray Stone Age man as grotesque, hairy and violent, but we have absolutely no justification, archaeologically or socially for such a portrayal. In fact, the reverse is more likely to be true, for in any of the more sensitive studies into the remnants of the Stone Age still living upon earth, their social conduct at least equals and in many cases far surpasses our own. Laurens Van der Post's famous book, *The Lost World of the Kalahari*, describes the life of the African Bushman and one is considerably humbled by their simple, natural and indeed instinctively spiritual approach to life. Their social and family behaviour far exceeds that of much of our own violent and divided society, with its incessant and childish demands for material possessions, power, 'comfort' and satisfaction of ego.

When we have wars, hundreds of thousands are killed, while in many of these so-called primitive cultures, fighting is a rare occurence and when it does (or did) occur, their weaponry is such that few are killed and with the exertion of hand to hand fighting and in the absence of modern armaments, the battle can only last a short while before the combatants are exhausted and some side has to give way. Likewise, from our excavations of Stone Age and prehistoric settlements, we have no evidence to suppose that their social structure and treatment of each other was either superior or inferior to our own. We are different, have a different emphasis, that is all; for man was always a man, composed of the five tattwas and thus endowed automatically with their characteristics.

Similarly with all the other species. Different species may have been present in greater numbers at different times according to environmental conditions and if one equates numbers with success (an idiom only of our modern thinking, perhaps) then those species were the most 'successful' at that time. But those roles, those species, the expression of life within those particular aspects of the energy fields of creation, are still filled even today. If the ecological niche disappears or changes due to natural events, including, in its widest sense, the 'interference' of man or other species, then either the species filling that niche have to adapt in order to survive, or they, become extinct. When new niches or conditions are created, existing species move in and adapt to the new circumstances – as we find with the urbanization of foxes, and in many other instances, including man himself.

If any one species overdoes its 'success' to the detriment of the ecological balance as a whole, then ultimately there has to be a backlash to restore the balance and, in terms of numbers, that species will go into decline. This is the case with humankind under present day circumstances, and unless we very rapidly learn to be a sensitive part of the total planetary ecosystem, a powerful readjustment of one kind or another is inevitable.

No energy system can keep going indefinitely in a yang state. There have to be times of yin, of receptivity and consolidation, of autumn and the discarding of what is of no value; of indrawing and reaching for the roots of our being, before the creative phase can once again be constructive rather than destructive. Too long a summer weakens the stamina and vitality of a species, and it is time for man to seek strength from quietness and peace within, to assess with all honesty where he really stands, and to act appropriately.

In this respect, the viral infection of AIDS would appear to be one of those factors that will actually bring man back into balance and greater harmony with his environment. AIDS is an imbalance in the body's natural immune defence system whose primary vibration lies in the tattvic energy domain of air. These protective and destructive aspects of the airy, heart and immune defence chakra have already been discussed. It is thus a disharmony or dis-ease in the energies of the airy tattwa which I would suggest are primarily at the basis of this condition. Interestingly enough, it has also been observed that the hearts of children born to AIDS infected parents, (and who have subsequently died of the AIDS virus), have been severely damaged.

Let me hasten to say that I do not consider AIDS as a divine retribution in the manner that some religious moralists have described it. AIDS is a tragedy that requires our intelligent resistance and response. It would be quite unsympathetic for it to be taken as an opportunity to peddle a religious morality at the expense of compassion. But all the same, it would seem to reflect an imbalance in our social and planetary ecology, that in terms of our group behaviour and conduct can be construed as self-inflicted. And I am referring here to far more general aspects of human imbalance than merely to our sexual proclivities, which are more a symptom than an underlying cause. Its positive aspect, however, is that it may force us to re-evaluate our approach to planetary harmony at a deeper level, and from this suffering will emerge inward growth.

Imbalance in one tattwa can be traced to poor energy tone in any of the others, because they are all interrelated, like notes in a musical scale. And this can explain why certain groups of people are at higher risk than others, since depletion of energies through drug abuse or over-indulgence in sex, or any form of disharmonious or unhealthy living can leave one energy field exhausted, drawing in pranic energy from other tattvic levels, in compensation.

These specific factors, however, would appear to be symptoms of a deeper pattern of present-day human expression with the primary problem regarding AIDS being a lack of nourishment to the airy centre. It is the heart centre that draws in this vibrational energy from the environment. This is expressed in such feelings as being a healthful part of one's community; an integration with the natural life of other species rather than a usurpation of their rights and territory; a warm, well-balanced, domestic, family and social existence and so on. These factors all contribute to the health and wholeness of any individual or group.

In our modern life, the power of travel and communications have stirred up the once more local vibrations and atmosphere of countries and communities, leaving us with little nourishment from the integrated emotional identification more readily enjoyed by a stable and familiar existence, where children were more like their parents than they are today. We even draw the food from which our bodies are constituted from multitudinous, international sources, complete with the vibrations of those sources and all those who have had a hand in its preparation and profit. In previous times, agriculture – and hence food supply – was essentially local.

In addition to this loss of personal involvement and identification – and in part because of it – man now sees no ethical difficulty in destroying his environment, especially if he shortsightedly sees it as someone else's! No one will destroy their *own* garden. But to disrupt the ecological and environmental balance of the atmosphere, rivers and oceans through industrial pollution, to destroy the natural ecology of the earth through massive aforestation, to force species into extinction and to contaminate our food and water through the abuse of chemical pesticides, herbicides and fertilizers, leaves us with a planetary atmosphere or vibration lacking in the subtle input of nourishment so necessary to our sense of well-being and therefore physical health.

We are thereby depleted by our own activities. Negative activity contains within it the seeds of its own destruction. And though the creative, yang or rajas aspects of man's great drive forward into the twentieth century has brought many benefits, we are increasingly entering a phase where the symptoms of a continuously yang energy system are being displayed in our running out of resources or energy – at all levels – to fuel the drive. In terms of physical health, this is expressed in such diseases as AIDS.

We desperately need, therefore, to move into an autumn or 'metal' phase, leading perhaps to a period of full yin or winter consolidation of our 'progress', where much of what is useless is gently discarded. And this would not be a time of coldness, but more a period of inner concentration upon deeper human values, relinquishing the restless and endless drive for material gain, comfort and satisfaction. This phase must ultimately come, though not in a purely idealistic form. Many financial experts, for example, who have followed the economic patterns back through previous centuries have predicted a falling off of financial value and prices during the latter years of this century – a depression or yin phase, which will further help to hold man's expansive nature in check.

Man is a part of nature and these cycles happen automatically. If an individual runs on and on continuously, his once healthy creative phase runs out of wholesome energy. If the person does not realize the need for consolidation and rest, they continue running on 'false fire', on nervous energy, on a draining of resources without recharging the energy banks from within.

Ultimately, the system can stand the abuse no longer and health breaks down, often suddenly. Thus, the heart attack victim may have boasted, "Never a day off work in the last fifteen years".

Similarly, with man's existence as a whole. Generally speaking, we have passed the true spring and summer of our existence in this major cycle and are into a 'false fire' stage where depletion of our resources, inner and outer, has set in. We thus become prone to such tragic diseases as AIDS. Whether it is the draining, nervous energies of our big cities or the disruption of cultural integrity in Africa and the Third World, the inner, nourishment-deficient syndrome is readily able to find a fertile resonance in which to proliferate.

In similar vein, numerous psychosomatic studies of cancer patients have shown quite conclusively that cancer takes root more readily in those people who have been deprived of warm domestic or emotional nourishment in their early, childhood years, leaving them with a dry, clipped personality that finds it difficult to draw in nourishment from their daily lives and environment. This is a further manifestation of modern, living conditions.

Even rats and mice when injected with cancer cells showed an increase of over ninety per cent resistance if they were also handled, cared for and loved. Similarly, mice that were permitted to suckle their young also shared a resistance to breast cancer not displayed amongst those in whom this natural, two-way nurturing process was prevented from continuing uninterruptedly.

That drug abuse, crime and cruelty manifest in the inner city areas of concrete, pollution, traffic and extensive human greed, exploitation and uncaring, requires no proof. It is self-evident. And the results are clear. I well remember the report of a sociological experiment in which two open-top, convertible motor cars were left with their tops down and under close, but concealed, scrutiny. The one was left in an unpleasant, urban environment and within a space of twenty-four hours had received innumerable attacks and acts of theft and vandalism. Tyres, wheels, bumpers (fenders), and engine parts were all successively removed, while the bodywork was slowly destroyed.

The second car, however, was left in a small rural environment, where people are generally more in tune with themselves, each other and with nature. After twenty-four hours, the only person who had touched the vehicle was a passer-by, who kindly put up the top, when it came on to rain.

Nature will therefore restore balance to man's insensitivity, and AIDS, cancer and heart disease are a manifestation of this corrective pattern *already in progress*. A disposition towards the development AIDS and cancer appear primarily to be due to inner imbalance and the lack of subtle nourishment, while one cause of heart disease seems to be a reflection of man's capacity to drive himself beyond the bounds of his harmonious resources. His inability to desist from 'running his motor hot' culminating in a seizure of his big end and severe curtailment of his activities. And although it is humanly tragic for those involved, it is nonetheless a part of a natural process.

But let us hope that an increasing number of people realize the positive aspects of the pattern that is being enacted and work along with it. It does not mean a return to the dark ages. Far from it. But it does mean an increase in spiritual awareness as we move into what astrologers call the Aquarian Age, and a greater recognition of the relative values of material existence and inner consciousness.

The Darwinian observation of natural selection will have its part to play too, for those who are aware of the destructive elements at work in man's planetary activities will have automatically, consciously or unconsciously, been observing better patterns of health, morality and lifestyle and be in a more inwardly nourished position to counter the effects of world diseases and conflicts. Thus, they and their progeny will be the natural survivors of world disasters, to continue on the human race.

In the broadest view, the speeding up and concomitant separation of extremes of polarity – the negatively destructive and the positively constructive elements at work on the planet today – are a necessary part of the progress towards the more peaceful phase yet to come. It is the swirling of energies required to pass back upward through a small, downwardly-directed valve and should be observed and entered into with constructive wisdom, rather than criticism or negative attitudes.

Neither does this enforced balancing mean the adoption of a defeatist approach to man's problems. Quite the reverse. For the meaning behind all of our struggles is inner, and it is from battling with the external results of his inner condition and realizing that he alone is the architect of all that happens to him, that man grows inwardly and spiritually. Indeed, with the cosmic brevity of an individual lifetime, and the resulting rebirth to continue on the same struggle with his own inner condition, man stands to lose nothing, but to only gain – ultimately – his own spiritual liberation.

Man, Animals and Eccentricity

We are all to some degree eccentric, most folk would agree. Eccentric means 'away from the centre', and when we begin to meditate we soon realize how far away from our thinking centre we have become. Those people whom we consider as genuinely eccentric, however, are those whose thoughts, and therefore actions, are motivated more particularly by one or just a few facets of life, to the exclusion of all others. To other people this facet may be seen as minor, but to them it is of supreme and mind-dominating importance, often to such a degree that their behaviour patterns become bizarre. Sometimes, the focus of their attention is directed more towards a particular way of doing things, due to psychological factors.

From a karmic point of view, each person is endowed with the mental, emotional and subtle tattvic constitution that enables them to do what they have to do and to understand things the way they do. As we pointed out earlier, this lopsidedness is reflected, holographically, in the astrological patterning, from where it can be read. The subtle tattvic constitution thus reflects outwardly in the life and psychological make-up of the individual.

It is only a rare person, indeed, whose tattvic constitution is evenly balanced. Amongst the lower species, the situation becomes even more pronounced for with only a limited number of active tattwas, they are inexorably predestined to a life of one-sidedness, that is: eccentricity!

The birds, to take an example, with their fire and air are the swiftest movers, greedily seeking out and pecking up food. And that, along with reproductive activity consumes almost all of their life. Clearly an obsessive eccentricity! The speed with which they live is demonstrated by their songs, some of which contain a compression of individual notes into just one second that is only apparent when played back at low-speed on a tape recorder. A wren, I have heard, sings up to twenty or more discreet notes in a single second.

All species are thus specialized by their limited and specific tattvic constitution, to a highly individual existence. Man possesses a far wider-ranging spectrum of potential as a species, but individually, he is nonetheless constrained to act in particular ways and to do particular things under the karmically predetermined mental and tattvic patterning.

Ecological Niches

I am often struck when travelling in different countries, how the basic economy of life is always so similar, though the niches may be filled by different species. Plant-life, of course, is always there, for without green plants, all other species will die. But while starlings strut about on our British lawns and raid the rubbish heaps, moving in quarrelsome flocks from place to place, the mynah bird plays the same role in India and in many other tropical climates, demonstrating a 'personality' immediately recognizable as akin to that of our starling.

Both are perky, sociable, inquisitive, scavenging and quarrelsome. Likewise there are always local species of wasps, ants, bees, butterflies, mice and most other creatures, with remarkably similar characteristics, the differences reflecting only the varying environmental vibrations and circumstances.

It is, in effect, nature's way of administering the play of

the tattwas. There is no point in all humans being the same, endowed with the same talents and propensities. The infinite variety permits all the necessary roles in life to be covered. We need the builders as well as the breakers, the intellectual as well as the physical, the administrators and the workers. All have an essential part to play.

Similarly, in the whole of nature. From a mystic point of view, all of the 'creation' is intended as an expression of life and consciousness. Immaterial dead and empty energy has no meaning. The Supreme Purush or Life Consciousness, the Ocean of Love, has manifested Himself, say the mystics, in order to play the game of Love with Himself, to "give Himself more meaning". He is beyond time, space, form and duality. His 'creation' is a projection from within Himself, bubbles on the surface of His ocean.

Structure and order, cause and effect, are the laws of this game and the manifestation of life. Even in the most stringent and difficult of conditions, we find life. From the burning deserts of Africa to the frozen poles of the Arctic and Antarctic, life takes form and lives successfully, too.

Similarly, with every niche – some life form has found its place – a manifestation of the vibration of that place and those conditions, and in tune with it, however harsh and uninviting it may be to ourselves or to other species.

In fact, some mystic philosophies say that there are species taking form within the subtle tattvic energy fields as well as in gross manifestation. Paracelsus and other mystics talk of salamanders, creatures of subtle fire, who live in the sun; undines – creatures of water, sylphs of the air and gnomes of the earth. These are the devas and the nature spirits, whose role is the administration of the subtle elements that lie as the blueprint to our world. Ghosts too, are a part of this subtle physical world – souls whose attachment to physical life was too strong to allow them to leave the environment to which they were so connected, following the normal course of either passing into sub-astral or astral realms for a while or of taking immediate rebirth. But even a ghostly existence is not forever, and they can often benefit from our help in escaping from their prison of attachments.

A Bit of a Dig at Darwinism

It is clear, then, that the Darwinian theory of evolution omits many essential aspects of life and begs the basic question of "Where does all this come from?" For this reason, many people these days find themselves unable to agree with such a theory in its entirety, and I count myself as one of them. It is altogether too superficial and furthermore the 'evidence', is far too flimsy – just a few fossils and a lot of thinking! Scientists who believe in it are often scathing of the alternative 'creationist' theory, assuming it to be based on a literal understanding of the Book of Genesis. But this is not the only alternative way of looking at things, as I have attempted to point out.

Indeed, as even modern Jewish Kabbalistic thinkers realize, Genesis is, in the eastern and middle-eastern tradition, simply an allegory or metaphor, requiring mystical interpretation for it to make any real sense. The spiritual literature of the east abounds with such mystic allegory. The problem is always that mystical experience and understanding is beyond words and that we, as humans, place far too much religious value upon words and intellect. But mysticism and western science are not at all at odds with each other. Rather, they are complementary aspects of human life.

Modern Darwinists, like Oxford zoologist, Richard Dawkins in his book, *The Blind Watchmaker*, do actually admit that it does seem unlikely that pure chance can have resulted in the intense variety, specialization and intricately integrated mechanisms observed in nature. They do, however, believe that it is possible for evolution to have occurred by slowly evolving towards a more perfect pattern, with each step, however small, being both mediated and preserved genetically. So while they do acknowledge that (to use the popular example) the odds against a monkey and a typewriter coming up with the complete works of Shakespeare, (or even just one phrase), are too far out to be seriously contemplated as a mechanism of evolution, given a perfect pattern towards which to evolve, adaptation will slowly get you there.

Dawkins gives the example of mimicry, where the hypothetical ancestor to the stick insect, for example, which looked nothing like a stick, is supposed to have evolved in, say, five per cent stages by random mutation towards an appearance more like that of a stick, with the five per cent changes selectively preserving the more adapted members of the species. But then he spoils his already suspect argument by suggesting that it evolved perhaps from something like a locust – one of the most successful insects on the planet today – which is already clearly well-specialized and has no survival need to look anything remotely like a stick.

Furthermore, there are no species that are *not* already specialized – neither living, nor in the fossil record. There are no vanilla or bland species. Every one of them is highly specialized, whether they are of the Devonian or present day era. Actually, the word 'primitive' is essentially an expression of an emotive, misguided and highly relative sense of present day superiority. It is not an objectively determined fact. The biochemistry, physiology and tissue structure would have been just as intricate as it is today.

Nature acts as a *whole*. It is our linear, conceptual, divided human minds which think they perceive specific cause and effect pathways. But whether we observe biochemical activity or ecological networks of symbiotically bound species, we are continually faced with complete and whole *cycles*. All of which are linked into one even greater whole.

If one part of a cycle were missing, *the cycle could not function*. And nature is one whole tapestry, a woven fabric of such 'cycles'. We could think of this 'part' as an enzyme, maybe, or a hormone, or on a larger scale it may be the sun, the moon or the nose on our face. But how can a whole evolve out of parts? When the whole has a greater autonomy than our analysis of its parts? What use would it be to randomly evolve three steps in a multi-step biochemical pathway? How can the whole even begin to evolve, piecemeal, in such a fashion, when the individual pieces would be useless – a liability even, during the process of such evolution? And when there is absolutely no evidence at the present time of there being *anything* extraneous or useless in nature, in the process of evolving into something else, just waiting around in order for it to evolve into something useful at some future scene in the drama?

What use is two per cent or even fifty per cent of an optical system such as the eye? A creature could not see anything with it. Functionally, its use would be zero per cent. What use is a biochemical pathway with a few enzymes missing? How could the majority of a complex system evolve spontaneously when all-important, key aspects that make it capable of performing a useful function were missing? What use is half a wheel? How could such a thing ever evolve, piece by piece? And what constitutes a 'piece' or a 'part'? When 'pieces' are concepts in our own minds and are defined according to almost arbitrary parameters which we humans have decided upon? We dream up concepts in our minds and then say that nature is 'obeying' these concepts! It seems to be us who are enslaved by these concepts and thoughts – not nature, who carries on sublimely indifferent to our ideas about her!

We should apply the important perception of quantum physics to the whole of scientific endeavour: that we only find what we are looking for, that the 'pieces' we think we perceive are determined by the concepts we have in our own minds. How can we say that it is nature that behaves in a certain way, when in fact it is our own minds that are behaving in that way? The more our own mind is divided, the more we see division in nature. The more our consciousness rises, the more we perceive that it is just one whole – one uni-verse, not a multi-verse.

So there is no method in nature by which such a multitude of mutations could ever occur or could continue to exist, in the absence of any useful function. The sheer detailed complexity of natural biological processes is such that every subatomic particle, every infrared emission, the structure and being of every vibrating, energetic molecule is in a state of maximum order. Where is the place for random mutation and evolution?

The whole may *adapt*, but only as a response within an overall system. The creature is also a part of nature's whole and responds accordingly to changes in the whole. But it does not self-create itself out of dust, water and electricity. There *is* a guiding intelligence in nature.

Presently, scientists are intrigued by the apparent ability of systems to 'self-organize'. But again, they are just looking at the rearrangement of energy patterns as they ebb and flow under the dominion of the three gunas, the attributes of the Universal Mind. The origin of the fundamental, intrinsic order and structure in the physical universe has yet to be understood. But simplicity is so easily overlooked by a complex mind.

Darwinists and conventional evolutionists actually postulate pure chance, chaos and randomness as the selective factors which move a species towards its perfect pattern. The admission of the existence of a pattern, however, especially if not yet even achieved and existing purely as a possibility, posits the existence of a non-random formative patterning process. For randomness can only be random within the constraints on limited and determined possibilities. Statistical analysis only works because of the assumption that there *is* an underlying pattern. But that in the absence of a knowledge of that pattern, the wealth of data can only be handled in a statistical fashion.

Indeed, the arguments or patterns put forward to establish Darwinism should surely be random if they are to be valid? For to use a pattern – in this case, an organized and rational mental conceptualization – to dispute the existence of a pattern-maker could be regarded as a self-conflicting process. But there *is* nothing that is ultimately random. Apparent randomness is actually conditioned by the constraints of the patterning process and only *appears* random if the total pattern cannot be immediately perceived.

Furthermore, the knowledge gained by mystical and yogic experience, if not from ordinary intuitive awareness, indicates that *life is prior to form.* That consciousness gives rise to biological complexity, not the reverse. Darwinist and neo-Darwinist interpretations of the fossil record presume that material substance is both self-created, self-organized *and* the only existent substance – ideas that run quite contrary to the inner wisdom and mystical *experience* of life.

Actually, evolutionary theory presents one of the most explicit examples of *a priori* reasoning, and even blind faith, ever seen in a supposedly scientific hypothesis. Books on evolution are full of the *prior* assumption that evolutionary theory is correct. The facts are then presented to fit the theory. And although many other interpretations of these facts are also possible, it is a rare biologist who dares to be a dissenter or to even suggest that other interpretations and explanations are also possible.

In its early days, Darwinism was embraced with a fervour that would have done credit to any religion, to the extent that evidence was even falsified in order to support the faith. The result is that we are all now taught it in our schools. And although such exposure to a belief system in childhood predisposes a person to believe it unthinkingly and to defend it vigorously in adult life, it is really no more than a form of conditioning. Much in the same way as a religious doctrine is propagated. It is just a mental habit, a groove in the energy fields of the mind. The very fact that beliefs, whether scientific, social or religious, are region-ally, geographically or culturally self-propagating shows the power of early indoctrination over supposedly rational and intuitive thought. Indeed, it is even able to colour the understanding of spontaneous, religious, semi-mystical experience. It is like those mediums who are supposed to be clear channels for communications "from the other side", but in fact are never heard to communicate anything that contradicts their own personal belief system.

So-called objective thought is riddled by subconscious, scientific, social and ideological conditioning, whether we realize it or not. Unless one's understanding is illuminated by inward, mystic *experience*, this will always be the case, to a greater or lesser degree. Mystic experience means an expansion of consciousness, and this happens only grad-ually. But even a mystic will only express that experience within the context and idiom of his times, according to the nature of the people he is addressing.

So evolutionists are observing just a horizontal slice of the processes involved in a vast and outwardly complex cosmological process. They are perceiving just a slit-window view of events that involve mind and conscious-ness, as well as material substance, as real entities, and which require understanding of mystic mechanisms that transcend and yet are responsible for the existence of the lower domains of thought, pranic and tattvic energy fields.

But there are many logical and scientific arguments to put against this evolutionist point of view, and in this respect I can highly recommend Michael Pitman's book, *Adam and Evolution* and Ian Taylor's, *In the Minds of Men*, where some of these arguments are very clearly presented.

Darwinists, of course, have a field day when dealing with arguments based upon religious doctrine and biblical creationism, because religious belief is quite a different animal to scientific theory (so they say). But there is a highly significant difference between inner mystic understanding and religious dogma. For while true mysticism – like all true science – is based upon *repeatable experience*, religious dogma closes down the avenues of free expression and inner spiritual development, as indeed does much of science. For science has many doctrinal aspects, as one soon discovers if any of its sacred cows are rigorously challenged with alternative and rational points of view.

But as I have expressed before, life is a personal adventure and each one of us is simply trying to comprehend what on earth it is all about. So all points of view are simply a valid reflection of our inner mystification. They are not something to be fought over. But some are more valid than others . . . aren't they?

A Biblical Digression

Like the spiritual writings of almost all eastern mystics, biblical literature is permeated with mystic metaphor. Story-telling is the great art of the ancient eastern writers and their saints have almost invariably used that device to explain their teachings. Even Christ spoke in parables. It was the idiom of the times. In olden days, too, it was also necessary for mystics to be more discreet, for 'heresy' was frequently punishable by death. Christ was not the only mystic to meet such a fate. Therefore, they put their teachings into allegorical form, so that only the initiated could truly understand, while others would derive benefit according to their inner spiritual stature.

The ancient mystics of Persia – Jalal'u'din Rumi, Farid'u'din Attar and Hafiz – the Kabbalists of early Judaism from whom are derived much of the mystical writings of the Old Testament, the yogis and munis of India writing in the Bhagavad Gita or the Ramayana, the Sages of China and the Far East – all these great souls put forward their teachings in the form of stories.

It is in this context that many of the Biblical stories must be understood. Now, with the passage of millenia and at the hands of multitudinous translators, transcribers, politicians and church councils, the message has become obscured. And man, in desperate search for meaning and truth, finds himself a slave to a story told long ago, to exemplify a reality long forgotten, and which was never meant to be taken literally.

The book of Genesis, for example, starts with the story of man's estate in this world. Adam is the primal essence, the 'first' principle, the soul. In his descent from the One Ocean, he meets Eve. Eve is derived from the same root as the Hebrew word meaning experience. So the soul, Adam, meets experience of life, as it leaves the Godhead. In Sanskrit or yogic thinking, Eve is Maya, the primal spinner of illusion. And since everything is derived from the primal essence, Eve is depicted as being created out of Adam's rib, out of the primal substance. But Eve herself is led astray by the serpent who tempts her to eat or become aware of the duality or polarity of knowledge, of good and evil, of the pairs of opposites, inherent in the mind regions.

The serpent is the mind, the principle by which duality is manifested in the materio–mental worlds. Knowledge is divisive, the attribute of mind. It assumes a separateness of knower and known. Love is the power of union of the soul with its source.

So the soul, Adam, portrayed as the 'first' man, the positive principle in creation, enters the world of maya, allegorized as Eve, the woman, the negative pole, and under the sway of the mind – the serpent – becomes aware of itself, its nakedness, putting on garments, vehicles or bodies for its functioning in the worlds of duality.

The biblical story continues and one can perceive the thread of mystic metaphor infused throughout. But to take such a tale literally was never intended. A child may believe fervently in Father Christmas, refuting all attempts to enlighten him and bring him into a wiser state, but that belief does not make the existence of Father Christmas any the less unreal.

Tattwas, Consciousness and Vegetarianism

Returning to our tattvic theme, the degree of consciousness of a soul when incarnate in a physical body is according to the number of tattwas active in its physical vehicle of expression. And man, with all five tattwas actively present, is the only species able to perform the highest function of consciousness, namely meditation, leading to self and God realization.

It is for these tattvic and allied karmic reasons too, that the highest spiritual paths insist on their practitioners being fully vegetarian. The less the number of active elements, then the less is the consciousness of the soul in that particular body. The lower the consciousness, then the less suffering is endured by that creature when its life is taken for the purpose of food. All suffering for which we are responsible, whether directly or indirectly, is due for later repayment through the operations of the law of karma, cause and effect. And since the purpose of higher forms of meditation and yoga is to clear the karmic debris of past lives which encumber the soul in its search for light, practitioners are therefore advised to feed only on life taken from the vegetable kingdom. Here, the suffering and karmic burden borne is likened to that of a light shirt rather than a weight of lead. The vegetarian diet is becoming accepted by increasing numbers of people as a far healthier diet, and good health is also a great help in meditation.

The Akash Tattwa, the Throat Chakra and the Thyroid and Parathyroid Glands

The subtle aspect, then, of the akash tattwa, is administered at the *vishuddha* (pure) chakra, also called the *kanth* or throat chakra. This centre has sixteen petals and is said to be of a smokey, dark blue-purple colour. Being the controller or mini-creator of the other chakras, we would expect to find a reflection of this status in the overall control of the body's physiological processes. And this indeed is the case.

The endocrine glands of the neck are the thyroid and parathyroids, with their management function of general metabolic controllers. In talking of endocrine glands one needs to be aware that further medical discoveries concerning their activities are constantly being made as research techniques are refined, and the importance of hitherto ignored or unobserved biochemical and bioenergetic interactions are appreciated.

Since from the eastern point of view, we are discussing 'specific generalities', it leads us to postulate certain areas of function that have not yet been identified in the western sense, but would be considered as likely, given the eastern understanding of the general funtionality ascribed to particular chakras.

Thus, the parathyroids are known to control the levels of body calcium through the medium of the *parathyroid hormone (PTH)*. This might, at first sight, be thought of as an earthy and non-general hormone to be emanating from the chakra associated with the akash tattwa. But the role of calcium in blood-clotting, nerve signal transmission, muscle cell contraction, cell membrane function, endocrine and exocrine cellular secretions and mediation of the action of other peptide hormones at their target sites leaves us with a clear impression of a mechanism which is highly integrated with all body metabolism. Just what we would expect to find from akashic reflections at the biochemical level.

Similarly, although it used to be said in endocrinology that there is no direct functional correlation between the parathyroid and the thyroid gland, the role of both these endocrine glands is clearly one of overall metabolic control. Functionally, they cannot be considered as separate entities. In fact, these days, with the role of the thyroid hormone, *calcitonin*, established as providing a directly opposing effect on calcium balance to that of PTH, we once again find a paired toning of polarities within one endocrine complex, emanating from one centre. My guess is that as endocrine research proceeds, the further interrelationship in function between these two glands and their secreted substances will become more fully understood. And that the parathyroid role of maintaining calcium balance will be seen in a wider context, in which calcium metabolism is just one aspect of general functional administration.

Furthermore, I am intrigued by the possible physiological correlations to the number of petals on the chakras –

each representing a particular function or modality. In yogic practice, each of these petals is experienced as a sound and as a colour. Sensory perception of energy vibration, in the subtle as well as the gross physical world, is the manner by which our inner mind and consciousness becomes aware of change in surrounding energy fields. Consideration of the actual number of these petals together with the tantric understanding that the petals relate to the pattern of the nadis issuing therefrom, leaves us with the distinct probability that each petal represents a particular energy control point for a particular physiological area of function or action. In particular, I have looked to see whether the number of petals is reflected in the number of hormones currently known to be secreted by each gland. Generally, however, this does not immediately appear to be the case, though the level of endocrine *intricacy* definitely increases from the bottom up, as does the number of chakric petals.

I will be returning to this analysis in a later chapter, but let us mention here that there are two lobes to the thyroid gland, making a four cornered structure. At each corner we find one of the four parathyroid glands. Four times four equals sixteen, the number of petals in this chakra, which leaves us with an interesting correlation in *shape* (something I discussed lightly in *Subtle Energy*), though whether it has any real meaning in this context I am unsure. I just found it interesting and noteworthy in case any future discoveries or thoughts should bring it into sharper focus. The fact that the parathyroid glands are often of a greater number and not so geometrically arranged is also an interesting part of the puzzle, since nothing is coincidental, everything reflecting the content of a more inward pattern.

This relationship may at first sight seem somewhat magical or too numerological for many tastes. But this kind of patterning may have some relevance and it is more closely examined in chapter eleven, within the context of the intricate biochemical organization characterizing living organisms.

Biochemical and Physiological Aspects of the Thyroid and Parathyroid Glands

At this point, we once again investigate some of the specific aspects of this centre and if you find it too heavy going then by all means skim through it to the next section, entitled, Akash and Discrimination.

The parathyroids, then, produce PTH, a peptide hormone that is closely linked functionally with *Vitamin D*, a steroid substance essential to the regulation of bodily calcium levels. Vitamin D needs to be either consumed in the diet or to be manufactured in the skin from a steroid precursor, in response to electromagnetic energy in the form of sunlight. Now the skin is one of the body areas governed primarily by the earthy tattwa, also responsible for the production of other steroids in the adrenal cortex. In this sense, therefore, vitamin D can almost be considered as a secondary hormone with the skin involved in the final aspects of its synthesis. One of its major activities is to increase the intestinal absorption of calcium, through the intermediary of a vitamin D dependent, calcium-binding protein found in the upper intestine.

PTH, on the other hand, promotes the synthesis of a vitamin D derivative (*1,25-dihydroxy vitamin D*) which, in its turn, stimulates the manufacture of this calcium-binding, intestinal carrier protein. But PTH also finds energetic sympathetic resonance at other areas in the body. In the kidney tubules, for example, it stimulates the cells to reabsorb calcium back into the circulation, while in the bones, PTH and vitamin D work in synchrony to permit the release of calcium into circulation when inadequate quantities are being consumed in the diet. These interconnections are simplified and summarized in figure 9-1. Dietary deficiency of vitamin D coupled with the lack of sunlight, thus results in the previously more common disease of rickets.

When it is said that a hormone has a certain action, from the biochemical point of view, this statement is a generalization of intricate molecular interchanges, some of which are understood, whilst many others are not. Remember the concept of the molecule as a vibrating energy pattern and consider that the whole body, (at a biochemical level of understanding) is completely made up of these interacting molecules. The resulting, highly interwoven and ordered combination of meetings and interactions can only be surmised. Who would be a biochemist!

Historically, the parathyroids came to fame when a link

was established between high blood calcium levels, gradual dissolution of the bone matrix leading to unexpected fractures, pain and shrinkage, and hyperactivity of the parathyroid glands or a parathyroid tumour. The parathyroids were then further linked with the dietary deficiency disease of rickets in which the role of vitamin D was established as an integral part of bodily calcium metabolism.

Since high or low blood calcium and calcium-related symptoms remain the major observable clinical symptom of aberrant parathyroid activity, medical research has tended to concentrate on this aspect of its function. It is, however, also known that PTH stimulates an increase in the electrically-charged, ion concentrations of sodium, potassium and bicarbonate in the urine, thus increasing bodily levels. Conversely, urinary levels of ammonium, hydrogen and magnesium, as well as calcium, are decreased, with PTH perhaps mediating some kind of ion exchange pump in the kidneys.

What this suggests, therefore, is that PTH is concerned with cellular and plasma ion concentrations – an integral aspect of all metabolic functioning within the body. PTH is also involved in the activity of *mitochondria*, small bodies within cells that act as the principle, intracellular storage areas for calcium along with a number of other little understood, cellular administration functions, including the synthesis of key enzymes. And this is all quite consonant with the role of the vishudda chakra and the akash tattwa as a manager of the business, but not the chairman or executive president.

Furthermore, the parathyroid glands consist of three major cell types, two varieties of *chief* cell and the *oxyphilic* cells. And while PTH secretion is clearly associated with one variety of chief cell, the function of the other is little understood, and though the oxyphilic cells are derived from the chief cells and seem able to synthesize PTH, their real function is still unknown.

The thyroid gland produces two known varieties of hormone. Firstly, calcitonin, which generally speaking provides the counterbalanced polarity to PTH. For while PTH promotes bodily calcium retention and increases calcium plasma concentrations, calcitonin inhibits the

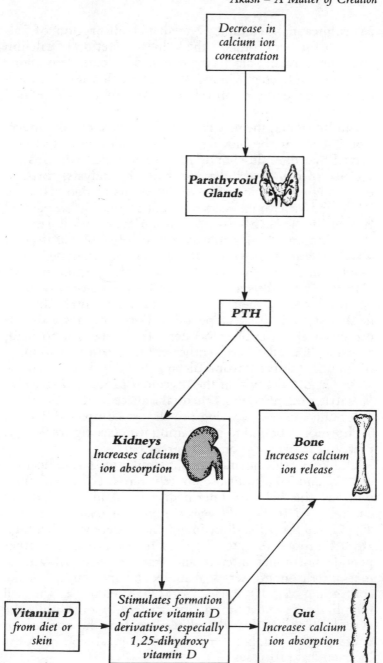

Figure 9-1. *Vitamin D, calcium and the PTH link-up*

gastrointestinal, vitamin D-mediated absorption of calcium. It further promotes the kidney excretion of calcium and other ions and blocks the release of calcium from bone cells into the general blood circulation. It thus decreases calcium concentration in cellular *cytoplasm* or intracellular fluid.

But like PTH, the mechanisms are only sketchily understood, even at the biochemical level, although it is suspected that the mitochondria are again involved, as is the activity of certain cellular enzymes or catalysts, through the changing of calcium levels. In terms of control, both PTH and calcitonin secretion appear to be influenced largely by the change in calcium ion concentration.

In addition to calcitonin, the two lobes of the thyroid gland produce the two metabolic control hormones of *tri-iodothyronine (T3)* and *thyroxine (tetra-iodothryronine or T4)*. Together with adrenaline, T3 and T4 are the only hormones produced by the six major endocrine centres that are neither steroids nor true peptides. For while adrenaline is produced in a number of steps from the amino acid, tyrosine, T3 and T4 are synthesized by a complex binding of iodine (derived from dietary iodide) with tyrosine amino acid units within the thyroidal protein, *thyroglobulin*. Structural alterations then take place within the thyroglobulin molecule leaving the almost completed T3 and T4 hormones bound to it, awaiting use, (see figure 9-2). A pretty neat system, you will agree.

Unlike peptide hormones, but similar to steroid hormones, T3 and T4 can diffuse directly across cell membranes without the help of intermediaries. And interestingly enough, *T3 is the only known peptide hormone to proceed directly into the cell nucleus*, interacting directly with a high affinity protein receptor attached to the DNA. All other peptide hormones interact and transfer their vibrational message through a series of molecular messengers to the controlling cellular nucleus of DNA either at the cell membrane (a most important structure) or within the cytoplasm, but *outside the cell nucleus*. It is the nucleus, of course, which appears to maintain local control over biochemical processes.

This particular power of T3, of containing a master entry key intrinsic in its energetic shape, is also consonant

242

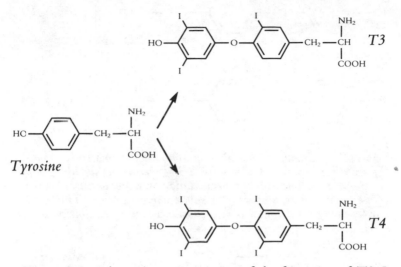

Figure 9-2. Schematic representation of the formation of T3 & T4 from tyrosine. Note the positioning of the all-important iodine atoms. This formation takes place within the far more complex pattern of the protein, thyroglobulin.

with the role of this centre as having command over the lower centres of activity within the body.

T3 is, in fact, apparently the more potent of these two thyroid hormones and within the peripheral bodily cells, outside the thyroid, only about twenty per cent of T3 arrives directly from the thyroid, while the remaining eighty per cent is synthesized from T4, on the spot. T4, however, is a hormone in its own right, with its own specific receptors and activities.

Furthermore, while the peripheral tissues can convert T4 to the more active T3, they can also dispose of T4 altogether by converting it to the biologically inert *reverse T3*, where the iodine atom removed comes from one of the other four molecular iodine locations, (see figures 9–3 and 9–4). That such a small change should have such consequences is similar in nature to the differing activity of stereo–isomers which we discussed earlier and shows how beautifully and finely tuned are our biochemical processes. It also allows the peripheral bodily tissues to themselves regulate the effect of the thyroid hormones, at a distance from the thyroidal centre, by varying the amount of T3

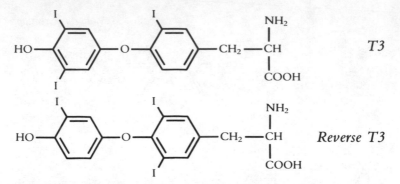

Figure 9-3. Showing the all-important, but apparently small, difference between T3 and reverse T3. It seems highly likely that this simple two dimensional representation on paper obscures the real difference at a more subatomic or subtle energetic level. This is the case for many very similar bodily substances which exhibit converse effects.

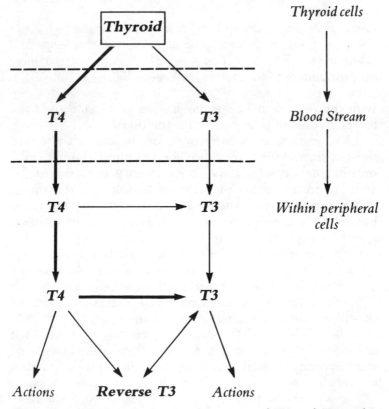

Figure 9-4. Illustrating the transformations of T3 and T4 within cells outside the thyroid.

244

and reverse T3 which are produced. The significance of this fine tuning and balance of bodily biochemistry is discussed again in chapter eleven.

T3 and T4 secretion and synthesis would appear to be primarily controlled by a familiar anterior pituitary/hypothalamic link, discussed in the next chapter, although there is also autonomic innervation to these cells whose function remains unclear.

T3 and T4 appear primarily to be involved with the control of general cellular metabolic activity, with the most well-documented and clinically observable effect being increases in the *Basal Metabolic Rate (BMR)*. Both anabolic and catabolic pathways are stimulated in almost all tissues with the exception of the brain, the central nervous system, the spleen, the lungs and the testes. In cases of T3 and T4 excess, this can be by as much as a hundred per cent, or in hypothyroidism, the decrease in BMR can be by fifty or sixty per cent.

The exact mechanisms by which this is brought about are little understood, but it is observed that, as with the parathyroids, the mitochondria and enzymatic pathways are once again involved. The mitochondria increase in size and number, exhibiting a greater content of enzymes. One can therefore understand *why* – though it is not known *how* – an increase of general bodily activity and heat should be prevented from affecting the brain and central nervous system (where activity needs to be controlled from a higher point), the testes (which are already kept outside the body in order to keep the temperature down), and the lungs (where the increase in cellular oxygen uptake will automatically stimulate the breathing).

Other observed effects include an increase in intestinal glucose absorption, as well as in carbohydrate synthesis and breakdown. Similarly, fatty tissue and protein metabolism are increased, both in synthesis, utilization and degradation. In this respect, the balanced operation of the thyroid gland is of particular importance during youth, when hypothyroidism will result in stunted growth if not properly treated.

The thyroid hormones, therefore, have a primary role to play in the growth and development of a child, not only in terms of physical growth, but also mentally, such that any deficiency needs to be corrected within weeks of birth. For in the absence of T3 and T4, the neurons providing the functional link between the akashic or vacuum state and its outward manifestations, do not develop correctly. The result is one of mental retardation, known clinically as *cretinism*.

Additionally, many of the other hormones are involved with an intracellular messenger, known as *cyclic AMP*, for the mediation of their effects and it has been suggested that T3 and T4 are involved in potentizing this aspect of intracellular biochemistry. The thyroid thus becomes a generalized manager and potentizer of other endocrine events.

It is very clear, therefore, that the thyroid and parathyroid glands are performing exactly the kind of role one would expect, if one accepts the possibility that they represent one facet of the outworking of the akashic tattwa.

Akash is the vacuum state of locked-in, energy potential. It is from this point that all the subatomic particles that comprise the other four gross tattwas dance into being. Control of akash, therefore, gives you control over all else, below.

So while the thyroid hormones have been known about for perhaps the longest period, historically, the complexity of their workings is one of the least understood. Even the medical textbooks admit their lack of knowledge of real mechanisms, because almost everything seems to be involved. And with vacuum being the substrate for gross physical reality, this is exactly as one would suppose.

The thyroid and parathyroid hormones, therefore, would appear to be molecules that represent the ability to shake up the three dimensional sheet of vacuum and all its subatomic patternings. Remember our illustration of the molecule as a vibrant energy dance, spun out of the akashic state, an effect upon the vacuum surface. Seen in this light, metabolism becomes the speed and complexity of this integrated and inwardly patterned dance. And control of overall function lies within the akash, with its close harmonics and tightly tied-in waveforms and patternings, appearing to us at the subatomic and molecular level of biochemical and bioelectrical activity.

Once again, then, the functional parallels are both intriguing and very clear and, I believe, worthy of further study and research, especially in the realm of establishing new therapeutic techniques.

Akash and Discrimination

As we discused earlier, akash is the element that gives us conscious reason and also the ability to meditate, to reach up within our consciousness to higher realms of vibration, experiencing reality from within. The integration into our conscious beings of the energy crossroads of this akashic tattwa provides us with an intelligence not possessed by the lower species.

Enlivened by its activity, the indriya of hearing is its subtle sense and the ear is its outward sense organ. The direct motor analogue of hearing is speech, with its activity in the mouth and throat, the centre of akashic administration. With akash playing such a vital role in the human constitution, its role is a frequent theme, which we will be returning to in the remaining chapters of this book.

The degree of akashic activity in an individual gives us our discriminative faculty, something distinct from the airy intellect of the conceptual man. While the conceptual faculty is manifested as the intellectual idiom known to us westerners, it is actually the good idea and light innovative touch that is the hallmark of air. Thus the quick-witted Stone Age men or women who figured out new ways of tool-making, or of stitching garments or of softening and decorating fabrics and skins, most probably had a good degree of active air in their make-up.

Akash is present throughout, and the airy nature may be as lacking in its manifestation as earth. Discrimination is obscured by the play of the mind through the medium of the senses, as the individual indulges and besports himself, playing amongst the tattvic energy realms. It is akash that gives us our sense of inner ethics and true morality. It defines for our inner, intuitive selves, the boundaries of correct and incorrect living, of truthfulness and dishonesty. Its manifestation is sharpened by meditation, and our conduct of life is heightened thereby.

Amongst the *siddhis* or miraculous powers that come to

247

yogis and practitioners of mystic spirituality – and which they are cautioned not to use – the power of everything said turning out to be true is the siddhi associated with the kanth or throat chakra. Deep inner honesty, with far-sighted wisdom and comprehension are the qualities of akash in its highest manifestation, providing a vision of patterns and events as they are going to be. Speech is the immediate manifestation of such discriminative intuition and with such impeccable honesty within him, the power of the words of such a one are considerable. They both reflect the inner truth and turn out to be true.

Just as you or I may see a ball falling and with a knowledge based upon past experience be able in essence to predict the future and to know that it will hit the ground, similarly the one whose wisdom and akash are awakened can see the obvious outcome of events which to others of us are obscured by the constant activity of our lower natures.

CHAPTER 10

Up to the Eyes

The Ajna Chakra, the Pituitary Gland and the Hypothalamus

Just as in any administrative system there are points of control carrying varying degrees and kinds of jurisdiction, so too in the inner realms and chakras. Whilst the akashic centre, therefore, maintains one kind of control and administration, the control exercised by the *ajna chakra* in the brain is of a different nature. If the throat centre is the general manager of bodily activities, then the ajna chakra is the president – who is himself answerable to the central government of the brain and higher centres.

The ajna centre is situated behind and between the two eyes. 'Ajna' actually means 'command', referring to this centre as the command or control centre of the other five chakras. It is also said to be so named because it is here that the command of the guru is received from within. It is also known as the *Eye Centre*, at which the guru instructs the disciple to meditate and focus concentration at the commencement of the inward spiritual journey, being the point at which mind and soul are knotted together. It is not, however, the true Third Eye, which lies further in, beyond the antashkarans, on the threshold of the astral world.

Being the focus for our thoughts, this is also the centre of mental balance. Mostly, our attention is scattered throughout the body and into the world. But when we can still our mental gyrations sufficiently, we automatically find ourselves back at this point. Even Thomas a Kempis comments, in the *Imitation of Christ*, "What can be more at rest than at the single eye."

The human quality of our thoughts is influenced directly by our level of consciousness. The higher our inner ascent and ability to withdraw consciousness and attention to the eye centre, then the higher the quality of our thought processes and the more control we can exercise over our emotions. Conversely, by controlling our mind, our emotions and our scattered thoughts, we automatically raise our consciousness towards the eye centre, because that is our focus of thought.

It is a two-way process. Just as mind affects biochemistry from above, so too do changes in biochemistry affect mental processes from below.

If this book were one on meditation, there would be much more to say concerning this and higher centres, but we are discussing here the physical manifestation of these energies and must proceed.

The ajna chakra is described as having two petals, one white and one black. These are the wings atop the Cadduceus (see figure 10-1), the staff of Hermes, the insignia of the wise physician, the ancient symbol of life portraying the six chakras in the physical body. Part of the gross physical reflection of this centre would seem to be a combination of the *pituitary gland* and the *hypothalamus*. These two glands between them are considered to be the control or command system for all the other endocrine glands in the body. Considering that the ajna or command chakra was so named perhaps thousands of years ago, it would seem a sensible move for modern life sciences research to at least investigate the expositions of both ancient and modern yogic teachings and philosophy.

Yoga, after all, is a far older science of life and has stood a greater test of time. And these days you can read books on yoga without being surreptitious about it or being considered weird. Many folk even respect it and certainly a scientist would not get burnt at the stake, or even lose his job, for taking an interest in the philosophy indigenous to one of the oldest cultures in the world. A philosophy that was being practised when our more recent British ancestors were still busy battling it out with the Romans.

The hypothalamus represents the most obvious point of fusion and functional contact, physiologically and anatomically, between the nervous and endocrine systems. Consisting of specialized nervous tissue, fed by nerve connections from the brain, and lying below the *thalamus*, it

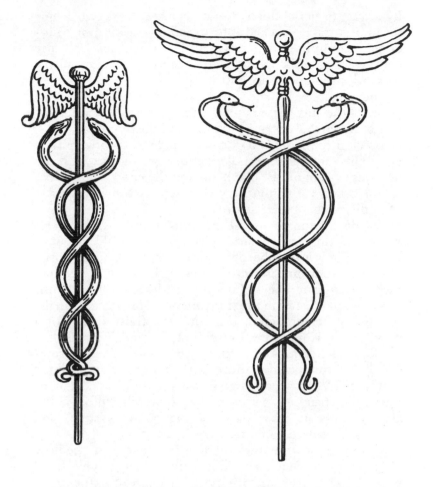

From: Polarity Therapy, the Complete Collected Works of *Dr Randolph Stone*.

Figure 10-1. The Cadduceus, the staff of Hermes, insignia of the ancient physicians. Different cultures have evolved different designs, but the underlying reality of the tree of life remains the same.

takes its primary orders from the mid-brain, by a nervous message encoding as yet unidentified. From there, hormones are carried to the anterior lobe of the pituitary gland via two portal veins that network into a blood capilliary plexus before exiting, (see figure 10-2).

The *posterior lobe of the pituitary*, on the other hand, is almost an extension of the hypothalamus in that it is 'fed' by a tract of nerve fibres down which at least two major hormones travel, packed into granules – a kind of endocrine quantum – for release upon a nervous impulse command from the hypothalamus, into a blood capilliary network in the posterior pituitary.

The possible existence of a parallel between the two petals of the ajna chakra and the two lobes of the pituitary – or between the anterior pituitary and the hypothalamus – is too clear to ignore and one is tempted to theorize on the possibility of an energy polarization existing between the nervous system on the one hand and the endocrine system on the other. Certainly, they represent two major aspects of bodily control mechanisms.

The distinction between these two systems is, however, not as distinct as classical physiology would have us believe. For it is now becoming clear that rather than just a few neuro-transmitting molecules such as acetyl choline, there are large numbers of neuropeptides and other chemicals that are integral in the transmission of nervous signals. It must be remembered, too, that the transmission of a nerve signal is infinitely more complex and ordered than the flow of electrons in a conducting wire. The information being conducted is more in the nature of an encoded radio or TV broadcast signal with a multitude of continuously changing patterns that represent information about events in other parts of the bodily system, and 'actions' that need to be taken as a result.

Moreover, a nerve impulse does not arise from the flow of electrons down a nerve, but from a change in electrical polarity across the membrane of a nerve cell (neuron). This polarity reversal results in the flow of ions (electrically charged atoms or molecules) across the membrane and down the length of the cell. Each neuron is able to transmit and trigger this information in the next neuron in sequence, thus ensuring a continuous flow of impulse, the energy flow appearing to rely entirely upon the electrical, ionic charges carried by electrons, as described in the classical picture of subatomic physics.

Furthermore, more modern theories in physics lead one to suggest that the activity of the nervous system – with its synapses, high speed polarity reversals across membranes and the flow of charged atoms and molecules – represents

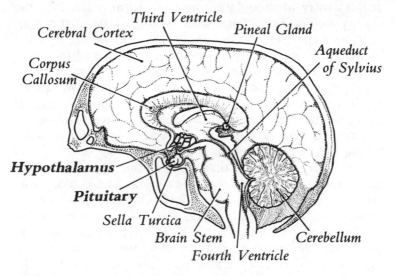

Cerebral Cortex
Third Ventricle
Pineal Gland
Corpus Callosum
Aqueduct of Sylvius
Hypothalamus
Pituitary
Sella Turcica
Brain Stem
Fourth Ventricle
Cerebellum

Adapted, with permission, from: Hormones: The Messengers of Life, *Lawrence M. Crapo,* W. H. Freeman & Co.

The thalamus and mid-brain are omitted from this drawing, in order to show the ventricles and the pineal gland, (see chapter 12)

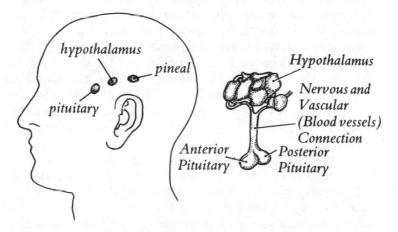

hypothalamus
pineal
pituitary
Hypothalamus
Nervous and Vascular (Blood vessels) Connection
Anterior Pituitary
Posterior Pituitary

After Evans: Mind, Body & Electromagnetism.

Figure 10-2. The location and connections of the hypothalamus and pituitary. Both organs receive chemical and endocrine messages from the rest of the body, via the blood stream. They are also intimately connectd by their own blood capilliary networks and nervous tract and both are linked into the higher brain stem.

253

an ideal way of modulating and being modulated by the energy-rich vacuum and more subtle tattvic states of matter or energy. That is, of directly connecting into the formative subtle energy blueprint in a process of two-way informational exchange. The electrical activity in nerve impulses, the bioelectric body potentials, the biomagnetic fields that result from cellular and atomic activity, as well as the electric fields of the brain itself are therefore seen as only one aspect of the energetic activity which is really taking place at both subtle and gross levels.

It is clear, however, that as with the Ida and Pingala nadis that carry yin and yang (or tamas and rajas) pranic energies around and through the chakras, meeting on either side of the ajna chakra, there is a polarization of function even at a biochemical level between the hypothalamus and the anterior pituitary. And there is an interesting polarity between the two hormones conveyed by the hypothalamus down into the posterior pituitary, which we will consider shortly.

Prior to the 1950's, the hypothalamus was thought of purely as a regulator of body temperature and autonomic nerve reflexes. Now it is understood as one of the major linkages between neuronal and endocrine activity. Within its tissues lie numerous groups of nerve cells, whose specific functions are far from understood. Many of their secretions are known to be peptides but for only a few of these has the specific endocrine activity been elucidated. In fact, only three have so far been isolated and their molecular structure described, while others have been demonstrated experimentally to exist, though as yet remain to be identified.

The role of the majority of hypothalamic substances is little understood. It is only those hormones that relate to the pituitary gland and to general control over the endocrine system that have received the most attention. In this category there are at least seven major hormones that either stimulate (yang) or inhibit (yin) the anterior pituitary production of further hormones. These then stimulate the other endocrine glands into production of their own particular hormones. The rising level of these hormones produced by the lower endocrine centres, then feeds back to both the hypothalamus and the anterior pituitary causing a fall-off in pituitary production of the stimulating hormone and a similar fall-off in the level of hypothalamic releasing hormone. Or conversely, they induce an increase in production of hypothalamic inhibitory hormones such as is required, for example, to prevent continuous pituitary production of *prolactin* which stimulates the production of breast milk.

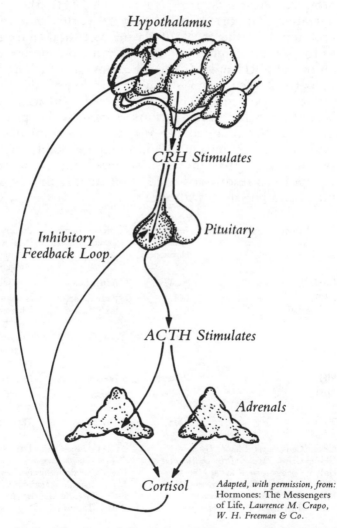

Figure 10-3. The hypothalamic – pituitary – adrenocortical connection

Adapted, with permission, from: Hormones: The Messengers of Life, *Lawrence M. Crapo, W. H. Freeman & Co.*

This may sound somewhat complex and is best illustrated by an example which – for the non-technically minded – may be seen simply as a part of the superb biochemical mechanism of fine-tuning, balance and control.

In the drawing (figure 10-3), we show how the hypothalamus produces *corticotropin-releasing hormone* (CRH). This then stimulates the anterior pituitary to produce *adrenocorticotropic hormone* (ACTH), the peptide hormone that stimulates the adrenal cortex into cortisol production. Rising levels of plasma cortisol then feed back to the hypothalamus and anterior pituitary inhibiting the output of CRH and ACTH. The consequent falling levels of cortisol then again stimulate the hypothalamus and pituitary into action. The polarity of the situation is thus beautifully balanced in a healthy system, whilst providing the flexibility required for adaptation to immediate environmental circumstances and changing bodily rhythms. Because of inertial effects, a stagnant and static system cannot be so readily activated as one that is already toned, tuned and pulsating with life.

Hypothalamic Hormones	Stimulates (+) Inhibits (−)	Anterior Pituitary Hormones	Primary Bodily Tissues Affected	Primary Response or Hormones Produced
CRH	+	ACTH	Adrenal cortex	Cortisol
GHRH	+	GH	Body tissues	Growth
Somatostatin	−	GH	Body tissues	Inhibition of growth
LHRH (GnRH)	+	LH and FSH	Gonads	Testosterone Oestrogen Progesterone
PIH	−	Prolactin	Breasts	Milk production
PRH	−	Prolactin	Breasts	Inhibition of milk production
TRH	+	TSH	Thyroid	Thyroxine

CRH   *Corticotropin Releasing Hormone*   ACTH *Adreno-Cortico-Tropic Hormone*
GHRH *Growth Hormone Releasing Hormone*   GH   *Growth Hormone*
GnRH *Gonadotrophin Releasing Hormone*   FSH   *Follicle Stimulating Hormone*
LHRH *Luteinising Hormone Releasing Hormone*   LH   *Luteinising Hormone*
PIH   *Prolactin Inhibitory Hormone*   PRH *Prolactin Releasing Hormone*
TRH *Thyrotropin Releasing Hormone*   TSH *Thyroid Stimulating Hormone*

Figure 10-4. The hypothalamic and anterior pituitary connections

Linkages of the hypothalamus with the brain provides for further overall coordination from the nervous system and the control circuit is completed, as far as present knowledge can say.

This mechanism or similar variations are played out for all the other major endocrine glands, and the anterior pituitary and hypothalamic hormones so far identified, along with the related pituitary hormones, are tabulated in figure 10-4.

One of the determining factors in the discovery, isolation and molecular identification of a hormone or any bodily substance is the quantity in which it is produced by the body. In any finely-tuned control system, however, it is not so much the *quantity* of a component as its *nature* which is of importance. A door key has to be exactly the right shape and size to perform its function. If it does not fit, simply bringing a larger key or more keys will not solve the problem!

Similarly with modern biochemical research. Techniques have traditionally been used that required vast amounts of animal tissue before just one hormone could be isolated. It took over a million pigs, for example, and a similar number of sheep from local slaughterhouses, plus the facilities of entire laboratories, to identify just three major hypothalamic hormones, during the 1950's, '60's and '70's.

More modern assays, however, are making it possible to identify far smaller quantities of substances in body tissue with the result that molecules exhibiting considerable biochemical capabilities are turning up by the hundred. And this is only the beginning. What this means is that even the endocrine glands, where it has sometimes rather naively been thought that most of the major research has already been done, will almost certainly turn out to have many surprises in store. With all these different molecules roaming about – all with some clear intent, though it is not at all obvious to us humans – it seems that the time is ripe for a new conceptual framework in which to understand bodily interactions.

Another Digression into New Paradigms

It is, as we suggested in previous chapters, a time for stock-taking and assessment. What began with the early chemists, biologists and physicists as a search for fundamentals has turned into a game of chasing endless and multiplying ramifications of cause and effect pathways. The true extent of this pandora's box is only now becoming clear. And this is still at the molecular level. Interactions at a subatomic level have hardly been considered. Biochemistry is thus – at its best – only an overview of energetic events, because the game is actually played out at a subatomic level, while biochemistry addresses itself almost entirely to the molecular domain. And the subatomic realm is itself only a dance, an effect, a tapestry, spun out upon the vacuum or akashic surface. *And within this dance, it is the implicate relationships within the whole which are of importance – not the observation of just a few linear, biochemical pathways.*

The game, as it has been played out so far has been invaluable, but it is now time to consolidate and to find some conceptual framework in which to hold all the contents of this amazing box of life that have been discovered. Even the magician knows that producing ten or twenty coloured hankerchiefs out of an empty box is entertaining and valuable, but after that it becomes at best, boring, and at worst – meaningless.

It means that the endless search for outer cause and effect pathways needs a context within a theory of energy that covers everything and puts simplicity, order and holism back into science. It is time for some true harvesting and for an autumn in scientific endeavour, perhaps a restorative, contemplative phase of receptivity and winter, from which can stem a higher and more wholesome scientific methodology.

Current biochemical thinking follows much the same pattern of explanatory thinking as that of the early chemists. $NaOH + HCl = NaCl + H_2O$, for example, perhaps with a catalyst (enzyme) over the '='s sign. This kind of theory or model is useful up to a certain point, but in physiological terms the necessary route maps would need not only to be extremely complex, but also multi–dimensional to accommodate the new discoveries concerning the biomagnetic, bioelectronic and similar energetic aspects of the body.

As with all good concepts, what is required is a theory which takes the common denominators out of the maze in order to provide a simple substrate or matrix into which all existing observable phenomena, with their particular modes of expression and conceptualization can be readily fitted. Some of these concepts can then be discarded, whilst others are retained for their practical value, just as the advent of Einstein did not make Newton obsolete, (just more relative).

Clearly, the basis of any such theory should be the established fact that all which we perceive (and I would include all which we do not perceive, as well) *is* energy. *Not contains energy, but IS energy.* The vibrating, scintillating dance of energy. From an eastern point of view, this idea is already well established and in some considerable practical detail, as in acupuncture and Ayurvedic medicine. Our western scientific thinking, however, requires us to be more analytical in our approach from without and I would suggest a model of bodily interactions which includes *energy pattern resonance and polarity* (in which are included molecular concepts, as one aspect). Thus, a molecular interaction now described in the conventional manner of molecular diagrams is 'floated' into a more composite and less straight-jacketed picture in which the molecular and atomic forces are given prominence in one's conceptual, mental image of the events and of the body itself. That is, *the body, mind and emotions – at both subtle and gross levels – are seen as one vibrating, integrated, energetic whole.*

Remember that a molecule itself is simply an integrated aggregate of subatomic particles and forces, spun out of the fabric of vacuum or akash and held together by movement and energy within the vacuum state itself. And in living forms, under the formative, pranic patterning from within, every subatomic particle, atom and molecule is moved in its own appointed manner.

The control network is complete, with no place for randomness or chance. Resonance and vibration or oscillation, together with polarized energy fields, also require mathematical formulation, bringing the molecular science of biochemistry and the expressions of modern theoretical physics into one fused whole, in a more basic understanding of energetic interactions.

I would also suggest that models should look for specific resonances related to the five subtle tattvic fields and pranic vibrations inherent in the role of the chakras, with some importance given to electromagnetic and magnetic properties of both biological substances and organisms as a whole. The work of John Evans, discussed in his book, *Mind, Body and Electromagnetism* is full of adventurous ideas which he has already taken into the realm of electromagnetism and mathematics. His largely theoretical mapping, using computer graphics, of possible electrical harmonics and waveforms in the spine are both fascinating and worthy of deeper, applied research.

I have, however, seen it written that prana and electromagnetism or kundalini and electromagnetism are equatable. This is, of course, incorrect as any serious student of yoga could point out, though electromagnetic energies are indeed getting close to the point of subtlety in matter where we could say that we are moving into subtle energy fields. But electromagnetic energies and all observable material substance or energy are manifested *out* of the vacuum or gross akashic state and the more subtle tattvic energy fields. They therefore bear a harmonic imprint of their immediately inward creative form.

The Anterior Pituitary Lobe

Returning once again to the endocrine aspects, the remainder of this chapter is somewhat biochemical in nature and may be read lightly if such details hold no appeal for you. The last section, however, does contain a discussion of the highly ordered state of physiological processes as well as an analysis of posterior pituitary function according to the fundamental principles of polarity. These may be of more general interest.

The pituitary gland, then – also known as the *hypophysis* – inhabits a small bony cavity at the base of the brain to which it is attached by a short stem or stalk. It consists, as we have said, of two lobes comprised of quite different cellular types.

The anterior pituitary is innervated with autonomic nerve fibres, though whether these are involved with direct endocrine control or simply regulate other physiological aspects of general cellular functioning, such as the blood supply, is not known. Similarly, although there are numerous cell types found within its tissues, their specific roles have only recently been identified with regard to which cells are responsible for the secretion of which individual hormones. The precise biochemical mechanisms are, as yet, little understood.

In addition to the hormones which are linked with the hypothalamic releasing or inhibiting substances in the overall control of the other endocrine glands, the anterior pituitary produces at least two hormones which have a primary effect on physiological processes, though both of these are linked to hypothalamic and neurophysical control.

These are *Growth Hormone (GH)*, also called *somatotropin*, and prolactin. GH promotes the proliferation of cells and hence growth in both soft tissues, as well as bone and cartilage. Hypoproduction in childhood leads to the classic case of dwarfism, whilst over-production results in giantism. In adult life, too much GH leads to tissue thickening and continued bone growth, the condition known as *agromegaly*, while under-production results in a wasting away of bodily tissues.

GH affects practically all aspects of metabolism, more particularly those processes that lead to synthesis of proteins, carbohydrates and fats. Sodium, potassium, calcium and other blood electrolyte concentrations are increased and almost the entire metabolic network is either directly or indirectly affected.

GH release is believed to be controlled by hypothalamic secretions which are themselves influenced by feedback from the body's autonomic nervous system. Hypothalamic *somatostatin*, which we previously encountered in the pancreas, is thought to be an *inhibitor* of GH release and a contrary *GH Releasing Hormone (GHRH)* is thought to have been isolated and identified. It is also known that oestrogen stimulates GH release, perhaps by altering the ability of hypothalamic hormones to influence the pituitary GH-producing cells.

Prolactin, on the other hand, is a polypeptide or protein with a very similar structure to that of GH. It is controlled, once again, via the hypothalamus, where the neurohormone dopamine has been implicated in hypothalamic inhibition of prolactin release. No role for prolactin has yet been established in males, but in women, prolactin release is mediated by nervous messages from sensory receptors, especially around the nipples of breast-feeding women.

Prolactin stimulates the production of breast milk, but even for this one function to be effective, the presence of many other hormones is required. These include oestrogens, the thyroid hormones, insulin, cortico-steroids, and with the high calcium content of milk, the parathyroid hormone and calcitonin will also be inevitably involved.

It has also been suggested that prolactin is quite generally implicated in reproductive function, and general metabolic effects that are similar to those of GH have also been observed, but the pathways, mechanisms and functions are not at all comprehended at the present time. It is clear, however, that milk must be one of the most carefully balanced and controlled secretions of the human body. The young infant is totally dependent upon this nutritional source for the ongoing development of its body. Every nutritional molecule that goes into its body comes from this milk. So its control from a high point, involving the integration of many other bodily processes, endocrine and otherwise, is just what one would expect.

Similarly, with GH, where the administration of overall body growth in all its multitudinous ramifications requires the unconscious formative intelligence of the higher subtle centre.

It is for this reason, I suspect, that while the endocrine activity of the adrenals, gonads and pancreas has been quite well defined, at least in essential outline, the finer and multitudinous workings of the three higher centres is only sketchily understood. The increasing detail of the intricately woven and airy thymus administration of the immuno-defence system, followed by the general metabolic control implemented at the thyroid centre, and the overall organization provided by the pituitary-hypothalamic link up, not to mention the involvement of the brain centres, leaves medical science only grasping at bits and pieces of the total mechanism. This is enough to identify the relationships of these activities to the more subtle centres, but in terms of understanding how the whole show is put together in its entirety, medical science has thus far taken only a few steps.

The Molecular Matrix and the Posterior Pituitary

Within the posterior lobe of the pituitary gland, there is an interesting polarity expressed which also allows us to speculate about functions beyond the current knowledge of modern endocrinology.

As explained, the posterior pituitary lobe is an extension of neurons from the hypothalamus down which the two hormones of *vasopressin* and *oxytocin* migrate for their release into the blood conveyor belt, through the posterior pituitary blood capilliary plexus. Both hormones are concerned with fluid control, and with water taking up sixty-five per cent of our bodies, providing a continuous and connecting matrix for biochemical and physiological activity, this is a major function requiring control from a point of high jurisdiction. Vasopressin is anti-diuretic in its activity. That is, it increases water retention in the body, thereby regulating the concentration of electrolytes and osmotically active substances in body fluids – sodium, for example, being one of them.

So while the thyroid hormones are concerned with the speed of molecular activity on the surface of the vacuum state, the posterior pituitary could perhaps be implicated in the concentration and positioning of active molecules within the watery matrix, the whole of which being manifested out of the gross akashic condition.

The total volume of water within the body has a direct effect upon blood pressure and hence upon the highly important movement of substances around the body. In fact, the increase in blood pressure induced by large quantities of vasopressin was its first outwardly observed function, and from which its name is derived. But such large quantities are normally produced in the body only in exceptional circumstances such as haemorrage, when a large quantity of lost blood requires the immediate participation of vasopressin to maintain blood pressure.

Again, picking up externally observable clues to the inner biochemical functioning of vasopressin, it has been seen to exhibit a stimulating effect upon the synthesis of pituitary adrenocorticotropic hormone, as well as upon certain behavioural influences related to memory and learning in rats.

Oxytocin on the other hand has as its established dual physiological functions, simply the control of uterine contractions at the time of birth and the ejection of breast milk, in response to tactile stimulation of the breasts, or suckling in the lactating mother. Beyond that, present research is at a loss, and in males, oxytocin is a hormone without a cause, though there is some evidence to suggest that it is implicated in male sexual arousal and ejaculation.

Lawrence Crapo in his marvellously entertaining book, *Hormones – The Messengers Of Life*, makes the comment, "God alone knows why these two hormones, so different in function, are so similar in structure and so intimately associated in the pituitary." I would like to suggest that a possible and simple answer is that oxytocin has a role in physiological water balance that is the polar opposite of vasopressin. Vasopressin is known to conserve water. In this respect it is yin. Oxytocin is recognized as acting upon what the yogic philosopy would call the procreative aspect of the jal or water tattwa. In this case, it is a mechanism of watery ejection, of yang – whether of uterine or mammary origin.

The mechanisms of bodily water balance are, of course, beautifully intricate and current medical knowledge is already aware of many factors which influence it. All the same, I would conjecture that oxytocin will be found ultimately to have a converse role on water balance at a very fine level within the body, to that of vasopressin. More particularly is this so, because up to the present time oxytocin has no known role in a man, who has no use for uterine contractions or breast milk.

However, there is another interesting aspect to all of this. The concept of bodily water as a matrix, formed out of the interlinking dipole molecules of H_2O, like iron filings in a magnetic field, is not without some scientific corroboration. Some scientists have suggested that water forms long and connected molecules in strings, through alignment due to the magnetic polarization of its simple, basic molecular structure.

The work of Russian scientist, A.P. Dubrov of the Acadamy of Sciences of the USSR, is of considerable relevance here. In his book, *The Geomagnetic Field and Life*, he discusses the effects of the earth's magnetic field upon water and has some interesting comments to make regarding the properties of water itself. Dubrov argues that what Russian scientists call the bio-plasma, and which I would call the pranas and the subtle tattvic states of matter, is responsible for maintaining all the water in the body in a *highly organized state*, such as is found normally only in superconducting materials at the extremely low temperatures approaching that of absolute zero.

Investigations into the thermodynamics of cellular metabolism shows that although the actively metabolizing cell should become increasingly hot, due to the work performed, it manages, in fact, to maintain itself at a highly specific temperature of 37°C or 98.4°F. Any deviations from this, outside a very narrow range, leave us feeling rather ill. The purpose or reasons underlying an increased body temperature during illness is itself of great interest, but it only takes very small changes – up or down – to result in death.

Dubrov proposes, with considerable experimental evidence, that the cell itself has a unique method of maintaining a constant body temperature, "involving continuous microphasic transitions of intracellular water and proteins from the liquid to the crystalline state". Since this process involves the absorption and liberation of heat, the body's ability to modify the frequency of this liquid-to-crystal and crystal-to-liquid oscillation therefore becomes a mechanism by which it is capable of finely tuning the regulation of cellular and hence total bodily heat. In conjunction with mechanisms related to changes in environmental temperature, the body is thus able to maintain an exactly even temperature. Dubrov also quotes another Russian scientist, Trincher, who asserts that the "water inside the cell is in a state of *maximum order*", pointing out that this state is only attainable in non-living matter at temperatures of absolute zero.

Dubrov summarizes his thinking quite succinctly, when he says: "Thus if we adopt as a basis the new thermodynamic concepts advanced by Trincher, we must assume either that biological processes take place, however paradoxical it sounds, at very large negative temperatures, or that in living systems, by the operation of a special mechanism of action of the biogravitational field, which creates specific conditions, there are effects dependent on molecular membrane biological superconductivity. This is not accomplished by the use of a complex cryogenic technique, of course, but by means of special processes in biological molecules, whose function is based on specific laws of living matter, which will be understood by science in the future."

The power to maintain this degree of order in a complex molecular system, well away from temperatures of absolute zero is provided from within the subtle energy fields under the morphogenic influence of the pranas. But at the biochemical level we can expect to find a patterned system that reflects this activity. Whether vasopressin and oxytocin are involved in this ordering of the watery and molecular matrix is open to speculation, but clearly there must be some outwardly observable mechanisms which specifically influence it.

Dubrov implicates the north and south polarity of the geomagnetic field as one factor and the bioelectrical and biomagnetic aspects of the body are no doubt, another. They are probably interlinked. But these factors are themselves operative only through the molecular, atomic and subatomic nature of material substance.

Actually, when one looks at the ordered structure of the macroscopic world, when one examines the detailed order that lies within the molecule and the atom, when one observes the amazingly complex, yet thoroughly integrated mechanisms of physiology and biochemistry, when one considers the brain and thought processes and bodily control – it becomes quite clear that a master intelligence is at work. It could be no other way. Similarly, the distribution of molecules around the body cannot be random. It has to have *maximum order* for that organization to manifest itself at more macroscopic levels.

"Not a leaf stirs, but by His order", says the Indian mystic, Guru Nanak. "Even the hairs of your head are all numbered", says Christ. Perhaps a modern science equivalent might be, "No subatomic particle spins into existence, but under His guidance".

It means therefore that the life force, manifesting through the pranas, holds every subatomic particle, every atom and every molecule in place. If there is a pattern, it has to be complete, even at the most detailed level. The organization has to very tightly controlled. And a control point from a high level of administration in the body for the oscillations and patterning of this linked bodily matrix would therefore be a necessity, and the vibrational structure of vasopressin and oxytocin could perhaps provide one aspect of this coordination, in respect of the molecular arrangement of bodily H_2O.

Like the two sides of a coin, these two hormones also have a very similar origin and final structure (they are both derived from similar precursor molecules), both containing nine amino acids each, the difference reflecting their functional polarity.

And note that their joint derivation from a common precursor is a requirement for any balanced energy equations expressing the polarity present between them. Thus, if the precursor is considered to be at zero, then the yin (negative) and the yang (positive) components are split off, each molecular change being mediated by a further vibrating molecular and subatomic structure, observed at the molecular level as an enzyme.

Represented schematically, this becomes:

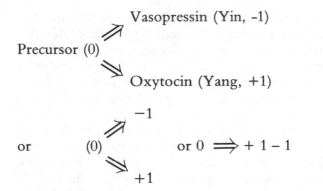

Overall balance is thus preserved. The exact nature of the energy involved in this expression of polarity remaining, at present obscure.

It therefore becomes almost axiomatic that balanced pairs of hormones with polar opposite effects will be derived from one common precursor. And we do most certainly find this to be the case in many, if not all, instances.

Thus, more generally, we have:

Yin Hormone, −1, Inhibits, Female

Hormone Precursor, 0

Yang Hormone, +1, Stimulates, Male

The sex hormones are another similar example, where the underlying polarity is even split between two types of physical body, appearing outwardly as the sexes. The natural attraction of the two poles, manifested as our sex drive or desire to be with the opposite sex, is nature's way of priming the energy system or recoiling the spring, so that procreation and reproduction will be assured of taking place.

In terms of molecular derivation and balanced equations of energy, both oestrogens and androgens need to have the same precursor – which they do in the molecule of cholesterol. The sexual polarity of the individual body determines which enzymes are present and the appropriately polarized splitting into predominantly male or predominantly female molecular patterns or hormones, ensues.

In fact, as we discussed earlier in chapters five and six, *all* steroid hormones have this same precursor, demonstrating that when energetically split, the one relatively inert substance of cholesterol is revealed as an inwardly balanced spectrum of possibilities, much as white light is split into a rainbow by the enzyme-like catalyst of a prism or of raindrops.

Perhaps, therefore, cholesterol build-up is also due to a failure in the energetic mechanisms by which it is split and modified into its full spectrum of possibilities. In modern therapeutic parlance, the phrase used is 'energy blockages'.

Where there is a correlation or a connection, there has to be an underlying 'reason', though ultimately it may not be couched in intellectual terms. So while Dr Crapo and many other scientists appear to be convinced of the horizontal evolution of life from innate dust and water (but how did that dust and water come into being?), I have always felt that the answer to such deep questions must lie in another, more mystical direction and that order and determinism underlie all the phenomena of our universe, perceived and unperceived. I cannot believe that life in *any* of its multitudinous and intricate aspects, is a function of pure chance. It is simply that in the presence of so much data and the absence of a knowledge concerning the underlying principles, a statistical approach based on the laws of chance (but how can *chance* have *laws*?) is the only way of determining or predicting what is likely to happen. It is possible, for example, to predict how many people will be in Cambridge on a tuesday afternoon in november, based on the laws of statistics and chance. But ask any one of those people how they came to be there and they will all have a deterministic answer.

Similarly, every subatomic particle, every force, every pattern and manifestation of energy exists by inward design, determinism and in a state of maximum order.

Therefore, even in simple matters such as why these two posterior pituitary hormones are similar in their amino acid content and arrangement, there has to be a pattern, the whole of which is simply unclear to us. And in this instance, there are other observable factors linking them together, so there has to be an underlying determinism.

CHAPTER 11

Energy, Language, Creation and Consciousness

Complex Energetic Ramifications

It is, I believe, important to realize that from without, we can only observe gross and obvious changes – getting fatter or thinner, bumps or swellings, blood pressure, skin texture and so on – while at a biochemical level we observe only the most obvious interactions. 'Obvious' being a somewhat relative word. And while medical research recognizes that the vast majority of the finer biochemical pathways remain unidentified, the still further detail, patterning and molecular correspondences are more or less an entire mystery.

But this does not mean that substances like vasopressin, oxytocin and many other of the recently discovered neuro-peptides are not performing vital roles that may not be understandable at all in terms of purely biochemical interactions. For their elucidation, even at a purely physical level, it may well be necessary to consider electronic, magnetic and subatomic aspects of molecular nature, a study for which there are few, if any, established methodologies or even adequate experimental instrumentation.

For if we really are dealing with physical manifestation as it first appears out of the vacuum condition, from a highly integrated formative energy state, then nothing can be considered either as random, nor as unimportant. Even the positioning of molecules upon the three dimensional surface of vacuum is of relevance. The patterning of dancing subatomic polkadots is both determined and of relevance in terms of outward understanding. And without any comprehension of inner causation – or even with it – one is forced to view this enormously complex molecular churning in a quantum statistical fashion. Thus providing yet another new and possible paradigm for the life sciences – quantum biology!

Body, Mind and Neuro-Endocrine Linkages

One is reminded, at this point, of molecular stereo-isomers, (see pages 31 & 133), where each (otherwise apparently identical) isomer has in some respects opposing properties to the other. Indeed, certain hormones are already known to be active only in their naturally occurring, stereo-polarity. So in respect of the response at target sites around the body, it becomes a question once again of energy patterning, the interplay of polarities as the driving force behind motion and manifestation, and of resonance or completion of energy patterns, somewhat like the fitting of pieces into a machine which will not work until the last component is in place. Though in this case there is a difference in that our human 'machine' is constantly moving and vibrating in all its many parts and aspects.

The neurohormone connection (inherent in hypothalamic and posterior pituitary activity) and its apparent polarity is also found once again, and quite clearly, in the adrenal glands where the medullary hormone of epinephrine or adrenaline is produced. Adrenaline is the hormone relating external circumstances which require whole body/mind action to inner biochemical, as well as mental, preparedness. The nervous system in its entirety – sensual, motor and autonomic – is thus completely involved both with the input of the original information leading to release of adrenaline, and in its response to adrenaline itself. In fact, in energetic terms, adrenaline would appear to increase the vibrational rate of self-preservative metabolic function by several harmonics, if not whole octaves. For this reason, therefore, whilst adrenaline is actually produced in the earthy, preservative, rectal centre, it is also found – and especially its analogue, noradrenaline – in the brain and throughout the nervous system. It is a key vibration related to survival within the energetic molecular complex of the body.

Similarly, there is an emotional aspect to almost all endocrine activity. Menstrual cycles and ovulation, for example, are affected by emotion and stress, whilst deficiency or overactivity in any of the endocrine glands leads to emotional modifications – depression, hyperactivity and instability of one kind or another.

Another example of a similar kind of linkage is found in patients with *Diabetes mellitus*, or an inability to store body fuels for later release of energy due to defective pancreatic synthesis of insulin. This would appear to be indicative of an imbalance in the subtle fire energy and an inability of this aspect of bodily function to enter the yin, or more specifically, in Chinese terminology, the metal and water, conditions (see pages 33–40). One would also expect to discover personality traits in diabetic patients which reflect this outward condition both in the present and during their pre-diabetic days.

The biochemical link between mental, emotional and physical energies via the subtle energy interface is thus highly apparent in endocrinology, feeding back through the subtle energy network into the vibrational nature of each molecule, as well as the central and peripheral nervous systems. The human being is one, whole integrated energy complex, as we have said many times!

Ordered Molecular Patterns and Biological Transmutation of Elements

There are a number of quite fascinating possibilities which emerge when one begins investigating the detailed ordering of biological systems and some of the bioelectrical and biomagnetic aspects were discussed in my previous book, *Subtle Energy*. But as we have frequently discussed, molecules and hence subatomic particles too, are more intricately ordered in living organisms than in dead matter, due to the presence of the life force. In inert objects, the creative power of the primal Shabda or Word is present only in a diffuse form, holding it together in organized, created manifestation, but without the expression of life.

Thus, when physicists study inert substance in particle accelerators, they are studying the manifestation of matter, devoid of the biogravitational life force of prana. And only at very high energies and under extremely artificial circumstances, too. No physicist has yet been able to peep in on the day-to-day subatomic activity in normal objects like this piece of paper you are reading, watching the interplay as a detached spectator. All current experiments at the subatomic level require intensely energetic *interaction* under very specific circumstances.

And absolutely no such experiments have ever been performed on living organisms, for very obvious reasons. Even modern medical techniques like magnetic nuclear spin resonance are only measuring general effects of atomic activity.

So the highly ordered structure of living matter remains a subject for scientific speculation, on the one hand, or subtle perception through yogic practice, on the other. Or a combination of both.

The Russian scientist, Dubrov, whom we mentioned in the previous chapter, possesses a penetrating insight into possible biological mechanisms and is, like myself, intrigued by the different effects and occurence of L and D isomers in nature. Dubrov sees this as related to the asymetry of the geomagnetic field (i.e. north is different from south), as well as its diurnal and longer rhythmicity, for the earth's magnetic field can couple to charged subatomic particles through the magnetic field generated by particle spin. He suggests that all these phenomena are related through biological and biochemical symmetry and dissymetry. That is, another form of energetic polarity.

His reasoning and evidence is exciting, though too complex to reproduce here, but he does raise the case of the French scientist, C.L. Kervran, who, as a result of years of detailed and painstaking research, demonstrated quite conclusively that living matter is actually able to transmute the atomic or chemical elements as they are known to Mendeleev's periodic table. The non-transmutability of the chemical elements, except at ultra-high energies or by spontaneous radioactive decay, is a sacred cow of science that we are all taught in schools, and I must myself admit to an instinctive rejection of the idea when first presented with the data. The evidence, however, is pretty conclusive.

Looked at from a subatomic point of view, with an understanding of the biogravitational force of nature operating as an 'understood' law, one can see how the *rearrangement* of the subatomic structure of atoms upon the surface of vacuum, under the patterning power from within, can readily come to pass. For, according to

Dubrov's analysis, those transmutations which are known to occur can be attributed to the fact that the atoms of the elements involved possess mirror symmetry, relative to each other. Such transformations include potassium to sodium, magnesium to calcium, iron to manganese, silicon to aluminium and so on. In fact, Dubrov points out that Mendeleev's entire table can be re-presented as sets of dyads or pairs of elements possessing mirror symmetry, which are thus more readily capable of transformation into each other.

Furthermore, in L and D isometric molecules it follows that the L form is comprised of L carbon atoms and the D form, of D carbon atoms. It seems probable, too, that the formation of L and D isomers may be due to subtle energy polarities, reflecting in the direction of subatomic, atomic and molecular spin. This would also explain the rotation of electromagnetic energy, such as light, as it interacts upon the vacuum surface with the spinning, subatomic 'particles' of matter. Stereo-isometry could thus be seen as another aspect of energetic polarity, of yin and yang. Clearly, particle spin and other aspects of subatomic polarity are of great importance for the balance of harmonious energetic function in living creatures. Interestingly, the north and south magnetic poles, which have yin and yang effects, respectively, upon living organisms, are also characterized by clockwise and anticlockwise electron spin within the magnetic field. This is discussed in greater detail in my previous book, *Subtle Energy*.

Kervran suggested that the atomic transmutations occur because there are certain, more stable atomic structures which are able to unite and separate without any change in the internal structure of the atom. He also speculates that the driving force effecting the change is the weak nuclear force, already known to be implicated in particle transmutations in inert matter.

And to this, I would of course add that it is the power of the life force which drives and directs all such changes from a more inward point, maintaining – as we discussed towards the end of the previous chapter – a state of *maximum order* in all living tissue.

These special, stable atoms possessing the power to transmute others are the commonest ones found within living substance. They include, hydrogen ($_1$H), oxygen ($_{16}$O), carbon ($_{12}$C), silicon ($_{28}$Si) and boron ($_{11}$B), whilst some examples of transmutations are:[1]

$$_{12}C + _{12}C \rightarrow _{24}Mg \qquad\qquad _{23}Na + _1H \rightarrow _{24}Mg$$

$$_{12}C + _{12}C + _{16}O \rightarrow _{40}Ca$$

$$_{39}K + _1H \rightarrow _{40}Ca \qquad\qquad _{24}Mg + _{16}O \rightarrow _{40}Ca$$

The full significance, therefore, of the organizing power of the life force from within has yet to be realized by modern science. For there is a tremendous difference between inert matter and substance bound into the external and physical vehicle of expression of a living soul within.

Consider, for instance, any of the apparently minor molecular changes which take place to make a previously inactive bodily substance highly energetically active. Have a look at figures 9-2 and 9-3 which demonstrate how the simple positioning of the iodine atom in the subatomic vibratory complex makes all the difference to the total activity of the molecule. Or study the similarities between the steroid hormones, especially testosterone and oestrogen in figures 5-4 and 5-5. Thinking of a molecule as an energetic, oscillating subatomic complex spun out of the tapestry of the vacuum matrix, one can perceive how our current manner of biochemical presentation is conceptually lacking. It is clear that the simple presentation on paper of the positioning of an iodine atom in the thyroid hormone, T3, for example, or the exchange of an OH for an O and the addition of a CH_3, differentiating testosterone from oestrogen, does not reveal the true energetic change that has taken place within that vibrating molecule and the manner in which it relates to other bodily molecules.

Perhaps, for example, the position of the iodine, OH, O or CH_3 is the trigger that reverses or resets the subatomic

---

[1] $_{39}$K = potassium, $_{23}$Na = sodium, $_{24}$Mg = Magnesium and $_{40}$Ca = Calcium. The number represents the atomic weight. This reflects the number of protons and neutrons in their atomic nucleus and, along with the surrounding electrons, is usually considered to be the factor which actually makes one chemical element different from another.

spin and oscillation into a totally different mode, much as a complex piece of machinery may move into another mode of operation at the pull of a simple lever, or the push of a single button. Or looked at inwardly, the patterning pranic vibration of the life force upon the vacuum matrix automatically results in the realignment of molecular vibration whereby iodine atoms are drawn in and repositioned, or testosterone is formed in preference to oestrogen.

In this context, too, it is also interesting to analyze our concepts of heat and temperature. Heat is essentially a sensory *experience*, a part of the sensation of touch, while temperature is a measure of the degree of molecular agitation that we experience as heat.

When this agitation, or vibration, is too much, then molecules are destroyed, which we experience and observe as being burnt. When this disturbance is too low, then not enough activity is present for bodily processes to continue and below a certain point the water molecules switch into the permanently solid lattice of ice.

At extremely high temperatures the agitation becomes such that the molecules break down into atoms and then the atoms break down into their constituent charged nuclei and electrons. This is known as a plasma, a whirling soup of charged particles, and is thought to be the material constituting the sun and most stars. In a sense, this is the pure fiery tattwa or state of matter, in its gross physical form.

At the lower end of the spectrum, there is a point at which the subatomic constituents of molecules are in their lowest state of energy. They cannot become less motionless or torpid. This is the temperature of absolute zero, equivalent to $-273.15°C$ or $-459.67°F$. The sun, on the other hand is thought to reach temperatures of around twenty million degrees centigrade (20×10^6 °C) in its core. So it is interesting to note that our body is sensitive to tiny changes in temperature of less than 1°C and is able to maintain itself at that temperature with tremendous accuracy despite a wide range of both environmental as well as biochemical changes. One wonders just what it is that is so special about 37°C or 98.4°F.

The speed of energetic transformations, however, within the molecules of living organisms even at these comparatively low temperatures is quite phenomenal. Energetic transfers and changes between molecules can occur in intervals of less than a nanosecond (10^{-9} seconds, or 0.000000001 seconds), while changes within a molecule, the movement of a hydrogen atom from one location to another, for example, and the associated restructuring of the bonds within the molecule may take only one tenth of a picosecond or 10^{-13} seconds.

The detail, the speed and the accuracy of biological mechanisms is therefore immense and it beats me how anyone can really think that the whole thing came into and is maintained in existence by 'chance'.

The presence of the patterning life force from within is essential for the continuance of life's processes.

Correlation, Complexity and Energy Models of the Body

I have done my best throughout the chapters of this book to describe enough of both the physiological and biochemical pathways, as well as the subtle and life energy aspects, to paint just a general picture. Too exhaustive a survey of endocrinological ramifications would have become boring to some readers and I only want to present enough of the known facts for any interested person to get an overall picture of what is going on. Beyond that there are many excellent books on physiology and biochemistry, though there are only a few really informed books on the inner practices of yoga.

As I commented in an earlier chapter, the yogic way of looking at the body from within-out and the modern scientific method of looking from without-in are both observing the same phenomena of life, the same energetic interplay. The method of observation, however, makes all the difference in terms of how we experience and describe it, and yet the parallels must be there if both are valid. It makes little sense for each to feel that they are on opposing sides of the fence. "East is East and West is West, and never the twain shall meet", is a fallacy, as this and other books by like-minded people are endeavouring to show. Indeed the inner yogic perception of the universe enhances and complements our western view of things.

It is clear, of course, that each endocrine gland is not a

pure reflection of the tattwa and pranic vibration that gives rise to its existence. The matrix of subtle tattvic energies are admixed by the point at which gross physical manifestation has taken place and certainly when they are bound up into complex organic life patterns.

Thus, for example, while the thyroid is generally the largest endocrine gland in the body weighing something like twenty grams, quite clearly it is not in itself comprised of pure vacuum or akash, but is, like all other bodily organs, an admixture at the physiological level of all the five gross tattvic conditions. Its *administration* and area of functionality, however, is derived from the akashic state – the gateway from the gross to the subtle tattwas, and then again from the subtle to mental level of thought and allied energies.

Similarly, we can see that the complexity of the roles played by these tattwas is reflected in the number of petals that are spun into the chakras by the morphogenic pranic vibration, creating the pranic pathways or nadis.

At the lower levels, there is some degree of correspondence between the number of these petals and the hormones produced. There are, for example, four petals to the rectal chakra and four main groups of adrenal hormones. But even this may not be a meaningful parallel, for we are dealing with *areas of functionality* that are administered through each chakra and though the endocrine glands represent a major aspect of this functioning, they do not, of course, represent the whole. It is possible, though, that these four areas of functionality are reflected in many different ways at the outward physiological level, the four main groups of adrenal hormones being just one of many.

At the sacral centre, which has six petals, the gonads are responsible for germ cell genesis and maturation, as well as maintenance of the reproductive organs and secondary sexual characteristics. The subtle watery tattwa also gives rise to the fluids in the body and their local organization. One could probably figure out six functional headings for this area, but I am by no means sure that this would be a valid way of understanding the manifestation of the more subtle pranic functionality. And the interrelationship of the tattwas and chakras would also require consideration and elucidation in any such model.

Then, proceeding higher, we find the eight-petalled fiery centre with part of its organizational reflection lying in the pancreas, also possessing both exocrine and endocrine activity. Above that, lies the airy centre with twelve petals and an even more complex and far reaching function. On the one hand, it is responsible for the distribution of bodily oxygen from the lungs to the tissues and the transport of carbon dioxide back to the lungs for elimination, and in the more inward biochemistry, the protective aspects of the immune defence system is overseen from this subtle centre.

Similarly, as we have described, the increasingly detailed and far reaching control of the akashic element is reflected in the sixteen petals of the throat chakra with its endocrine aspect of general metabolic rate control, its finger resting upon every molecular and subatomic button. Here the complexity is such that the endocrine function is separated into two glands containing opposite polarities, as we see in the converse roles of PTH and calcitonin. At present, no other parathyroid hormone has been found and there may be none, but if found one would speculate on its possession of a converse role to that of the thyroid hormones, T3 and T4.

In the ajna chakra, we are presented in most yogic texts with just the major polarity inherent in its twin petals and reflecting in the endocrine and neurophysical linkage of the anterior pituitary and the posterior pituitary/ hypothalamus. Leadbeater and other theosophists have claimed, long before the advent of current knowledge concerning these glands, that each of these two lobes are themselves split into forty-eight further sub-lobes or petals. Bear in mind the complex interactions of these two endocrine centres with each other and with the lower centres. Then add to this, our knowledge concerning the host of recently discovered neuropeptides in both of these glands, plus the multitudinous neurophysiological aspects of hypothalamic and posterior pituitary functioning, and one can readily see how two times forty-eight or ninety-six petals or functional aspects could be defined for the outwardly manifested activities of this centre, if not as specific hormonal molecules themselves.

The white and black colours ascribed to the two petals

of this chakra also reflect its commanding position. For just as white light contains within it the vibrations of all the colours of the full spectrum, so too does the ajna chakra contain within it a reflection of all the varying colours of the five lower chakras. And just as white light is our experience of this admixture of electromagnetic vibration at the physical level, so too is it the way we experience the energetic aspects of this chakra as the vibrational source of all the lower chakras, with their coloured petals.

The differentiation of this chakra into white and black presumably reflects the manner in which the inflow and outflow of energy are experienced when consciousness is focused at this point.

Actually, these petals make an interesting study in a similar direction. Look for a moment at their mathematical sequencing:

$$2(96) \quad 16 \quad 12 \quad 8 \quad 6 \quad 4$$

Twice 4 (earth) makes 8 (fire) and twice 8 makes 16 (akash). Similarly, twice 6 (water) makes 12 (air).

Musically, this represents a *harmonious* partial chord, thus:

$$(C) \quad C \quad G \quad C \quad G \quad C$$

The total number of petals equals 48, with the ajna chakra containing within each of its two petals or polarities a resonance to each of the other chakras. And this is exactly what happens when the endocrine activity of the lower glands feeds back to the pituitary/hypothalamic centre. There is an energetic response or a resonance, resulting in inhibition (yin) or stimulation (yang), depending upon the direction of molecular activity, to or from the higher centre.

John Evans, in his book *Mind, Body and Electromagnetism*, takes this mathematics some considerable way further and it is worth deeper study.

"As above, so below." Just as the thousand-petalled lotus, the Sahans-dal-Kanwal at the heart of the astral realm, (sometimes referred to as the crown chakra), is the energy powerhouse of all below, yet it has itself come into being as a result of interaction in the more inward energy currents of which it is itself comprised.[2] Similarly does every molecule or energy pattern in the body arise due to interactions at a more inward or subtle level. Each molecule arises, moves and has its being because of the structure and relationships within the more subtle energy fields. Each molecule bears a harmonic relationship to inward function and energetic activity.

If the specific nature and structure of *these* energy fields could be modelled, *then* we would possess a model of body function that would be of inestimable value.

A Natural Language in the Akashic Fields

There is one final and fascinating aspect of these chakric petals. As I mentioned earlier, each petal represents an energy vibration which can actually be experienced when the attention of the individual is focused within in specific yogic practices. That experience is made possible through the inner indriyas of sight and hearing. That is, each petal has both a visible and an audible aspect.

It is said that the ancient rishis and yogis, hearing these sounds used them for the fashioning of the language known to them as *Sandhya Basha*, described by some scholars as the *Twilight Language*.

In this language, it is also said that there are no words for material and physical objects, but only for spiritual and higher subjects. Whether this is true or not I have no idea, but its final physical outcome has become Sanskrit, with which is it very similar. And in the Sanskrit language there are 48 major sounds or letters[3], each derived from one of the petals on the six chakras within the physical body. It is for this reason that Sanskrit is often called the "Language of the Gods".

This idea of what is essentially a natural language encoded into the akashic level of man's existence, reflecting the patterning of physical life, below, and linked into the patterning of his antashkarans, ready for conscious use, is quite fascinating, for it means that given a higher

---

[2] See the prologue to *Subtle Energy*.
[3] Some texts say that there are 50 or 52 characters in the Sanskrit alphabet, those would presumably include two sounds not normally written, and two 'breathings' or sound modifications.

consciousness, man would possess an *instinctive* language; that we have not been born into a Tower of Babel, but have only made it so by our lower consciousness.

Indeed, in the mystic cosmology of the Vedas it is said that man progresses cyclically through four ages or yugas – *Sat Yuga, Tretar Yuga, Dwarpar Yuga* and *Kal Yuga*. Of these, *Sat* means truth, and *Kal* means the Universal Mind, Time, Death or the Negative Power.

At the present moment in history we are at a point of up-turn in the Kal Yuga, where man's lifespan is short due to the low conditions currently prevailing and to our low level of consciousness, creating disharmonious and hence diseased conditions. But during the Sat Yuga, man's inner estate was of a far higher and finer vibration. This was reflected in his level of spiritual awareness and consciousness of the higher realms within himself. And if man ever had a natural language, it would have been spoken or used almost telepathically at that time.

And this explains, too, why there are so many words in our various languages that quite clearly have the same root. Language is something we all use constantly without ever really attempting to understand where it came from. Linguists have, of course, attempted to trace back whether there is one common origin for all language, though inconclusively, for the time scale has become so long and the trail of progression, so obscured. The existence of a natural language could further explain why words and phrases often possess a most revealing meaning above that which we normally ascribe to them. The word 'human' itself, for example, comes from the latin 'hominus', possessing a possible arabic derivation meaning soul (hu) and mind (man). And in both Hindi and Sanskrit 'man' also means mind, whilst 'homen' is the word for ego, a built-in characteristic of both mind and man.

Similarly, with the origin of many expressions, a few of which I have used in this book to demonstrate an intrinsic knowledge. 'A dry fish', 'have a heart', 'dis-ease', 'uni-verse' and so on. The derivation of the word 'universe' is of particular interest. Literally, it means to 'turn on One' or to 'turn (or move) as One'. Clearly, the originators of the word had a more holistic perception of life than our science of today!

So the possibility of a natural language as an intrinsic part of the mechanism which gives us intelligence does make considerable sense. For if birds can possess an instinctive subtle pattern for migration or nest-building, and if so many abilities both in humans and other species are an integral part of the subtle energy matrix with which both we and they are born, then why should there not be a natural patterning or language encoded into the subtle akashic field of our beings? But since we operate mostly at a low level of consciousness, we are out of tune not only with this pattern, but with many other aspects of our inner life, too. Quite simply, because our attention is outward, we cannot perceive the inner energetic mechanisms that constitute our beings – spiritual, mental, emotional, subtle and physical.

How is it, for example, that a human child aged but two or three years can speak a language, using all the complexities of syntax and grammar that permit the expression of inward meaning? A mental skill that entails considerably more logical structure and detail than the understanding of differential calculus. It is clear that a pattern must already exist within, requiring only the learning of various means by which such inward mental meaning can be given utterance or 'outer-ance'. And one form of 'outer-ance' is speech.

Akash is the energy field that provides us with our inward speech and hearing capabilities and in this age we have to learn language, because our inner mind cannot automatically read the vibrations within. All the same, the basic human ability to grasp and *understand* the meaning of concepts is *above* language, per se. We often, for example, find ourselves mentally searching for words to describe an experience or concept. It means that the understanding or meaning is *prior* to the words and their verbalization through speech or writing.

This natural language could therefore be seen as the unconscious and subtle blueprint whereby we learn all other languages, the pattern to which we unconsciously refer all mental concepts and ideas. Communication with it could be seen as the unconscious process of intellectual realization, the 'Ah-ness', the 'Of course-ness', the 'Eureka' which sweeps through us with a wave of both relief and certainty, when we recognize the inherent and simple truth lying *behind* some mental formulation that slips into our mind during moments of repose, (such as in the bath!).

For being the source of all the vibrations which pattern the physical universe, the subtle akashic field contains within it a reflection of all the processes of manifestation, available to our mental understanding, if we are only quiet enough to listen.

Many folk who receive just one such good idea, not really understanding its source, dine out upon it for the rest of their life. The processes of ego and excitement that wrap themselves around the one idea automatically preclude the infiltration of further realizations. The individual is unaware that there is a gold mine of such understanding awaiting the more humble and quiet approach that is more interested in seeking reality than in making one good idea into a platform for a lifetime of personal promotion.

Language, Learning and Instinct

One has to assume from observation that a child has *an instinctive ability to learn* the details of language, for example, or the finer mechanisms of walking or the ramifications of any skill. That is to say that there is a subtle energy patterning associated with any species, which is apparent physically as the characteristics of that species itself. And while we do not question the details of the anatomy and physiology, feeling that they are governed by the genetic mechanism, we do feel a lack of comprehension at the instinctive behavioural patterns which give that species its own character. In fact, I believe that we should feel equally amazed by both the genetic and the instinctive behavioural mechanisms, since the genetic material is itself not a *primary*, self-existent energy field.

Indeed, though there is clearly a connection between DNA encoding and outward form, it is a fallacy to believe that science understands how DNA, the genetic material, 'results' in the form and behaviour of a species. It does not. The observation that DNA is intimately *associated* with this process is clearly correct and the unravelling of a few of the biochemical pathways is creditable. But a knowledge of a few biochemical pathways does not constitute an under-standing of how total form, behaviour and instinct come into being.

We must, after all, remember that all species, (including ourselves) are *alive* and that life is a finer essence and experience within. It is *this* which is of such importance both to ourselves and to all species. And it is *this* which constitutes the real creature. It is *this* which patterns the outer form merely as a vehicle of expression upon the physical plane.

I would suggest, therefore, that the primary patterning for a creature lies in the more subtle tattvic realm which manifests outwardly in the cellular and genetic mechanism as well as behaviourally within the instinctive intelligence of the species, depending upon its subtle tattvic constitution.

The difference between instinctive and learned be-haviour represents the ability to adapt that is required of any energetic system if it is to be successful in a complex and varied environment. A deer, for example, is instinc-tively able to walk. It does not need to learn. It may even have an instinctive fear of anything shaped like a lion. Yet it does need to learn the nuances of walking and finding its way over the terrain into which it is born or of where lions may be hiding in its particular territory. Similarly, swal-lows may be *instinctively* and subtly patterned to migrate north or south on a particular magnetic or stellar bearing. But they have definitely *learnt* to find that same place under our eaves where they have nested for the last several years.

Or again, the natural and instinctive energy field of man's linguistic capability is present in all of us. Yet, we have to learn the particular local noises and their vocaliza-tions as language which are given their life and meaning by the more inward energy field within the subtle akashic domain, and which provides us with our higher intelli-gence.

Interestingly, the ratio of learned response to instinctive behaviour and capability amongst the species increases with the degree of intelligence or the number of subtle tattwas active within that class. And in terms of fine tuning – within each species and indeed within its individual members. A plant, for example, while still able to adapt to changes in light or temperature has little ability to really learn. But a bird, while following its instinct to find food or build nests, definitely learns to use local foods and nesting materials and to find its way around its own home territory.

Man is the most versatile of all, even appearing – and definitely *feeling* – that he posseses a level of free-will, though heavily conditioned by environmental, geographical and genetic circumstances. His ability to use his intelligence for 'good' or 'bad' is also far in excess of that exhibited by any other species. At one end of the scale it gives him the capacity to seek inward enlightenment, while conversely his mind can turn to destruction of a most horrific and inhumane nature.

Within the lower species, language or communication is instinctive, with little learnt behaviour. A duck, for instance, will still go quack, though raised by a farmyard hen. It does not need to learn its natural language. I would suggest, therefore, that it is an inherent part of the subtle matrix forming that creature. In man, however, unless he rises to higher levels, linguistic communication requires learning. At those higher levels, one assumes that there must be a natural language with an increasing degree of fineness and telepathic content as one rises up. For descriptions of mystic experience all speak of a communication wherein 'spoken' language is increasingly minimal, but where even such outward forms of soul to soul discourse are naturally available to consciousness, as a means of communication.

This thinking also provides us with an understanding of how some quiet and tuned-in individuals, living with nature, have come to comprehend the simple language of birds and animals. For when the awareness of subtle patterns falls into our mind, we automatically perceive meaning, where previously was dullness and ignorance. Understanding is thereby caught, not taught.

The Collective Unconscious

Finally, Jung's concept of a *collective unconscious* and racial memories become seen in terms of an encoding of the subtle energetic substructure or vibration of a place, a country or even our entire planet. There is no doubt that there exists a wave, a karmic pattern, upon which we all ride. Thus do scientists and writers follow the same themes, and 'discover' the same things, though previously unaware of the other's existence, often publishing their results almost simultaneously, yet quite independently of each other.

Serendipity is at work, too, the coincidental or accidental discoveries of scientists are too well-timed, in terms of their global or social context, for one to contemplate the existence of pure chance as the underlying factor in their occurrence. Or, one can say that all the answers are constantly staring us in the face, but only within the context of the currently prevalent planetary atmosphere are we able to tune in, read and express such discoveries or realizations.

Those who are ahead of their time are the path-beaters, the ones who tread and form the energy patterns of the collective unconscious, such that the habitual resistance of their contemporaries to the new concepts is slowly and unconsciously broken down, though its full effect may not be incorporated as 'general knowledge' until the maturity of the next or succeeding generations.

Whether this patterning spreads out in a specific fashion is open to speculation and experiment. There is, for example, Rupert Sheldrake's hypothesis of *morphic resonance* which suggests that if humans (or any other species) solve a problem in London today, a similar group can elucidate the riddle more readily in New York, tomorrow, without any conscious communication between them. And within the context of the energetic mechanisms expressed herein, this would seem quite possible. The real learning and change, however, that affects our social, philosophical and scientific outlook is in the more subtle realms of ideas and attitudes, spun out over the span of years, as concepts, thoughts and understanding spread into the subtle planetary energy fields, slowly affecting us all, in one way or another.

Pralaya or Dissolution

The Sanskrit and mystic literature speaks not only of the four yugas, but also of vaster aeons of time, taking in many cycles of these yugas. Into this structure, it is said, is built an automatic ebb and flow of creation and dissolution or *pralaya*. That is to say that the physical and inner universes possess a day (creation) and a night (dissolution) in which they are first manifested and then drawn up within, into potential form. The souls inhabiting these regions at that time are said to be maintained in a 'comatose' state, though those of a higher consciousness are immediately able to take their conscious place in the more inward regions.

There are said to be two degrees of pralaya in which either the three mind worlds – the physical, astral and causal – are dissolved, or the spiritual regions above them, too. The existence of the three mind regions, terminated by their subsequent dissolution up as far as the level of Brahm or Universal Mind, the causal or primal pattern world, is known, for example, as a *Day of Brahm*. After that follows an equally long period of 'darkness' or 'uncreation', the *Night of Brahm* – a sleep, a period of recovery for the Universal Mind, itself.

These yugas, pralayas and creations represent the in-breathings and out-breathings of the Universe, the slow but inexorable underlying patterning and polarity, spread out over a vast time-scale. Within this we have lived, taking on innumerable forms, moving through this amazing panorama with a tunnel vision focused largely upon just our own tiny slice of current experience. And for the maintenance of sanity at our low level of consciousness, this is no doubt essential.

But the mechanism of pralaya is of interest, for each tattwa is said to be drawn up or transmuted into the one above and thence into the particular sky or akash of that region. Thus, at the gross physical level, earth gains in energetic content and becomes liquid. Liquid, similarly, is drawn up into the fiery and airy states. The akash or vacuum barrier then takes all of that manifestation back into itself in potential form. No energy is lost, only transmuted.

Synchronously, within the subtle physical realm, the same process again takes place for the complete dissolution of the physical universe. And, similarly, with the astral and causal realms, for these three comprise an integral whole. All things undergo pralaya. They come into being (rajas), have their existence (sattvas) and are destroyed (tamas).

This is the manner of all transient phenomena. Nothing lasts forever amongst created forms. Permanence is not a built-in part of the picture. And this is true as much at a horizontally causative level, as within the vertical energy spectrum.

When we die, the soul is disassociated from the body. The mind goes with it and the pranic patterning is withdrawn, leaving an uncoordinated tattvic shell, which rapidly disintegrates.

In our physical environment, 'inert' matter is being spun out of the vacuum, created from within. And although the subatomic particles are moving incessantly, the molecules are 'comparatively' still. In the presence of the pranic life-patterning vibration, however, the molecular complexity and the movement, the pathways and the associations are formed into a most wonderfully integrated and intense mosaic of organic life, which continues for as long as a soul is linked with that complex, and is giving life to the pranic vibration and the mind within it. As soon as the soul withdraws, life departs – quite suddenly – with no hope of resuscitating the now quite dead body.

Yugas, Evolution and the Fossil Record

There is another interesting and speculative aspect to the interaction and evolution of the five tattvic fields and the four ages, as described in the Sanskrit literature. It is said that during the Sat Yuga, the vibration of the physical universe is extremely subtle and fine in nature. Man's estate at that time is essentially of the subtle tattwas, the density of gross physical accretions being minimal. In modern terminology one could say that his physical form possessed only a light concentration of physically man-ifested subatomic particles.

This means that when he died, his physical residue would have been minimal and have left no remains, while his subtle form would have been drawn up in a pralayic manner into the next level of akash, within, at the base of the astral region or sky of the physical realm. And naturally, *he would leave behind no fossil evidence* of his etherealized existence!

If this then is man's estate during the Sat Yuga, what is

the condition of other species, with only the other four tattwas active within them?

Descriptions of inner, mystic experience all give reference to there being creatures, in addition to man, in the higher realms, and which are something akin to those of our familiar physical world. One imagines that their forms are spun out of the finer tattvic matter of these astral and causal realms. The first tattvic manifestation, remember, arises in the causal region. And just as our physical creatures possess activity in a varying number of tattwas, so too do those in these inner mansions. Indeed, even the polarity of sexual differentation is prevalent in descriptions of inner experience, all the way up to the level of the Universal Mind. This, I imagine, is the mystic origin of such beings as angels and archangels, seraphim and cherubim, some of whom are 'male' and some 'female'.

So during the vibrationally subtle era of the Sat Yuga even the higher species would be more subtley constituted such that little material remains were left.

And this would be yet one more explanation as to why there are such 'anomalies' in the fossil record. Anomalies, mind you, which are only perceived as such when one attempts to fit the Darwinian theory over the extremely scanty fossil record. Without the attempt to fit the evidence to the theory there are no such anomalies – only a very sketchy record of a tiny part of our planetary history, which is quite naturally difficult to interpret.

In fact, while the fossil record is thought to span over 400 million years, the cycle of the yugas is said in yogic texts to take only 4.32 million years to traverse from the Sat Yuga through to the Kal Yuga. This period is known as a Maha Yuga. The fossil record thus spans many such Maha Yugas. And, interestingly, most fossilized remains of man, (of which there are only *very* few), are dated at a maximum of two to four million years, relating only to the last cycle of yugas. At least one human skull has, however, been found in completely mineralized form in coal deposits near Freiberg in Germany, said to be over 100 million years old. Then there was the 'Lady from Guadeloupe' – a female human complete, except for the feet and head, found embedded and fossilized in Miocene limestone, over 25 million years before man was supposed to have appeared on the scene. These finds, in themselves, put paid to Darwinian theory concerning the origin of man and other species.

Even these very approximate estimates, however, assume that our scientific methods of dating are accurate. Something we are quite unable to verify, scientifically.

Actually, the Sat Yuga is a long and necessary period of spiritual renewal for the physical plane, for it is life, the spirit or consciousness which enlivens mind and matter and permits the physical universe to exist at all. At such times, man is even said to have a lifespan of 100,000 years. 'Impossible,' our conditioned mind wants to say, but does anybody understand why, having come into existence, this most amazing of organic constructions, our own body, should actually only live for only a hundred years or less? In the Sat Yuga, the harmony of the physical creation is such that the aging factors of the present times do not exist. It is our lack of spirituality and the dominance of our unbalanced minds that wears out a human frame within such a short span of years.

During the Sat Yuga there is a closer conjuction, so to speak, between the physical realm and the astral and causal domains. The effect of this re-spiritualization every 4.3 million years upon biological systems can only be surmised. But surely the physical processes of nature would be quickened and would flow more readily than does the dense material with which we are presently familiar? Nature would be like an old man suddenly receiving the elixir of eternal youth. The bent and tortured frame is renewed with inward life and vigour, the troubles of the ages fall away.

The cycling of the yugas is a real cycling, and when the spirituality, the real inner life, begins to wane, the quality of life on the physical plane goes into a steeper and steeper decline. Ultimately, conditions become untenable and there is a spring upwards once again, a phase-jump to a new beginning. Memory and experience of spiritual consciousness begin to emerge spontaneously from within, and then to dominate life once more.

Some modern evolutionists, realizing that there is no evidence in the fossil record of the species doing any really serious evolution at all have suggested that all the major evolutionary jumps occurred over relatively short periods of time, of which no evidence actually remains. This is the theory of *punctuated equilibria*. That is to say that nature is mostly in a state of equilibrium, but occasionally (geologically speaking) something happens which sets the evolutionary process in rapid motion, leading to a renewal of the species. A sort of evolutionary musical chairs with an 'all change' on the short occasions when the music stops!

In a strange way, these theorists are probably right, for it is said to be during the Sat Yugas when species renewal takes place as a direct result of the closer conjunction of the physical with the astral and causal realms. The greater flow of the inward life force could well be the factor which brings new forms of existing species into being, according to the tattvic niches present at those times. And the reason why there is no fossil evidence of these changes is because of the spiritually more vibrant condition of matter at those times. Does all that sound bizarre? Yet it does not sound one half as bizarre as the theory that consciousness has arisen from subatomic particles which came out of nowhere in a Big Bang long, long ago.

Actually, this subject requires a far greater elaboration, which will be appearing in a future book, and I may have already overstepped the bounds of my readers' credulity! But let me add just one final thought. Given the quite different quality of vibration present during the Sat Yuga, then the 'laws of nature' known to science would also quite probably be different.

That is to suggest, for example, that the values ascribed to universal 'constants' would also change, cyclically, over long periods of times. They – like everything else – would be subject to the ebb and flow, the cyclic patterns in nature. After all, if there are natural cycles of which we are aware, all the way from the split-second periodicities within atoms and molecules, to the twenty-four hour cycle, the rotation of the seasons or the length of a lifetime, then there must be other, vastly longer cycles too, of which – being longer than the span of a lifetime or human memory – we are quite unaware.

But I will return to this topic of nature, the species, natural cycles, the life force and evolution in a future book and I must apologize if I have left certain statements hanging without greater elucidation or discussion.

It is worth pointing out that it was not until the last hundred years or so that western man relinquished the idea that our universe was just a few thousand years old. Yet the yogic writers of the ancient Hindu Shastras have written in some detail concerning the cycles of the yugas, estimating that the present age of the universe, since the last pralaya, is about two billion years. With current scientific hypotheses placing the age of the universe at about fifteen billion years, (but changing frequently as new theories are put forward), the ancient sages are seen once again to have been somewhat ahead of us in their perceptions.

And for those who are dismayed by tales of the end of the universe being just around the corner, let me say that these ancient yogis write that the physical universe goes through about 1000 cycles of the four yugas before dissolution, a total of 4.32 billion years[4]. So with 2 billion already passed, we still have 2.32. billion years left to go!

But this is a wide and controversial subject and just a few paragraphs cannot do it justice. It has to be conceded, however, that within the history of life upon our planet, not only those events have happened which lie within our imagination and comprehension. Many things must have taken place in the last several hundred million years which we have simply failed to think of and are probably quite unable to imagine.

So it is better to say that we do not know than to adhere to a theory that is so fundamentally flawed as to be maintained more by faith than by sound judgement.

I refer, of course, to Darwinism as an explanation of the origin of life. For, as I have said, it so clearly fails to observe the distinction between life and form, taking form to be the origin of life and consciousness, rather than the reverse.

Nor has the flimsy nature of the evidence gone unnoticed by the academics who perpetrate such theories upon an unsuspecting public. Indeed, at the Huxley Memorial

---

[4] *Padam Purana.* The Puranas are Sanskrit writings not included in the Vedas.

debate held at Oxford University in February 1986, when the motion debated was: "The doctrine of creation is more valid scientifically than the theory of evolution", although the evolutionists 'won', the margin was by only 198 votes to 115. More than a third of the scholars present did not accept Darwinism as a valid hypothesis. Oxford zoologist and Darwinist, Richard Dawkins' reaction to a possible defeat was interesting. He declared that it would indicate a poor selection procedure for Oxford undergraduates. In other words, he makes the a priori assumption that his scientific theory is correct and that all intelligent people would believe it. An attitude which is surely more suggestive of dogma than scientific method.

In fact, some of the evolutionists in the U.S.A. are presently taking the creationists to the high court, because they are outraged that creationism should be taught in schools alongside evolutionary theory. I wonder, is that a *scientific* attitude or an *emotional* reaction to a belief system under serious challenge? The creationists, on the other hand, are content that both should be taught, though perhaps that is purely a pragmatic approach to modern circumstances.

Live and let live, as well as true democracy, are not only unattainable ideals amongst humans, as we are presently constituted, but are also an impossible dream. For man is given only that much understanding as is required for him to complete his pralabdh karmas or destiny. He does only what he is meant to do, according to his actions and thoughts in previous cycles of his physical existence. At best he can be said to possess only the most conditioned and circumscribed elements of free-will, both in his actions, as well as thoughts.

States of Consciousness

Man has the capacity to function in four primary modes of consciousness.

1. Super-consciousness or mystic experience, above the eye centre. This includes some *near-death* and *out of the body* experiences.
2. Waking consciousness, at the eye centre.
3. Dream consciousness, at the throat centre.
4. Deep sleep, unconsciousness, below the throat centre, operating in the lower centres.

Super-Consciousness

In this condition, the mind is completely withdrawn from the world of the senses and the physical tattwas, working through the astral and causal bodies in their respective regions, finally leaving behind all traces of mind when it rises into purely spiritual domains above the causal realm of the Universal Mind. For this practice, a perfect mystic adept or master is required both as an instructor on the physical level, to impart the technique and answer practical queries on how to concentrate and withdraw the mind, and as a guide on the inner planes so that we do not get lost there or misguided by other well-meaning, but unenlightened souls inhabiting those regions.

The life energies or pranas continue their link with the body, thus preventing death, while the soul flies within. This link is mentioned in the Bible as the *silver cord*. And it is only at death that it is broken, when the physical body, no longer maintained by the life-giving pranas and the presence of the soul within, immediately begins to decay.

This silver cord represents the flow of life-giving, pranic vibration, taking its existence from the soul and maintaining the body in living condition until the return of consciousness. Glistening and vibrating, it is said to be visible to inner sight, in the manner of all energetic vibration. Its colour is sparkling white or silver, carrying within it the full spectrum of the vibrations required for the maintenance of all unconscious bodily processes.

But during life, the soul is ultimately drawn back to the body from the higher spheres to continue the play of destiny karma. Waking consciousness thus ensues. Depending upon the person's spiritual development, these mystic states may last no more than a few minutes and be purely a grace or a gift from within, not under the control of the individual. Or they may be the hard-won fruit of years of meditation. In this case, the soul goes within at will and returns only to continue the play of life in the physical world, according to its individual karmas. At death, when the energy of the pralabdh or destiny karma is finished, such a soul lays down the physical body with thankfulness and in full consciousness, more than ready to continue its life on the inner planes.

While within the astral and causal regions, the soul works through an astral and causal body and possesses an astral and causal mind, analogous to the physical body and human thought processes with which we are familiar. But they are comprised of a far finer quality and vibration of material or energetic substance. From the very threshold of the astral plane, the soul is illuminated by inner light and enlightened by the inner power of the vibrating Shabda or creative Word of God. Mystics describe the power of this increasing light as being equal to that of sixteen of our physical suns by the time the soul lays down its causal garment on leaving the realm of the Universal Mind and moves into the purely spiritual regions. At this stage, the soul knows itself for the first time as soul. This is true *self-realization*, which has nothing to do with the psychological realization of facets of our personality which we experience as struggling human beings.

Beyond the spiritual regions, say the mystics, lies the Supreme Being, the undivided source of all being, consciousness and substance.

It is clear, therefore, that as humans, when someone experiences some small inner illumination, their attention is mostly either within the subtle tattvic realms of the body below their eye centre, or at the most they have risen up to the sky of the body wherein the antashkarans are located. All these experiences can be infused with intense inner bliss, depending upon the inner devotion and love of the individual. They can also be accompanied by visions of light and sound or even of events reflecting the past or the future, derived from the antashkarans where our destiny is stored in potential form.

From a human point of view, these experiences are wonderful and can change a person's life if they come upon one spontaneously and without prior understanding of the inner mysteries. Indeed, even amongst those who have studied such things all their life, but have never had such an experience, they can be life-changing, as theory becomes the long sought-after reality.

Such inner illumination may come simply as a lucid moment or in a sudden and intense realization that life is a mystical phenomenon whose source lies deep within and where some great power vibrates through every atom of our universe and every part of our inner being. These beautiful moments comprise the religious experiences of the devotees of the many world religions, where the inner spiritual truth at the base of all religions, behind all the outer rituals and ceremonies, is momentarily grasped. They also give power to the visions of the great poets, musicians and artists, whose inspiration is always drawn from within themselves. Even a belief in religion or God is not a prerequisite for the inner soul within each one of us to make its plea for recognition. Spiritual moments or experiences have thus visited people of many ways of thinking and all walks of life.

The point to be understood, however, is that such experiences are only the tip of the tip of the iceberg. They are an incentive to us to rise higher and to sharpen up our seeking for the greater reality. The human tendency can be for our ego to feed on such experiences, feeling that we are a little superior to our fellow humans and indulging in clairvoyant and psychic glamour, or feelings of spiritual superiority. Then, we lose what we have and, spreading our energies horizontally, lose the inner intensity of life which can take us higher and is, ultimately, of greater value to us.

The full story of the mystic path is not however the subject of this book and reluctantly we must leave this fascinating and all-absorbing topic.

Near Death and Out of the Body Experiences

In recent years, scientists and doctors have been taking more seriously accounts from their patients that they have left their physical bodies during times when they nearly died due to illness, accident, childbirth and so on. One American doctor, setting out to show that such experiences were really derived from imagination, hallucination and the memory of television hospital scenes and dramas, was set back on his heels when he found that folk who had had such experiences were frequently able to describe details that were unique to their particular circumstances and could not have been generalized from such memories. It is a credit to the open-mindedness of the doctor that he was then able to reverse his opinion on the matter, as well as writing a book and appearing on television about it.

These experiences have been classified as *near death* or *out of the body* experiences and broadly speaking, they appear to fall into three main categories. Firstly, there is a disassociation of the mind and its sensory analogues (the indriyas) from the physical body. The attention, however, remains in the physical world and is able to perceive events as one would with one's physical senses. Characteristically, the individual leaves the confines of the physical body and floats up to the ceiling where he or she observes the attempts to brings them back to life.

Proof that these experiences have really occurred is revealed when the patient has described in detail the efforts of the doctors and nurses to resuscitate them. For example, "You tried to inject me in my right arm and failed. So you went round the top of the operating table to my other arm and were then successful." Or they have provided descriptions of clothing being worn by individuals who could not have been seen prior to the loss of consciousness or even from their particular viewpoint in bed, but only from the ceiling. In a recent BBC TV scientific documentary, for example, a gentleman related how he had seen through panes of glass high up upon a wall, permitting observation from the ceiling of events in the adjoining corridor, which he later accurately described.

Such experiences have been known about for as far back as one cares to make a research and have usually been described as 'astral projection'. But as I described earlier (see page 81), they are actually subtle physical or 'etheric' experiences. This is the region where ghosts and nature spirits reside, too, and in mystic parlance it is still a part of the physical realm. It is not astral at all.

Souls who were very attached to this world or who had had little preparation for death, as in an accident or warfare, may reside in this area for a greater or lesser period. Or you can say, that it may take some time for such souls to die completely to the physical world from which they have so suddenly been snatched away. In the case of warfare, anger at being unexpectedly deprived of a gross physical body together with attachment to their previous home, now destroyed by bombs, for example, holds the souls in the vicinity for some while until they either take another birth or pass into some lower astral zone, awaiting rebirth.

The second kind of experience related by those who have been through near-death experiences is that of passing through a 'tunnel'. This tunnel is the soul's experience of passing through the veil which separates us from the lower astral realms. It is also known as the inner 'sky' of the body or the subtle physical akashic gateway. In Indian mystic terminology it is called the *Bunk Nal*, usually translated as the *crooked tunnel*, because it is not 'straight'. Doctors who are studying these phenomena could well increase their understanding of what is going on by studying what the experts at meditation have to say about it. For these adepts have mastered the art of dying while living, of passing through this narrow gateway or crooked tunnel as and when they please, and of returning to this world as required.

Finally, a few souls have passed through this tunnel into a bright, self-luminous world, where they have even met other souls and conversed with them before, often reluctantly, they are drawn back to their physical body by their destiny karmas which still need to be undergone, returning to 'consciousness' with the nurses and doctors standing around them. The Brazilian-Portuguese translator of my book, *Subtle Energy*, Beatriz Sidou, once wrote and told me that an accident had thrown her into a "dazzling world". Almost without exception, this experience possesses clarity and often great beauty and is taken by the individual as an experience whose higher reality is self-evident, unquestionable and life-changing. Much as one knows that a dream was only a dream as soon as one awakens.

Waking Consciousness

Man, if he is a true man with mystic knowledge, operates in this world from no lower than his eye centre, working through the sensory and motor indriyas and the tattvic fields for the outworking of his karmas and his physical life on earth. The rest of us operate partially from this centre and partly from the attention playing within the body. We are thus emotionally-orientated beings and suffer a variety of ills. All lucid moments, all mental or intuitive revelations of science and the things of this world, all human understanding, all the great creations of literature, art and music – all the highest parts of man's endeavours have arisen from attention rising to its true human focus in the thinking centre, flavoured by the individual's karmic orientation of national culture, as well as mental and emotional inclinations.

The mystic, therefore, possesses the greatest capacity not only for enlightened cosmic understanding, but also for the highest of human comprehension, formulation of ideas, and their practical manifestation in this world. For he works from a point of real *inner knowledge and experience* of how the universe is constructed. Moreover, he appreciates the true and limited nature of outer knowledge and acts accordingly.

The Dream State

In sleep, our attention slips to a point of focus in the throat centre or lower. At this level, our will-power or ahankar is in abeyance and in the absence of the cohering force of our mind at its centre behind the eyes, the subconscious images (comprised of energy patterns in our mind), float into a state of dream-awareness, connections between these events being made purely by association, similarity of conjunction, or the depth of such impressions in our mind-stuff. Our subconscious mind thus becomes our reality and we experience all the normal human emotions in response, awakening with fear, happiness, lust or desire – or any other admixture of feelings – just as we experience them in daily life.

Our dreams thus convey to us a muddled and incoherent patterning of our subconscious mind, often reflecting the current events in our life and sometimes possessing an origin which we cannot readily determine.

Dreams, too, may be good dreams, of a spiritual nature, when we awake in a state of bliss or grace which lasts with us for some while. Sometimes, too, snatches of our pralabdh karma, already patterned into our antashkarans or thought centre, are filtered into our dreams and we receive dream-visions of the future. These may, however, be only partially correct, since they are liable to interact with the hopes, desires and impressions of our subconscious mind, forming distorted images on our inner mental screen.

This, in fact, is true of all psychic and clairvoyant visions and messages, so that all such intuitions are liable to be only more or less correct depending upon the experience and inner ascent of the individual. Mystics do not normally inform people of their destiny, because it helps them very little and may only engender deeper attachment. They can, however, provide much inner guidance at every step in life, so that life proceeds in an orderly and relatively easy fashion. Psychics and clairvoyants, on the other hand, usually work from below the eye centre and like all of us, are prone to human weakness and error.

Dreaming also appears to be a necessary process in our night-life, without which we become mentally disturbed. This has been demonstrated by awakening subjects during the dream state, identified by the brain-wave patterns characteristic of the dreaming condition. Presumably, dream is required to sort out the multitude of impressions, thought-grooves, emotions and experience that we receive on a daily basis and in an almost random fashion. Without this re-processing and organization we become increasingly disturbed, leading to increasingly emotional behaviour patterns, as our rational mind at the thinking centre loses more and more of its control.

A similar situation can arise due to the pressures of everyday life. Then, if we cannot remedy the situation or help is not forthcoming, the energy patterns can become so disturbed that our attention is caught up in them to the exclusion of outer events and our neuroses or energy disharmonies become the focus of our identity. A nervous breakdown or even psychosis can be the result, when extreme care and nourishment at all levels are required to nurse the patient back to a healthful mental and emotional condition.

The attention of the true mystic, however, never falls below the eye centre. Therefore, when he lies down to rest, the body sleeps while his consciousness goes into the higher realms. The dream function of ironing out the fibrillations and experiences of the previous day is no longer necessary, for in the waking state, the mystic holds his mind at a higher level than the rest of us. In consequence, the plethora of subconscious activity is largely eliminated and far less mental rest is required.

Deep Sleep, Unconsciousness

Whilst dreams or a form of consciousness is possible with attention at the throat centre, when the focus slips below this point to the heart or navel centre, we experience deep sleep and complete unconsciousness of our surroundings. Though we can be awoken by sensory input, through activation of the mind at the higher centres of the body. As mentioned above, it sometimes happens that while under anaesthetic, the soul goes within and becomes conscious of the physical universe through the faculties of the inner mind, watching the operation from a distance – seeing the nurses and doctors performing their tasks.

These states are actually an operation of the mind and soul within the subtle tattvic fields of the physical plane. Consciousness of the astral level is not attained. Thus, a person who is in a coma could be either conscious within or completely unconscious, with our possessing no outward way of knowing their true condition.

It is clear, therefore, that there is a distinct difference between deep sleep and an unconsciousness produced by injury, illness or anaesthesia. For in the latter, the pathway by which consciousness manifests is biochemically or physiologically ligatured and the person cannot be simply awoken.

There are, in fact, many different varieties of sleep which vary from person to person just as much as our waking states differ from day to day and between individuals. For the point at which the attention hovers within the body and the nature of the subconscious images which manifest in our dream life, remembered or otherwise, varies continuously, as we observe in the changing quality of our sleep and the content of our dreams.

Similarly, unconscious states – characterized by our inability to return to a conscious state upon external stimulation – differ in their nature. Loss of consciousness caused by accident, anaesthesia, mesmerism or hypnotism all vary in the means by which the pathways of physical awareness are disrupted. Anaesthesia is due to chemical or electrical disruption of the central nervous system resulting in an inability to maintain the transformative links between mind energies and sensory physiology. Many carbon-based gases – chloroform and ether were two of the earliest ones used – displace oxygen from the blood stream and hence the tissues, the resulting depression of nerve function leading to unconsciousness. Dr Stone suggests that oxygen is a conveyor of prana and certainly oxygen presents a life-supporting vibration to the body, a positive polarity at the level of molecular activity.

Similarly, whenever there is mechanical injury to the head, disruption of brain function and hence unconsciousness may occur, depending upon the severity. Likewise, various toxins can cause loss of consciousness through biochemical disturbance to nervous tissues of the brain.

Mesmerism and Hypnosis

Mesmerism and hypnotism, too, are interesting forms of semi-consciousness. In mesmerism, the mental energy normally focused in the brain is dispersed to lower areas of the body by passes of the practitioner's hands, sometimes in conjunction with magnets. This is reminiscent of electro-sleep devices which use a sudden change of electrical polarity across the scalp to induce an unconscious condition.

The hypnotist, on the other hand, engages the mental attention of the subject. Through strong suggestion, often accompanied by focused concentration on a particular object or a soothing voice suggesting sleep, he maintains the thinking mind of the subject in a state of consciousness while unhinging the awareness from its association with the senses, as it slips to lower centres within the body. The senses still operate, but the hypnotist's own control is now latched into the mechanisms of the subject's mental awareness and cognition.

In both cases, the subject's will-power (ahankar) is in abeyance, as is his control over and appreciation of sensory function, and hence the various bizarre phenomena of hypnotism become possible. In fact, the hypnotist takes over partial control. The subconscious mind can be impressed to react in particular ways to certain stimuli upon return to the waking condition, or the mind can be made to over-ride sensory input such that heat or cold, for example, do not become uncomfortable. Or conversely, the subtle sensory mechanism of the indriyas can be activated by suggestion to produce the apparent sensation of heat or cold when no such physical stimulation has actually occurred.

The cooperation of the subject is, however, required and weak-willed people make far better subjects than those of a strong-willed nature. In fact, mesmerism and hypnotism essentially manipulate the will power and mental integrity of the subject. As such, they are usually advised against by true mystic practices, where full presence of mind is required for successful meditation, personal control and integrity of one's own mental processes.

Everyday States of Consciousness

For most of us, our waking state is not focused in the thinking centre, but is spread out through association with the indriyas of perception and action – the sensory and motor aspects of our human constitution – into the physical world of the five tattwas. We thus experience emotions and our centre of thought is disturbed. The more scattered into the world and the lower down in our body our attention is active, then the less conscious we become and the more enclosed and circumscribed is our ability to perceive, to observe and to think clearly and consciously.

So, although we are awake, we are in many respects asleep and living unconsciously. Reactions become instinctive and emotional, sometimes violent. Even a veneer of intellectual rationality is often underlain with a deeply emotional response, especially to ideas which conflict with the habitual patterns of thought. The manner of expression in the refutation of new ideas may at first be intellectual, but on examination, the reasons are found to possess no really logical or open-minded basis. On further discussion, many such people become emotionally agitated and even angry, wishing to either terminate the conversation or blast the other into submission by a continuous stream of verbal pressure. In some cases, the threat of insecurity engendered by new or different ideas will even result in physical violence, especially with emotionally, rather than intellectually, based ideologics, as in much of politics. It is in this way that peace-loving peoples can be led into war by the emotionality of their leaders.

Our human constitution, therefore, provides us with the capacity to be an angel or a devil, to rise to the heights of spiritual and mystic transport or to descend to the depths of human depravity and low consciousness. But for most of us, we operate in the middle ground with a greater or lesser urge to seek the higher and more inward places of our being.

Poetic Interlude

INDWELLING

If thou couldst empty all thyself of self,
Like to a shell dishabited,
Then might He find thee on the Ocean shelf,
And say, 'This is not dead,'
And fill thee with Himself instead:

But thou art all replete with very THOU,
And hast such shrewd activity,
That, when He comes, He says, 'This is enow
Unto itself – 'Twere better let it be:
It is so small and full, there is no room for Me.'

T.E. Brown

CHAPTER 12

Physical Control Centre – Brain and Mind Relationships

Sensory Input and Motor Output

In the brain lie the mechanisms by which mental energies are first manifested at the physical level. First, I have a thought of going for a walk. Then it is manifested in the brain as nervous impulses, and my legs, back, arms and so on, perform the necessary functions for the achievment of that aim. But without the continuing *will* to walk, the legs and arms immediately cease their activity. The intention to be walking must always be present; the subtle, mental indriya of 'walking' or 'going' must be active however much of a background thought it may become. Without the image of walking present somewhere within my mind, walking ceases, as would be the case if I fainted or lost consciousness.

In the brain are located the linkages through to higher consciousness as well as the integration of all the complex activities of the body and the more physical aspects of sensory perception. Nervous, endocrine and probably other forms of energetic message are all passed through the brain where cognisance is taken of their meaning and they are integrated into one functional control centre with motor action and response output being taken as the yang balance to the sensory, receptive, yin input.

Just imagine the brain function for a while. Indeed, our centre of thinking and consciousness is located in our head and we can imagine the activities of the brain by just being at our inward centre, observing and considering the multitudinous input and output signals. Some signals are automatically available to our being, though it may need our directed attention for them to be brought into our consciousness. This is the case with most *sensory input* – we are not actively aware of every detail in our surroundings at all times, but only that which is currently the centre of our attention. The rest is present and available, but peripheral to our central awareness. We can direct attention to it, as and when required.

Then there are our *motor responses* to this sensory input. We move our head, arms, hands, legs, feet and other muscles. Just as there are only five real categories of sensation, there are only five real modes of action, the indriyas, as we discussed earlier.

The yin and yang of sensory input and motor action is enough to absorb the conscious activity of most folk for much of their life. Indeed, it requires a conscious effort of will to step back, inwardly, and perceive the panorama of life's activity as a detached spectator. But then, usually, something else catches our attention and off we go again. Actually, these moments of pause are stepping–off points in our life to higher aspiration and should be taken advantage of and encouraged.

Memory

In addition to our sensory and motor activity, we have *memory*. This links the moments together, through the apparent separateness of observer and the observed, and gives us our sense of time. If we had no capacity for memory, we would live a strange existence, totally in the present moment. All our sensory impressions become meaningful, only due to a past knowledge of them or things like them. Our present thoughts are based on conscious and unconscious memories of past events, experiences or other thoughts and feelings. All actions, all language, all modifications to mental energy due to the changing tide of circumstance would be lost from view if our capacity for memory ceased.

Psychologists have identified two aspects of memory, designated according to their characteristics as *short-term* and *long-term memory*. Short–term memory lets you remember enough of your sensory input to function without much difficulty. It lets you remember a telephone number long enough to dial it, for example. For this we hardly use our higher mental capacities and may often find ourselves repeating it in our mouth, audibly, in order to hold it in semi–consciousness for just long enough.

Short-term memory also helps us to make sense out of our sensory input. Imagine, for example, how you would function if there were no short-term memories of your sensory input. You would be continually forgetting where you were and why you were there. You would hardly be able to cross a room without bumping into things. Almost unconsciously, we maintain a visual mental image of our surroundings and a memory of our intentions for just long enough to be able to move about coherently.

Long-term memory is the mental filing system that retains impressions long after the event or experience has passed. It usually requires either an effort of will to retain a memory, or the retention comes as the result of something that really attracted our attention at the time – a frightening, beautiful, strongly emotional or otherwise impressive experience. Alternatively, the impression becomes fixed in our mind because it is a memory we use automatically every day, becoming ingrained through repetition – the names of relatives and friends, where we keep our shoes, more intricate aspects of our day-to-day jobs and so on.

Memory is stored in the antashkarans where the new impressions of our present life, as well as those from the past and which make up our current destiny, are lodged. Being non-material, it cannot be erased by physical means and this is actually born out by brain research where large sections of people's brains have been damaged or even removed without their loss of long-term memory. In certain instances, depending upon the exact location of the brain damage, the ability to store new sensory and experiential information in long-term memory is impaired, indicating that the physical through-route to the mind-stuff of the antashkarans is damaged, though those impressions *already stored* in long-term memory are not disrupted. The antashkarans themselves, being immaterial, cannot be damaged by physical agency alone. We will be examining the anatomy of brain function shortly, where it becomes comparatively clear, in a very general way, which parts of the brain are responsible for which functions.

Speech, Reading and Language

Following on from, and closely associated with memory, we have the faculties of *speech*, *reading* and *language*, involving the integration of many other faculties for the three phases of *sensory appreciation, intelligent understanding* and *outward expression*. This inflow and outflow is a reflection of the separation of polarity between the sensory, yin input, the more inward thought processes and the subsequent yang or outward action of communication. The sensory input is first processed by little understood brain energies, before moving up into the higher mental level of the antashkarans for intelligent appraisal and a sense of personal consciousness. After that, any outward responsive action, if any, is made. The speed of mental activity is so fast that we can appear to perceive and act almost simultaneously, but this apparent simultaneity is due to past experience and habit, the inner mind following grooves in the antashkarans, barely, if at all, above the threshold of consciousness.

One might, in fact, think that these three phases are synonymous, but accidental damage to particular areas of the brain leads to reasonably well documented and repeating patterns of speech and language difficulties which point to a differentation between them. Sometimes, there is perfect *understanding* but difficulty in correct grammatical *expression* – connecting words like 'if', 'but', 'the', or 'and' all get missed out, for example, and speaking is slow and laboured. Or the speech may be quite fluent but almost meaningless, (a kind of politician's syndrome?). It means, therefore, that damage or disruption to the energy pathways can occur at any point in the process, due to physical or psychological accident or disease, thus displaying a wide spectrum of possible impairment depending upon the nature of the damage and the individual himself, his own physical and mental constitution.

Unconscious Integration and Control

The brain is also involved in the *control and integration of all the unconscious activities* of our bodily organs through the autonomic nervous system as well as bioelectronic and biomagnetic energy patterns currently just on the borders of scientific understanding. This is no small feat!

The *subconscious* ramifications and activities of our mind and personality as they interact with the lower energies of our body and run around in complex patterns within our thinking processes and below the threshold of consciousness, are a further area for consideration and one which neurologists and those involved with brain physiology and anatomy usually appear to ignore, due to lack of any real method or paradigm for approaching the subject.

That the subjective approaches of psychology, let alone mysticism, spirituality and yoga etc., are hardly integrated with neurology is indicative of the fact that the classical neurological explanations of biochemical and electrical brain activity bear little or no relationship whatsoever to the subjectively and objectively observed manifestations of the human psyche. The few neuroscientists who feel that mind and brain are separate entities are small in number. To those people who practice meditation with any degree of success (and many others too), the concept that their blissful inner experiences, their personal growth from unconsciousness into consciousness, their development of understanding, and their growing appreciation of life and beauty are simply the expression of biochemical changes in the brain is quite simply, ludicrous. They *kmow* without a shadow of doubt that they are, in their being or consciousness, not their physical body at all. This is a totally unscientific attitude, of course, from the point of view of the one whose attention is so spread throughout every pore of his body that his consciousness of higher aspects of being human is quite severely curtailed. In terms of detached appreciation of experience, however, such an attitude, though personal, is quite logical and scientific.

One must remember that the scientific approach of intense intellectual analysis is only an idiom, not an absolute reality. What is important is *life* and – since we will all face it – *death*. What happens after that is also most important. The span of one lifetime is, after all, only a fraction of a cosmic second. What a fuss we make about such a small matter! But then perhaps, the stakes are high. Higher, even, than we imagine.

Consciousness too, clearly has a point of focus in the brain, without which only the autonomic nervous system continues to function as in sleep or coma. But let us now examine some brain anatomy and identify what little is known of brain function, according to area. This contains some interesting surprises.

Brain Anatomy

The brain, (see figure 12-1), or *cerebrum*, consists of an outer *cortex* and an inner core containing the *thalamus* and *hypothalamus*, as well as the *pineal* and *pituitary glands*. Leading off from this *centerencephalic* region or mid-brain is the brain stem which runs downwards becoming the *spinal cord*.

Large areas of the cortex can be damaged or removed without the loss of life or consciousness and even in some cases with very little permanent loss of the functions peripheral to consciousness – use of the sense organs, language, memory etc. – though initially the injured patient no doubt feels quite weird and spaced-out. Any injury or lesion, such as a tumour, to the higher brain stem, however, results in unconsciousness, while severe damage to any of the central brain areas, especially the thalamus, hypothalamus or pituitary glands and brain stem (but not the pineal gland), results in rapid, if not instantaneous, death.

It is fair to say, therefore, that the centre upon which mind and consciousness focus their more inward energies is the higher brain stem, which in consideration of its close proximity and linkage to the hypothalamus, pituitary and pineal glands makes considerable sense of our thinking thus far.

This does not mean, of course, that the mental energies only impinge upon this one area of the brain. There is, as we have been discussing, an entire network of subtle energies which act as the blueprint for the complete body. But just as there are organizational or focal points in the spinal chakras, so too is the brain a focal point. Within it lie even more intense points of focus and organization – such as the mid-brain – which relate to more inward mental and subtle energy organizational and focal centres. It is just like any organized system in this world – there is an entire hierarchy of control, sub-control and distribution etc.

The mid-brain, (see figure 12-1), is the area upon which all the functions of the nervous system converge. From below, through the lower brain stem, come (and go) the connections to the spinal and cranial nervous system, both motor and autonomic. From in front come the optic tracts

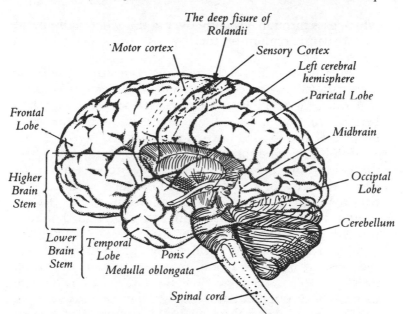

Figure 12-1. Overall brain structure, showing the mid-brain and brain stem within the cerebral hemispheres. The cerebral cortex is 'divided' into the various lobes by deep fissures in its surface.

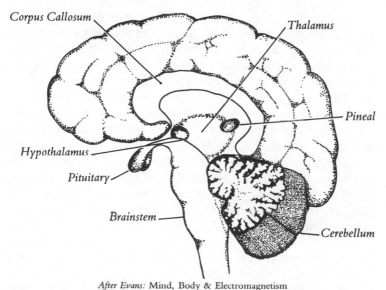

After Evans: Mind, Body & Electromagnetism

Figure 12-2. Brain structure in longitudinal section

which pass through, crossing over at the *optic chiasma* in the hypothalamic region, on their way to the visual cortex at the rear.

Similarly, branches of the auditory, olfactory (smell) and gustatory (taste) nerve tracts are all sent specifically to the thalamic area of the brain. The central area of connection between the two halves of the cortex, known as the *corpus callosum* is also located in the mid-brain.

Within the higher brain stem and associated areas, then, there must be a focus at which the nerve signals are understood by or transformed into more subtle energy patterns bearing a 'harmonic' relationship to the electro-chemical nature of the sensory input and presented directly to the indriyas and antashkarans. In converse manner, the mental energies transmit their instructions downwards and the thought becomes action. Without thought, however fleeting or subconscious, we will not act. The mind remains in control throughout, though whether our higher consciousness is in control of our mind is another matter.

A Diversion Towards Consciousness

In the perfect spiritual man, the soul or consciousness merged in God, the Supreme Being, controls the mind and the mind controls the senses. Love – the quality of soul, and rationality – the quality of mind, are beautifully mingled into perfect human expression, be it man or woman. Such a being operates, in the physical world, from behind his eyes and the quality of his gaze is quite unique, especially as it strikes upon those who themselves aspire to mystic and higher spiritual experience. For such a Perfect One, there is no fear, no confusion, no lack of understanding or comprehension of anything; there is no doubt. All is clear and all is possible. The relative limits of intellectual understanding are comprehended. The human mind is used as a vehicle, just as we ourselves use our bodies – but with full consciousness of its limitations. It is simply a tool for use within a certain sphere; not a means for grasping the Universal, but simply a part of the human apparatus required for life on this plane.

How clumsy one feels when one straps on oxygen tanks, control valves and gauges, oxygen jackets, lead weights, flippers and mask when scuba-diving into deep water. And how difficult it is at first to manoevre, even to swim. But how beautifully coordinated is the expert instructor in whom there is no fear or apprehension and who with great patience and tolerance instructs us how to handle ourselves and our apparatus, in order that we may become expert divers ourselves.

Similarly, is the perfect man, the mystic. As for the rest of us, we flounder. The lower the centre of attention in our body, the greater the area of mental activity that is *subconcious*. All the thoughts, impressions, experiences, actions, moods and desires that have ever crossed our mind leave their impression on our *chit*, part of our antashkarans, our mind. And without any focus of attention or conscious control, they go on chattering away without our knowing about it, determining most of our attitudes and thoughts. Our attention, attracted by life in the physical world through the senses, and our desire for enjoyment and self-indulgence, sinks down, away from its natural centre within the brain. With this sinking, we lose consciousness of who and what we are. Then we are totally the victim of our subconscious mind. Our 'conscious' mind is so deeply conditioned by its subconscious muddle of impressions that consciousness is often hardly the word for it. Small wonder then, that we sometimes come to think of ourselves as just the body, and our thoughts, memories and consciousness to be no more than electrochemical activity in the brain.

Similarly, do we conceive of all life originating by chance from dust, because our experience contains nothing more than material substance. And yet we do not relinquish our search for understanding. We are often afraid to say of such theories, that which vast numbers of people already think: that they just do not make any sense.

I believe, however, that it is time for a breath of fresh air, of *true* philosophical and scientific 'democracy', when even scientists (supposed to be the most open-minded of all thinking people!) can express their personal opinions without the fear of losing their livelihood. But social and psychologically conditioned pressures are so strong. And to admit total ignorance of all deeper issues after a lifetime of study is no small step and takes inner courage and an understanding of life as an adventure towards truth, not as a competition for success or achievement or intellectual knowledge.

Brain Anatomy Continued – The Cortex

The mid-brain, then, appears to be the central control unit with links to higher mental functions. We need now to discuss the specific roles of the outer cortex.

The cortex itself, is divided more or less centrally down the middle, longitudinally, creating two hemispheres, known even in neurological circles as simply the *left* and *right brain*. Note, however, that these are really the left and right *cortex*, omitting the major centres associated with consciousness in the mid-brain. In the cortex are found the areas associated with the general physical integration of sensory and motor function, as well as those more particularly involved in the linkage of mental energies to the motor (vocal) and sensory (hearing) aspects of speech and language control.

The spatial arrangement of the cortex appears to be of considerable importance to its function, for it is deeply convoluted and fissured, resulting in an extensive surface area of which only about thirty-five per cent lies directly beneath the skull. This fissuring, up to an inch and a half deep, provides us with the major landmarks by which the cortex is anatomically described – the *temporal lobe, parietal lobe, hippocampus* and so on, (see figures 12-1 and 12-3).

All life possesses consciousness and all vertebrates possess a spinal cord terminating in the brain stem. But it is only amongst the higher mammals and especially man, that the extensive elaboration of the cortex has taken place. This would appear to imply that the greater subtle constitution requires a larger physical system for the outward implementation of its increased repertoire of intelligently directed, physical capabilities.

Much of our limited knowledge of brain function according to area is derived from either the study of the effects of accidental brain damage or brain surgery, or from the work of such neurologists as Wilder Penfield. Penfield has conducted brain experiments on epileptic patients, removing sections of the skull and stimulating

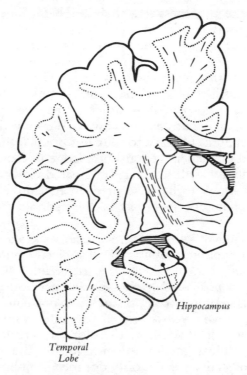

Figure 12-3. The deeply fissured structure of the cerebral cortex. The view is a frontal section of the left hemisphere.

the underlying areas with a small oscillatory current, *while the patient retained full consciousness* – without the aid of a general anaesthetic. The surgeon and patient are thus able to 'explore' the brain together and Penfield has caused some disturbance in scientific circles by his conclusion that the mind and brain are separate entities, a conclusion also reached by one of the great pioneers of brain research, Sir Charles Sherrington.

Penfield reached this point of view after his repeated observation that whatever muscular, sensory or cerebral stimulation occurred, the patient always remained a passive *observer*. The patient's sense of mental identity or consciousness never became *identified* with the effects that were being created. From a subjective point of view, it is this feeling of being separate from one's body and the objects of sensation, even from one's thoughts, that brings people to the awareness that their real being and essence is something different from the body, as we have already discussed. It is this same awareness that allows us to disbelieve the evidence of our senses when our rational mind knows that what we are apparently perceiving is an illusion. This is our experience, for example, when we are seated in a stationary train and feel that *we* are moving when the train next to us pulls away. We *know* that we are not moving, but still have to look out of the other window to confirm our inner mental knowledge of being stationary. Similarly with artificially created visual illusions which we know to be false or even meaningless from a structural point of view, as is the speciality of certain painters.

The pursuit of knowledge, science, makes a great mistake by attempting to obliterate all subjective information, because *nobody actually lives an objective life.* Our living is essentially *subjective.* Our own experience and interpretation of it is very important to each one of us and it colours all we do, all we perceive and all we think. It is the essence of our being. The attempt, therefore, to create a system which is almost totally given over to the pursuit of apparent objectivity is not only doomed to failure (because all those participating bring in their own subjective approach anyway), but it is also so constraining as to be life-destroying, in the inner sense. Moreover, it engenders the self-deception that one's apparently rational thoughts are free from all one's subconscious and emotional conditioning. It is reminiscent of a tea-party in which the manners, forms and social customs are so all-important that nobody actually *communicates* anything to anybody else at all. It is dead. Everyone is afraid to speak their own inner thoughts and indeed have played the game for so long that they have totally lost touch with what they really feel or think. The result is an occasion of apparently good order and decorum, but which actually means nothing at all, from any higher point of view. Such, I feel, is the state in which much academic research finds itself, today. It has become a ritual in which the excitement and adventure of discovery have largely been lost.

Returning then, to the brain. The research of Penfield and others demonstrates that there are two main categories of effect which result from either excision of parts of the cerebral cortex, or its electrical stimulation with the patient remaining conscious. These categories are associated firstly with sensory and motor functions and secondly with more inward psychological aspects concerning the way the subject is feeling – strangeness, familiarity, fear, memory flash-backs, deja vu and so on.

But while there appears to be a general functional mapping of cortical areas which is more or less constant in all normally constituted people, (see figures 12-4 and 12-5), it is also well-known that patients may have large sections, or even an entire hemisphere removed and yet regain full use of their faculties. If the excision was small, this may be within just a few days or weeks. If large, it may take longer or, depending upon the damaged area, may never fully return. If it occurs during childhood, then the return of full function is particularly likely. There are many such case histories of children from whom one hemisphere has been completely removed and the full cortico-cerebral repertoire has been relocated into the remaining half. There is even the celebrated case of the Oxford don who was born with only a small section of his cortex intact and yet went on to lead a normal life in which his intelligence and intellectual capacities were quite clearly unimpaired.

Electrical stimulation of the cortex in the sensory areas results in flashes of light, sounds, smells, taste or tingling sensations, but never whole pictures or complete perceptual hallucinations of objects or events. Stimulation of areas associated with motor function can result in unco-ordinated limb movements over which the patient has no control, or in vocalizations such as a long, drawn out vowel sound (Aa . . ah! or Oo . . . oh!, for example), but no integrated movements or explicit words and phrases are ever elicited.

With small sections actually removed, there can be temporary loss of function or *aphasia* which is often regained quite rapidly. The nature of the aphasia produced by removal or electrical stimulation of particular cortical areas tells us the function ascribed to or connected to that area. The occipital lobes, for example, at the rear receive the crossed-over nerve tracts from the eyes after their

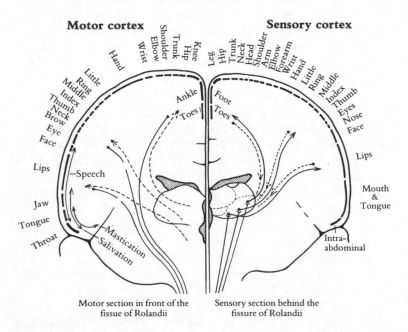

Figure 12-4. Functional mapping of the cerbral motor and sensory (tactile) cortex. Two vertical sections, looking from in front, also showing nerve tract pathways, passing through the higher brain stem and centrencephalic regions, to and from the cortex[1].

[1]Just as the inner mind structure is organized such that the antashkarans (memory, intellect, identity etc.) are deeper within, with the mental indriyas, sensory and motor, forming as the mind plays against the subtle tattvic energies, so too are the more central brain functions contained deeper within, in the mid-brain, with the yin and yang, sensory and motor, tattvic interplay located peripherally in the cortex.

The mental functions of the indriyas are thus mapped or projected outward, like a holographic, image projection system, forming the motor and sensory areas of the cerebral cortex, with overall control lying within the mid-brain. The brain, possessing a nervous correspondence to all parts of the body, is thus another reflex centre within our complex body hologram, the most powerful of all, for it is the one by which we drive our body functions from our inward mind centre and receive sensory impressions from without, with corresponding capability for psychosomatically inducing health and disease.

The sensory cortex really refers to the tactile (touch, including pain) sensation, ubiquitous throughout the body, in particular the hands and fingers, (note the large area devoted to them). Other areas of the cortex are devoted to the other senses – sight, hearing and so on. But the yin and yang polarization of sensory and motor function is even projected as a physical division within the cellular structure of the cortex, for the motor areas are at the front, while the sensory areas line the posterior flank of the fissure of Rolandii, as it runs from side to side, transversely, through the cerebral cortex.

The whole body is actually formed in this way, as a projected image from within–out. It would make a tremendous piece of research to show how the projection and intermingling of the energies within actually result in the detailed form, structure and dynamic functioning of the physical brain and body.

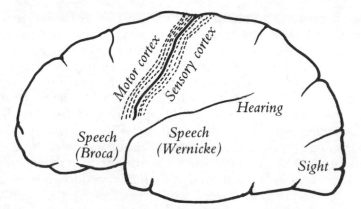

Figure 12-5. General cortical areas. The cortex, generally, seems to be the elaborator and synthesizer of informationally encoded energies concerning the physical aspects of life – motor, sensory, speech and so on – for the purposes of integrated awareness within the higher energies of mind and consciousness.

passage through the centerencephalon or mid-brian. Removal of the areas on either side of the *calcerine fissure* (see figure 12-6) results in blindness, with the exception of just a small central 'disc' of sight. Each side is related to the opposite eye, so that removal of one side results in the loss of vision in just that one eye. But excision of or damage to the surrounding *secondary optical cortex* leads to only relatively small visual impairment, which is not related to a particular eye.

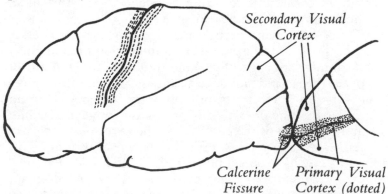

Figure 12-6. Location of the optical (visual) cortex. The internal mapping of the area is shown on the right.

This pattern of *primary* and *secondary* areas for localized sensory and motor function is repeated for all our major senses and for our voluntary muscular or motor system. While damage to the primary area results in loss of function (which may later be regained), excision of the secondary areas results in little or no aphasia. The function of the secondary areas would appear, therefore, to be connected with further integration of the particular sensory input or muscular activity into the total human energy system. Thus, excision of the supplementary motor area from just one side may produce no great disability, but only a decrease in the capacity for rapidly alternating movements of hands and feet.

Man has the largest cortical area of all creatures and it seems that rather than being the seat of consciousness and intelligence itself, the cerebral cortex is the site of integration at the physical level of the far greater repertoire of actions and perceptions which our higher intelligence makes possible.

Man, for example, has no primary survival need for extreme athletic skill, and yet he can train himself to climb mountains or execute the creation of physical artefacts with a range of skills far surpassing those of any other creature, ranging from the construction of the pyramids to the manufacture of microchips. He can paint pictures, play music, cook his meals (some of us!), and perform amazing gymnastic and athletic feats. He further possesses an ability to communicate, using language and gesture in an almost infinitely complex manner.

Think how many verbal languages our earth possesses and of the height of gestural communication found in deaf and dumb language. Speaking requires integration of mouth, throat and language faculties. Hearing introduces the ear and auditory stimuli into the schema. Writing includes the fine operation of hands and fingers. Reading requires the use of the eyes. And when we speak, we also listen; when we write, we read what we are writing. This kind of intelligence, supplied in the subtle fields by complex, integrated activity within the subtle akashic domain, requires a high degree of elaboration at the physical level for its successful outward manifestation. And this function would appear to be the responsibility of the cerebral cortex. And with all of this cross-integration going on, it is not surprising that cortical centres possessing a totally exclusive function do not appear to exist.

The neuronal pathways, themselves, do provide us with some clues to elucidating the manner by which these faculties are integrated both at the physical level and into the higher levels of mental functioning. I imagine, though, that the vacuum and more subtle fields which pattern and give life to the physical brain are built upon more integrated and holographic principles than our purely mechanistic electrical and computer models. Consciousness, is able to maintain many simultaneous and integrated areas and lines of activity and function – an entire mind-emotion-body complex and much more besides. In comparison, even our most advanced computer and electronic technology appears no more sophisticated than a simple child's doll.

From the sense organs and the musculature, nerve tracts pass first to ganglions or synaptic junctions in the mid-brain. And remember that each separate nerve fibre may have up to 100,000 further synaptic links to other nerve cells. From thence, the tracts fan out to the particular area of cortex dealing with that function. Nervous impulses pass both ways along these tracts and hence we have a picture, (see figure 12-4), in which nervous messages are passed from sense organ to mid-brain where mental levels of energy are first imprinted from below with the energies of perceptual input. From thence, energetic patterns, in the outwardly observable form of nervous impulses, pass to the cortex for synthesis of the data. On its return to the energy focus in the mid-brain, the now more integrated sensory pattern is transmuted into the higher level for the mental and subjective experience of perception.

At this point, the mind may be passive, recording the perceptions (manas and the indriyas) as memory (chit) or it may decide (buddhi) on action (ahankar), in which case the mid-brain is impressed with the will to act in a particular fashion. The physical coordination of this envisaged action is likely to be highly complex, involving speech as well as motor action, plus further and continuous perceptual activity. The eyes and head may be moved, the legs, arms and body are brought into action and both speech and hearing may be simultaneously involved. And while the mid-brain appears to be the focal point for the link into consciousness, the inward subtle blueprint is no doubt involved in the entire brain patterning, just as it is with all of the body.

For the physical integration and execution of all of these faculties, already existing as an image in the mind, the mid-brain sends messages to the cortex, which – guided by the higher will of the mind – performs its task, sending back the right nervous signals to the mid-brain where the mind is kept informed concerning the details of the physical side of events and the impulses carry on to the muscles and organs involved.

All of this is actually happening continuously and simultaneously, as we live each moment. For the purposes of simplicity, it is described as a linear process, whereas in reality it is the enaction of the one complete human energy system, subtle and gross. And though we have the will to see or move a hand, we do not have the consciousness of the physiological mechanisms by which such activity is made possible. This is the function of the pranas, themselves patterned by the mind and working through the subtle tattvic fields both within the body as well as in the physiology of brain function.

The mind is quite unable in its normal conscious state to appreciate the compexity of biological mechanisms. But no wonder that someone with damage to certain particular sections of the brain may try to speak, but cannot find the words associated with a particular concept or perceptual image he has in mind. Or conversely, the one who tries to understand speech but cannot relate the words to his inner understanding of concepts. Such aphasias, however, are quite localized in their effect, for the patient can readily demonstrate that he recognizes and knows what objects are used for, and he is still able to learn and remember.

But no cerebral excision ever results in the loss of *portions* of memory as would be expected if the theory that memory was due to a neuronal and synaptic encoding were correct. No blocks of words, concepts or memories ever go missing after cerebral surgery.

Interestingly enough, however, Penfield has found that electrical stimulation of parts of the temporal lobe of the cortex (above the ears) occasionally results in the patient experiencing a vivid flashback to inconsequential and long forgotten scenes. These are more real than simply the remembering of events can be and are more in the nature of a waking dream, with the patient fully and simultaneously aware of both his past memory and his current existence. But as Penfield himself points out, this only shows that those parts of the brain are implicated or linked with the functioning of mind and memory. That memories are stored in the physical matter of the brain is not thereby demonstrated, for the electrical stimulation of the cortex will reach into the thalamus and the mid-brian and from there can spuriously activate a memory pattern within the subtle energy field of the mind itself, which is then played back from within the chit, for the subjective experience of the subject.

Similarly with all other psychological feelings induced by surgical and experimental techniques. It is no more surprising, for example, that emotions of fear are elicited when certain areas of the temporal lobe are electrically stimulated, than it is for a person to take fright at a loud noise or at any disturbing visual scene.

For just as the adrenal glands are also associated with the reflex emotion of fear, so too can parts of the brain be involved in its integration into appropriate physical action, without the need to conclude that fear is actually located in the temporal lobe. It simply indicates that the brain, the body and the mind are one integrated whole, not a sum of the parts.

There is also the case of a gifted BBC music producer and choral conductor who received damage to his temporal and frontal lobes during a viral infection of the brain. He is left with an inability to remember any event that happened longer than a few minutes ago. He constantly feels and reiterates that he was dead and has just returned to life, that his senses have only just returned to function, that previously he was blind, deaf and had lost the power of all his senses. And yet his intelligence and linguistic ability are quite unimpaired. And though he has no memory of being able to do so, he can – when presented with written music – still play the piano. He was even able to conduct his old choir with correctness and enthusiasm, when the members were reassembled for his benefit. A little later on the same day, however, when shown a video recording of his playing and conducting, he had absolutely no memory of having done so. His wife also comments that despite this loss of memory, the same basic personality is present. So it means that the memory of events and happenings is stored and accessed differently from our capabilities, talents and 'basic' personalities.

Actually, the inability to recall the details of events just passed is common to all of us. Few, if any, can recall the details of a conversation, certainly not verbatim, that has only just taken place, let alone after a passage of time. Similarly, most of the minutiae of our daily lives is apparently forgotten quite soon after it has happened. And with the exception of a rare few, our memory of past lives is completely blocked off from our consciousness by a natural, protective mechanism at the time of birth. But total loss of normally accepted recall is, of course, unusual.

So the integration of subtle energies into physical manifestation and with consciousness is clearly complex and beyond the purely mechanistic paradigms of conventional science.

In some modern theories, concepts of the brain as a hologram are employed to explain such problems as non-localization of memory and other mind functions within the physical brain, and to comprehend its clearly integrated activity as one whole. But even such a hologram would need a point of projection, creation and organization, because it is not a static system like the stored and fixed holograms of science, which can only reproduce one particular image – though even they require creation.

So intricate energy relationships at a subtle level are no doubt involved, but the higher patterning of the antashkarans is an essential part of the mechanism.

I do realize, though, the deep implications that this way of thinking has for one who has been taught and continues to believe that man is a chance and fortuitous arrangement of molecules that have bootstrapped themselves into existence out of nowhere in a Big Bang, many millions of years ago. The philosophical implications in even beginning to accept that man has a mind, let alone a soul, which are at fundamentally different levels of energy manifestation from his normal physical awareness, shake the roots of his being and sense of ease. Because he wants to feel that he is doing okay and does not need to change either his thinking or his behaviour.

The result is always the same. In previous times, such 'heretics' who challenged the current convention were at best ostracized and at worst imprisoned or even executed. Even now, in many parts of the world, we find one group of humans oppressing another, permitting no freedom of expression. In our own western culture, prejudice is only legally expressable by ridicule and rational argument. But in the supermarket of scientific and philosophical ideas, if a scientist backs the wrong horse, he can find himself out of a job. So fear of academic opinion keeps him upon the straight and narrow, if indeed he ever feels inclined to stray. It is only those who are already acknowledged experts in their fields and possess the necessary personality to carry it off, who can become accepted deviants from the current idiom. But even they may be ultimately pushed out from any central academic position.

Returning, then, to our discussion of the brain, what all this evidence means is that while certain areas of the cortex are characteristically used by the thalamus and central brain area for elaboration of particular functions, in the absence of these areas, other parts of the same cortex can – to some degree – suffice. The cortex is, therefore, a sort of universal area or scratch pad for working things out at a physical level. This would either be prior to action, after deliberation in the higher mental energies, or prior to shifting the information up into the higher levels within the mind energies for the purposes of memory, awareness, decision making and considered (however briefly) action. And it would be an integral part of vacuum and the more subtle patterning of pranic and mental activity into physical manifestation.

The actual positioning of the cortex, on the exterior, protecting the central area of precious, irreplacable thalamic and allied brain material is also a practical arrangement, so that a bang on the head does not automatically mean death. Furthermore, there are within the brain, something in the order of 10^{11} or 10^{12} neurons or brain cells, not all of which are used at any one time. In fact, the brain appears to be the one bodily organ where cells cannot be replaced when damaged or when they die due to old age. They are replaced by fatty material (the origin of the expression 'fat head'?), but the remaining neurons can, it has recently been discovered, grow new connections. A single neuron is likely to have up to 100,000 synaptic connections to other neurons, so you can imagine the complexity.

It is often said that we actually use only a small percentage of our brain cells. What is really meant, I suppose, is more that we only use a small part of our potential as human beings. We have the potentiality for super-consciousness and God-realization, but live most of our lives below the eye centre in an emotional and only semi-conscious condition. To say that we use only a fraction of our brain cells may or may not be true, but without any real understanding of how the intricacies of brain function are worked out, we are quite unable to say how the brain is impressed from within and performs its amazing functions.

The Non-Linear Relationship of Mind and Brain

We must always remember that the patterning and precipitation of energy from the within to the without is non-linear. It does not operate on a one-to-one basis, but on a more holographic principle of interwoven relatedness. Consider, for example:

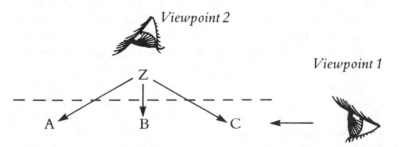

Viewed horizontally (1), A, B and C may appear to be unrelated. They are seen in a truer perspective, however, when viewed vertically (2) from Z, their point of origin.

Furthermore, both A, B and C automatically contain an imprint of Z's nature and are related, even at the horizontal level. This may or may not be outwardly apparent, though if it is, it is ususally inexplicable in conventional, linear and horizontal thought.

This is why, for example, oestrogen and testosterone are clearly related, being so similar, and yet biochemistry has no good reason why this should be so. On the paradigm presented herein, one would actually predict that the subtle patterning that relates to sexual polarity would be reflected in just such a fashion at the manifest level of molecules, tissues and organs. For opposite polarities are recognizably of the same nature. 'Up' relates to 'down', and a north pole to a south pole, not to any odd mixture of these dualities.

This mechanism of manifestation is true of all body function and becomes an essential aspect of understanding the energy flow when we come to appreciate the way that the mind patterns the whole brain, both simultaneously and specifically. Thus do we observe both localized areas of the brain with specific function and yet the ability to shift functions to alternative locations in the event of damage.

Some Simple Experiments with the Brain-Mind Interface

When we write a sentence, we have an idea in our mind and words appear upon a sheet of paper, through the medium of our fingers. But the mechanism or miracle by which this happens is not at all clear to our conscious experience. We lose sight, so to say, of the mental energy when it dips down into the realm of unconscious activity, reappearing to our sense of sight as we write.

It is in this scientifically uncharted and unrecognized area of subtle energies that interface with the brain actually takes place. This is why one sometimes makes linguistic mistakes when speaking or writing. Sometimes, even if the mind is clear, one's thoughts have moved ahead, faster than one's ability to write or speak. So one writes, for example, "The cat sat on the the mat", instead of "on the mat". The mind's controlling focus of attention is temporarily and partially unhooked from the lower brain energies which therefore slips into 'automatic' mode, producing odd or uncoordinated results.

There are a number of simple experiments you can try out to highlight your own awareness of your perceptive and mental experience in any activity. Try writing:

The cat sat on the tdxbnlhcm mat.

Or see how long it takes you to memorize, (so that you can write them down), the two meaningless words:

tdxbnlhcm taxbanhum

Try writing with your eyes shut or – even more difficult – decide upon a short sentence to write and then try writing it while looking to one side and reading something else. Be as aware and observant as you can, of all your mental and physical actions and note how *familiarity* is of great help. These everyday tasks will give you a very simple idea of mental, sensory and motor connections.

But note that in every instance, the mind is quite unconscious of the energy pathways between your thoughts and your action. You cannot consciously control your individual muscle cells or your physical brain physiology. This is the area of mind-brain-body interface.

The Brain as a Vacuum State Computer

As I have intimated it seems likely that the primary level of brain function lies in the vaccuum state, with the physical brain itself being a vacuum state, bioengineering unit. The overall structure, style of synaptic interconnections, electrical and magnetic properties, the biochemical and molecular activities, as well as the arrangement and structure of brain cells, all point to their being a part of an integrated *Vacuum State Computer*, both reading data from and encoding it into the vacuum or akashic condition. The brain itself consumes vast quantities of nutritional fuel, relative to its size, something like thirty per cent of all available body glucose, for example, and no doubt it requires all of this energy for driving the translation of energies into and out of the subtle state.

In fact, I imagine, that as a new generation of vacuum

state, energy-source and information technology devices are developed, it will be 'discovered' that nature has yet again beaten us to it and that our brains have been at it all along.

Actually, Sir Charles Sherrington, mentioned earlier, whose book *Man on His Nature*, is written in a most endearing and poetic form, believed that mind is essentially of another nature altogether to that of the matter and energy of the conventional physicist. But what it is, he did not know. In the context of the thinking expressed herein, mind is simply a more subtle and inward field of energy. The natural, subjective experiential aspects of the patterning inherent in the physical outworkings of such faculties as memory, speech, sensory perception and so on, are found in the akashic and subtle tattvic energy realms, leading inwardly to the central human mind or antashkarans. The brain is thus seen as a two-way (in-out and out-in) neurochemical vacuum and more subtle state computer or organizer of the inner matrix.

The active presence in man of all five tattwas gives him his superior mental apparatus and higher capacity for consciousness, while in lower species the increasing lack of active states within the subtle tattvic tapestry results in mostly instinctive behaviour, modulated by only a limited capacity for learned responses. Naturally, the greater the subtle tattvic complexity, then the higher the potential intelligence and consciousness of the creature.

That even plants have subtle aspects to their life experience is evidenced by their response to human care and vibration in other than the more mechanical ways of correct feeding and watering. Experiments have shown that plants do indeed respond to human emotion and that they also possess that indicator of subtle to gross activity, changing electrical fields and potentials.

Electrical Brain Activity

Much has been written in popular science concerning brain wave patterns. Most people know, for example that alpha waves are associated with meditation and relaxation, whilst beta waves are present during sensory or motor activity. And while this is interesting, medical science is still far removed from any coherent theory of brain function and its electrical activity. Indeed, Dr Paul Nunez in his book, *Electric Fields of the Brain*, comments in his opening chapter: "What is badly needed in EEG[1] is a comprehensive theoretical approach in order to obtain a rough idea of answers." That is to say that by conventional scientific method, no-one has any idea what on earth is going on. The idea must, however, have occurred to many scientists and others that simply examining the complexity of physiological and biochemical pathways in greater and greater detail, is not going to provide the answers which are sought. What is required first is a major shift in paradigm.

But without an understanding of mind, consciousness and the subtle energy domains, the state of bafflement will continue. At the most it will be possible to observe the brain's physical behaviour in greater detail. But no-one will ever dissect a thought. Our subjective sensory experience will never be caught under a microscope. The aesthetic sense of beauty, poetry and meaning will never be localized to the functioning of a few brain cells. Experience of being lies quite beyond the domain of the electrobiological and the biochemical, though its activity may be reflected therein.

The brain is simply the elaborator of mental, sensory and motor function at the physical level. It is the crossroads from gross to subtle and subtle to gross, in respect of subjective experience, consciousness and the higher controlling aspects of the physical body.

The electrical brain fields are measured on the scalp through interaction between the experimenter's instrumentation and the varying electrical potentials found upon the outside of the head. Basically, there are two kinds of activity. Firstly, there are rhythms and waves created from within the brain which relate to the individual's mental and emotional state, including sleep, rest, meditation, physical activity and so on. Secondly, there are potentials evoked by external stimuli. An auditory stimulus, for example, subsequently produces electrical variations within the mid-brain that spread out and can be measured

[1] Electroencephalogram or brainwave patterns

on the scalp with appropiate instrumentation and techniques. But the exact sources within the brain are little understood. Clearly the millions upon millions of brain cells, each with their thousands or hundreds of thousands of connections to other neurons are deeply implicated. The cortex alone contains ten thousand million (10^{10}) nerve cells within its two to three millimetres of outer thickness.

Certainly, it is observed anatomically that there are tracts of nerve cells radiating out from the mid-brain linking it to the cortex. But that tells us little concerning the details of this electrical activity. One imagines that it plays a part in keeping the brain integrated, so that all its parts work in synchrony, are informed of what the rest is doing. And this is born out by the effect of brain injury where selective damage can cause bizarre behaviour and experience, as we have discussed.

Conversely, it has been convincingly demonstrated many times that a subject can influence his brain wave patterns by conscious effort. By performing, often self-taught, mental exercises that relate to relaxation, a person can, for example, induce alpha rhythms. And when this effect is made visible to him through lights or audible tones, it can be used as a means of promoting relaxation. This is the basis underlying all biofeedback equipment. And interestingly, it has been observed that those who are most in tune or in harmony with themselves, more aware of their own existence as a conscious being and are in touch with their own feelings and thoughts, are the most readily able to control their own brain wave patterns or work successfully with biofeedback equipment.

Generally speaking, those who practice meditation are readily able to exert such control. That is to say that consciousness, awareness and control of the mind are totally dependent upon each other. And this is the basis of all eastern yogic philosophy. All eastern meditation is aimed at raising the level of consciousness by controlling the mind. Whether, ultimately, one needs biofeedback equipment is highly doubtful, but since meditation can be so difficult and tasteless for many beginners, the goal-oriented approach of biofeedback instrumentation is clearly of value, for those drawn to it.

In fact, in the early days of this kind of research, back in the 1960's, Joe Kamiya started out by paying his subjects. Quite soon, however, he had a long waiting list of volunteers who had found this technique of relaxation to be of such value in their lives that they wanted to return for no charge.

The mind, therefore, quite demonstrably affects brain physiology, both biochemically and electrobiologically, just as it does the rest of the body – consciously through motor and sensory activity and unconsciously through the patterning by the pranas of all unconscious bodily processes. And note that most of the motor and sensory systems are actually unconscious. Within ourselves, we are unconscious, for example, of the biochemical and physiological mechanisms by which nervous impulses travel and by which muscles contract.

Brain Polarity, Habit and Consciousness

In recent years there has been considerable talk concerning the polarity expressed between the left and right hemispheres. Normally, the left hemisphere in which functions concerning the right hand side of the body are formulated is spoken of as yang or male, responsible for the rational, analytical and executive aspects of one's being, while the right hand cortex is assigned the role of yin and is supposed to contain the more feminine faculties of intuition and synthesis.

Although there is no doubt that, generally speaking, rationality and analysis are more normally associated with men, whilst women are often more intuitive and synthetical in their approach, there seems to be little evidence to assign this polarity to particular parts of the physical brain itself. The yin and yang aspects of mental function are more correctly assigned to areas of mental energy higher up and more within than the brain. Though this needs to take expression through energy at the brain level, there is little real research to associate it with the right and left hemispheres.

According to conventional brain research, the left hand side of the body is controlled from the right hand cortex, and the right hand side is administered from the more dominant left hand cortex. And this also appears to be the same whether the person is left or right-handed.

Being dominant over the right hemisphere, the left cortex does express a polarity, a tension necessary for good tone and function, and in this sense it is yang or positive regarding the more yin or receptive right brain. But this is the same for both men and women, not the reverse. And there is also some electromagnetic evidence indicating opposing magnetic polarities between the two hemispheres.

The severing of the nerve fibres comprising the *corpus callosum* which connects the two hemispheres above the mid-brain region has been performed in certain epileptic patients, resulting in separation of certain sensory and motor functions. The dominant side continues its role, with the physical aspects of memory and mental processes clearly being continued from within its boundaries, while the other hemisphere assumes a more automatic functioning. As an interesting example of this, if the images entering each eye are carefully screened such that each hemisphere receives different visual input, it is possible for the right, yin hemisphere to receive written verbal instructions and communicate actions to the left hand without the conscious mind of the patient being aware of it.

That is to say, that (since it has been cut) the corpus callosum can no longer function in its role of transmitting information to the mid-brain and hence up to the higher area of mental function and awareness, but that in the vacuum and more subtle states, the information is still being transmitted, horizontally. And hence the patient moves his hand without *knowing* it or experiencing it within consciousness.

The brain itself naturally possesses other polarities of function – the motor and sensory cortex being but one example. The manner in which the optical nerves cross over from left to right, for instance, is also of interest and must clearly have some purposeful function, but apart from that associated with stereo-imagery for understanding where you are in a three dimensional world, I am at a loss to understand the deeper function behind it or its real significance.

Some theories of brain function assume that the conscious mind cannot work fast enough to perform such tasks as playing tennis where, in fractions of a second, decisions are made as to where to place a ball, how fast to hit it and so on. Scientists have therefore evolved theories of complex biochemical pattern-making and retrieval programs invoked from outside our consciousness, to explain such phenomena. But no physiological basis has been determined for such a notion, for the mind is swifter than any energy of the physical world and does provide the necessary thought. It is, indeed, almost at an instinctive and subconscious level, in that there is no time for rational, ordered thinking, but the spark of discrimination is definitely there of what to do with the ball for best advantage.

Habituation and reliance on previous patterns is, of course, essential, hence even the most gifted players of any sport or art, must practise. Habit is required both in musculature as well as in physical brain functions; but it is also required in the finer energies of the mind for the conscious, discriminatory process to take place. The motor and sensory indriyas, the tattvic energy fields and the antashkarans will all be involved. So in this sense, theories of complex, habituated energy paths are entirely correct, but more than just the biochemical is involved.

Actually, this same speed of the tennis player, making things up out of a inner library of learned or habituated responses as they go along, is employed in all of us all the time as we walk around and function in this world, avoiding this, doing that and so on.

Similarly, having learned to write one's signature with a pen, if one then tries to write it on a board with chalk or in the sand with a stick, using totally different muscles, the signatures are all identifiable and bear the same personal hallmark. It means that there is a pattern in the mind energy, upon which we draw when using new muscles to create a familiar pattern. It is just like a musician who has already learnt to play the guitar will then find it easier to play a lute or a banjo, rather than a wind or keyboard instrument. The similarity makes it possible for him to use already habituated mental pathways, of both a conscious and unconscious nature.

Inward Patterns, Instinct and DNA

Certain patterns are clearly built into the being that we are. Some young birds migrate independently of their parents, without ever being shown how or where to go. A baby deer or calf can walk within minutes of being born. The pattern is already there – instinctive, not learned – but then so is the whole subtle pattern that makes a deer a deer, a calf a calf, or a bird a bird. It is no more remarkable that a deer can stand soon after birth than that particular arrangement of energy or molecules and so on, has taken on the form of a deer at all. We may trace a part of the causative biochemical patterning to DNA, but where and out of what does the embryo really develop? What patterns the DNA? Where do its subatomic particles come from? Even embryologists have to admit defeat in the face of the final questions. And these questions do require answers if the structure in which our scientific knowledge is formulated is to be considered as valid.

It is a mistake to think that geneticists actually understand the processes by which they assume that the DNA code generates the form and structure of a creature. In terms of the minute biochemical and bioelectronic detail, the relationship of DNA to form is not at all understood. Nature may operate under the law of cause and effect, but the pattern of connection is not as linear as our intellectual minds would like it. It is one functioning whole, not a complex series of straight line or circular pathways, like we see in science books.

DNA is not the primary pattern. It is simply a point of focus upon which the more inward pattern is impressed. It *reflects* and is *involved* in the process of creating the form and physiology of a creature. But it is not the creator of form itself. If this were so, how could the absence or overproduction of a single molecule such as pituitary Growth Hormone override the genetic code for height, producing giantism and dwarfism, simply by its injection into otherwise normal and unsuspecting laboratory animals?

In the developing germ cell, as well as in the whole organism, DNA would appear to be a primary point of focus for the more inward life force. It is a part of the 'brain' of each cell. It is a window, a channel or a gateway through which the more inwardly directed energy may flow. The result is a molecular patterning which we mistakenly read as the formative pattern itself, not realizing that it is only a reflection of the subtle pattern which lies within. Its mechanisms are only a part of the process by which the inner blueprint manifests outwardly.

The existence of all aspects of instinct, therefore, would also seem to indicate that there is a patterning in the subtle fields that is transmitted from parent to child, just as the DNA, at a biochemical level, is also derived from the parents.

The Pineal Gland

Right in the centre of the head, (see figure 12-7), associated with the mid-brain, we find the *pineal gland*, the subject of much occult speculation and some little advance in scientific understanding during recent years. The size of a large cone-shaped pea, more usually called the *pineal organ* by modern medical research, it sits in the gateway between the third and fourth ventricles, washed by the cerebrospinal fluid as it flows from the two lateral ventricles into the third ventricle. From thence, via the *Aqueduct of Sylvius*, this fluid passes over the pineal gland and into the fourth ventricle.

Over the centuries, the pineal has been the subject of considerable speculation. Herophilus, the Greek anatomist, thought that it was a valve, regulating the flow of thought. During the seventeenth century it was considered that the pineal regulated the flow of cerebrospinal fluid, but by the end of the nineteenth century, after the discovery that a number of boys with pineal tumours had experienced premature puberty, it was assumed that the pineal had some relationship to ovarian and testicular development. In the mid-seventeeth century, the philosopher Rene Descartes, published his book of human physiology in which the pineal gland was first described as the seat of the 'rational soul'. There was (and still is), however, no evidence to support such a notion.

The theosophists took up this theme, however, around the turn of the nineteenth century and proclaimed the pineal as the seat of consciousness and the Third Eye, through which the inner regions of the soul are reached. Theosophy, until recent years, being the greatest body of occult literature in the west and from which many authors

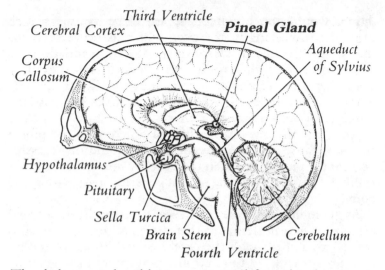

The thalamus and mid-brain are omitted from this drawing, in order to show the ventricles and the pineal gland.

Adapted with permission, from: Hormones: The Messengers of Life, Lawrence M. Crapo, W. H. Freeman & Co.

Figure 12-7. *The location of the pineal gland.*

have derived both information and inspiration, has spread its ideas far and wide. These days, in certain circles, it is often taken as *sine qua non* that the 'Third Eye' has its point of operation from the pineal gland, or that the pineal gland is the seat of the soul.

This has always seemed remarkable to me, when the brain itself, and particularly the higher brain stem, would seem to be the primary brain area through which mind and consciousness manifest. The true Third Eye, being further in than even the antashkarans, would appear to have no direct correlation whatever with the pineal gland.

Modern studies of the pineal organ link part of its functioning with that of the body's circadian rhythm, through the intermittent and cyclic secretions of its hormone, *melatonin*. In certain reptiles and amphibians, the pineal is indeed a third light receptor, located under a patch of thin skin, while in man and mammals it has a link with the exterior light conditions via a neural link in the *superior cervical ganglion* (in the neck). This direct knowledge communicated to the pineal concerning outside light conditions would not, however, appear to be its only source of informational input, for even with this nerve severed, the twenty-four hour cycles of melatonin production are not immediately disturbed. Nor indeed are they lost altogether after removal of the pineal (in lower species) when melatonin levels continue in a rhythmic pattern, though of reduced amplitude.

Note that the removal or loss of function of the pineal does not cause death, an event which would of necessity occur if the pineal provided the primary link with the inner realms of being or was the seat of consciousness within the body.

As I mentioned earlier, recent research in cranial osteopathy has determined that there are distinct physical waves flowing through the cerebrospinal fluid, created by or at least correlated to rhythmic movement of the cranial vault, involving both musculature and movement of cranial bones. Cranial osteopaths are trained to feel these rhythmic expansions and contractions while holding the cranium in their hands, readjusting the rhythms as required.

The pineal is situated in a duct, an organ-pipe, which would make an excellent point of resonance for the creation of any oscillation or vibration, being a confined space. Its relationship to both body rhythms and cerebrospinal fluid suggests quite strongly, therefore, that the pineal gland could also be both an emitter and monitor of vibration or oscillation within the body, providing part of the overall control of patterning or rhythm in physiological functioning, especially at an endocrine level.

Whether these waveforms are like sound waves or whether they are electromagnetic, electron plasma, scalar wave or some other rhythmic energy variation is open to speculation and the energetic resonances inherent in the shape of the melatonin hormone molecule might provide some clues.

Melatonin (see figure 12-8) itself possesses a unique shape and structure of molecule, quite unlike that of any other hormone in the body, and related more to *serotonin*, *dopamine* and other neurotransmitters.

One is, therefore, led to speculate that just as adrenaline and noradrenaline have similar structures and perform analagous roles in the endocrine and autonomic nervous systems, respectively, so too might melatonin (the hormone) and serotonin (the neurotransmitter) be expressing a similar neural to endocrine polarity, though the current language of biochemistry does not give us a terminology in which this may be expressed.

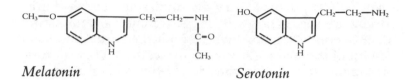

Melatonin   *Serotonin*

Figure 12-8. Melatonin, an unusual hormone, showing its similarity to serotonin.

It is also possible that the inner resonances and structure of melatonin could hold many pointers to pineal function, perhaps even to atomic wave patterns or oscillations hitherto undetected in nature.

And this is born out to some degree, not only by the rhythmic secretion of melatonin, but also by suggestions from pineal research of recent years that melatonin and/or the pineal are in some way connected to the patterns of secretion of other bodily hormones and chemical messengers. Noradrenaline, serotonin, acetyl co-enzyme A, oxytocin, a vasopressin-like substance, prolactin, testosterone and gonadotropin releasing factor (a pituitary hormone) are all implicated in lower species where the pineal clearly has a role in the seasonal control of sexual activity related not only to light and dark cycles of the sun, but also to the considerably weaker light of the full moon. Melatonin, for example, blocks the LH surge in rats that leads to ovulation, whose oestrus cycle is also affected by changes in the light and dark cycle. Many of these substances as well as LH and somatostatin, are also found in human pineals, but the same kind of research that is conducted on animals, cannot of course, be performed upon humans. So it is difficult to get direct information regarding human pineal activity.

Similarly, urinary and blood plasma levels of testosterone are suppressed in blind men, as are levels of thyroxine

(T4), where the link is thought to be via the pituitary gland. Again, the pineal seems to be involved in the thermoregulatory, behavioural patterns of terrestrial ectotherms (ie. cold blooded creatures that use the cyclic availability of the sun to warm up), though whether this function is present in warm-blooded species is unclear. In fact, seals have the largest pineal organ amongst mammals, whilst penguins carry the similar honours for birds. Both these species have a wide geographical and migratory distribution in locations where both the temperature and length of day and night vary considerably. These factors, in addition to requiring considerable physiological adaptability in themselves, also have a direct bearing on the timing and geographical location of reproductive functioning.

There is considerable evidence, too, that melatonin may not be a primary endocrine secretion of the pineal but only a link in the chain of activity. Melatonin is also known to be produced in the retina of the eye, in *enterochromaffin* cells and in human red blood cells or *erythrocytes*. It is also found in very small concentrations in the peripheral nerves of man and other species.

The pineal organ itself consists of four main cellular types and melatonin synthesis is only implicated with two of them – *the noradrenergic sympathetic nerve fibres* (part of the neuronal input) and the indigenous *pinealocytes*. But these two cell structures are themselves involved in considerably more than just melatonin synthesis, in processes as yet unravelled, while no specific function at all has yet been assigned to the *glial* tissue and *pineal nerve cells* which connect to the central nervous system. Nor is there any scientific explanation offered for the electrical activity within the pineal, which, in the thinking of this book, is associated with the vacuum and subtle state interface.

Furthermore, much of pineal research has focused upon melatonin only because the *indolamine* group to which it belongs has been the subject of much previous research and because another of this group, serotonin, is a neurohormone with known activity in other parts of the brain, even being implicated in certain mental disorders. And serotonin is an immediate precursor of bodily melatonin synthesis. There are, however, many other active substances in the pineal upon which little research has yet been conducted, as researchers will readily concur.

The pineal organ responds (in animals, at least, where research is easier) to thermal, auditory, olfactory, visual, nutritional and stress-related stimuli, where the links may be via other bodily organs and systems rather than directly upon the pineal. Stress responses, for example, are primarily mediated via the adrenal medulla, as is evidenced by the fact that stress-related changes in the pineal are prevented by removal of the adrenal gland.

The pineal also has receptors for sex steroids and is influenced by other endocrine glands, a fact which has led researchers to postulate a pineal role as an endocrine to endocrine transducer, helping in the overall neurohormone integration. Within the brain, research data suggests that it has a close working relationship with the hypothalamus. There is increasing evidence, for example, that both melatonin and serotonin influence hypothalamic releasing hormones. The hypothalamus, too, forms concentrations of melatonin which have been injected into the blood stream. And the hypothalamus, like the pineal, is physically in very close association with the third ventricle.

Considerable research remains to be done, but there is accumulating evidence for a complex, reciprocal relationship between the central nervous system, the endocrine system and the pineal, including some intriguing research on the patterning of its electrical activity. It is, after all, very much a part of the brain, where electrical activity is already an observable aspect of its functioning, though the role it plays and its significance are far from understood.

For as much as it is worth, therefore, I would put my bet on the pineal being both an originator and sensor of energy patterns (molecular and otherwise) governing and monitoring physiological rhythms with linkages to endocrine, neural and other systems in the body by energetic mechanisms as yet undiscovered. And since rhythm, pattern and polarity are essential in any energy system, this gives the pineal a uniquely powerful function. This conjecture also makes sense of the pineal tumour and early puberty syndrome (an upset to the rhythm of sexual maturation), as well as of the evidence of medical research that pineal activity is linked with the rhythmic output of other bodily hormones. Perhaps the pineal works in close concert with the hypothalamus and the pituitary gland, imposing a rhythmic and generally integrating control over their releasing-inhibiting feedback loops.

The presence of a multitude of other hormones within the pineal, representative of all the major endocrine glands and its role in the administration of bodily rhythms leads one to speculate on the possibility of molecular resonances as a part of the mechanism by which this rhythmic control is effected. If each molecule is a vibrant lower harmonic of higher energy within the vacuum and subtle states and if hormones are seen as epitomizing the modality of a particular energetic function, that is – as a keynote – then the integration of rhythms by the pineal could occur by resonance or by activation of vibration within the molecules that are 'waiting around', ready for energizing. That is, the pineal could be channelling into itself patterns that reflect the rhythms abounding within both the body and the environment. These could be electrical, electromagnetic, molecular, electron plasma, scalar wave, gravitational or any other form of energy manifestation with which, as yet, we may not even be familiar. Certainly, seated below the mid-brain, the crossroads of the central nervous system, the pineal is uniquely situated for the performance of such a role.

These rhythms and energy patterns would then selectively activate, by resonance, the hormones already attuned to that sphere of energy vibration and from that resonance and activity would be derived a knowledge of the incoming pattern and, from the function of the hormone, what to do about it.

From a tattvic point of view, one can speculate that each endocrine gland takes its associated chakra and tattwa as a dominant theme or vibration out of which are spun or woven the molecular structure of the individual hormones, modulated by the different petals or energy characteristics within the chakra, and influenced to a smaller degree by other tattvic vibrations. Thus, for example, the adrenals also produce small quantities of steroid hormones normally associated with the watery, sacral chakra, as well as blocking the pancreatic secretions of insulin through the activity of cortisol.

The brain ventricles previously mentioned are also likely to be implicated. They constitute a comparatively intricate arrangement of interconnecting lacunae filled with cerebrospinal fluid. This fluid, which bathes the pineal gland, also surrounding the brain between the inside of the skull and the cerebral cortex, is generally considered to provide protection, nutrition, support and a means of removing metabolic waste products. In content, it is somewhat similar to blood plasma but is less concentrated, possessing fewer potassium and calcium ions and less proteins. On the other hand, it contains a higher concentration of sodium, chloride and magnesium ions. Its suggested function of carrying vibrational impulses has already been discussed and it would not be surprising if it were also found to carry energy patterns from place to place in the shape of neurohormones.

CHAPTER 13

Mental States and Disturbances

The Recurrence of Themes

One is continually struck, when attempting to unravel the
multitude of data presented from biochemical research, by
the recurrence of themes. It is as if one is presented with a
computer-generated graphics pattern of complex interconnecting lines, displayed on a video terminal, but viewed
through a cardboard panel with holes in it. The data seen
through the individual holes have similarities with each
other and the mind is led into feeling that all would be
revealed if only the obscurities between the holes could be
removed. The research becomes all-absorbing, since patterns are found to continually re-occur, leading one to
believe that the complete answer will be discovered simply
by removing more and more of the cardboard between the
holes.

The fact is, however, that the pattern of apparently
causally connected lines is only an effect, an illusion even,
created by the computer program, where the primary
causative pattern is actually to be found in a quite different
energy field to that of its visual representation on screen.
Similarly, the outward manifestation of atoms, molecules,
subatomic particles, electromagnetic forces and the like
are simply bubbles or patterns on the surface of more
primary, causative, energy fields, within.

Mental and Psychological Disturbances

Given a complex energetic mechanism and structure containing both physical subtle, emotional and mental energies, some within our consciousness and others at unconscious levels, it is easy to understand how imbalance and
malfunction at any one level or point can result in symptoms of ill-health at any of the others, whether of a

physical, psychological or mental nature. For the system operates as a whole.

Imbalance and malfunction can be biochemical, from dietary, genetic or environmental origin. They may be electrobiological, due either to defects in subtle energy manifestation mechanisms or to external electromagnetic factors that are particularly allergenic or disharmonious to that individual. The source of energetic disturbance may be in the subtle tattvic domains – over or under-activity of one or more tattwas or a lack of coordination between them. Flows of subtle energy patterns around the body may be blocked, or they may be too yin or too yang. Pranic patterning, too, may be blocked or impeded, resulting in a loss of mobility in particular areas of one's being, physical or psychological.

Particular gates, valves, pathways or through-routes and focal or resonance points, such as the chakras or endocrine glands, may be at fault. Disturbance in endocrine function, more than any other non-neural system in the body, results in emotional and mental changes. Practically all endocrine secretions have both subtle and obvious effects on emotional life and conversly, emotional and mental energies change the pattern of hormonal activity.

Damage to areas of the brain, whether arising from accident, haemorrhage, tumour or some other physiological disorder will modify both the bodily and the finer energies of our human constitution, while disharmonious energy complexes in the through-route to the antashkarans can result in disturbance to mental function, leading to emotional frustration.

Energetic disturbances within the antashkarans arising from activities and impressions of the present or previous lives can lead to problems of communication, where the ego becomes centered upon energies, memories and activities within its own mental patterns, with little outward activity or direction of attention. This perhaps is the area of schizophrenic disturbance, where the individual becomes withdrawn into his own mental world and where the apparent causes of withdrawal can be any of the factors mentioned above. Bizarre behaviour patterns will naturally result since the focus of attention is within, not under meditative and conscious control, but in a contorted and troubled manner.

In fact, mental energy vortices could occur in the patterning of the antashkarans, as the sense of identity moves between such vortices, uneasily seeking coherence and integration, appearing outwardly as the split personality or extreme swings and changes in mood and behaviour. There have even been cases recorded of schizophrenic individuals oscillating between not just two or three 'personalities', but between ten and twenty.

An understanding of inner energy patterns provides a comprehension of how these states can occur and how environmental, dietary, physiological and all other energy interchanges will affect the patient.

A medically oriented approach of blocking the manifestation of behaviour patterns by drugging or electrifying the areas of the brain responsible for the most obvious motor action and behaviour will therefore do no more than ligature the pathway between the problem and its outward manifestation, making the patient more amenable and easy to handle, but doing nothing but further damage to the patient himself.

Psychotherapy is more likely to have some success, but where the patient is too withdrawn into their own inner world of mental gyrations and uncoordinated energies, or locked into habituated behaviour patterns, none but the most sensitive of therapists may ever reach them. Dietary changes, too, can modify and enhance bodily biochemistry, toning up the energy pathways through which the higher energies are manifested, and much good work has been done along these lines. A superb and highly nutritious diet should automatically be provided for all mental (indeed, any kind of) patient, as a basis for further treatment, preferably balanced for each individual. An administrative nightmare, no doubt, but trials have shown considerable improvements in hospitals and care units where these methods have been tried. Just the atmosphere of loving care, itself, can work wonders, creating harmony where once was discord.

Then, the work has to be at a subtle level. I cannot see how drugs can really help a patient whose primary problems are clearly in subtle levels of energy. At best they will block off the expression of symptoms which those who have to deal with them find socially disturbing, but they will not help the patient at a deeper level.

Mostly, this kind of deep patterning, like personality, is so deeply ingrained into the energies of the antashkarans and patterned into the subtle tattwas that at best one can only hope to ameliorate the condition, not cure. Just as one rarely sees an individual's personality change so much that they become unrecognizable. The basic karmic patterning of that life is always there, expressed in physical terms as the constitution, and emotionally/mentally as the personality.

Polarity therapy, which works directly on the tattvic fields, homoeopathy, Bach flower remedies, gem remedies, crystals, Pulsors, colour therapy, acupuncture – all these and more – do work and can provide help at the subtle energy level. Recently, my acupuncturist has been using a technique based on a fusion of acupressure and other subtle energy balancing techniques and known as *Zero Balancing*. The originator, Dr Fritz Smith M.D., is trained in acupuncture, osteopathy, rolfing and cranial osteopathy, as well as having a conventional medical background. This technique, like many others, works on the subtle energy interface and has a considerably relaxing, calming and balancing effect. The originator is also conversant with both yogic and Chinese philosophy of the kind that is discussed herein and has written an interesting book, *Inner Bridges*.

Molecular and Energetic Relationships

Many neurologists and endocrinologists, when confronted with a particular molecule performing apparently different, or even related, roles in different parts of the body, miss the obvious connection and decide that it is parsimony on the part of evolutionary nature which lies behind it. Thus, for example, we find hormones such as adrenaline not only performing their classically understood functions as messengers from the adrenals, but also behaving as neurotransmitters in neurological tissue, including the brain.

Bearing in mind the image of the molecule as a vibrating energy pattern, it takes very little imagination to perceive how similar vibrations and resonances will occur at various points in an energy complex and how similar functionality is likely to possess similar vibration or energy patterning. Though the outward manifestations of the function may *appear* to be different.

Taking this one step inwards, where spatial relationships are likely to have different characteristics to those of the gross physical world, we perceive with our subtle senses, that the vibrational interaction of the five subtle tattvic fields, through the intermediary of the vacuum or gross akashic state, causes nodes, and points of confluence and divergence. These are perceived outwardly as subatomic particles, atoms and molecules themselves. This is much in the manner of sand, which organizes itself into intricate and symmetrical forms when placed on a plate that is vibrated with a violin bow. Or it is like the complex patterning formed by the combination of varying electronic wave-forms on an oscilloscope or on our TV screens, producing the illusion of real scenes with such intensity that even our emotions are aroused and we weep or laugh. Indeed, mystics have always maintained that this world is an illusion, Maya, spun into existence by the vibration of energy beyond our perception. Like a TV screen, it is a dancing mirage that grips our mind and emotions, but ever changes, finally disappearing from view only when we die.

In the context of this thinking, therefore, coincidence and patterns would be nodal points, points of specific or particular interaction, places of energy confluence or depletion within the interplay of tattvic vibration. They are like the discrete tunes that attract one's attention, emerging from the (organized) background of a symphony.

Similarly, we often observe that the same biochemical constituents which are found in lower species are also found in higher animals. This, too, is put down to evolution from common ancestors. An alternative theory, however, would be that we are constituted from the same subtle, tattvic energy fields as the lower species. Therefore, the inter-actions and patterns formed by their vibrations as the dense precipitations of *physically observable energies come into being*, would predictably be similar. In fact, on this hypothesis, it would make an interesting corroborative survey to check for the relationships between the biochemistry of different classes of species according to which tattwas are said to be active within them.

Mental Handicap and Autism

The problems of autistic and mentally handicapped people similarly pose us with difficulties in understanding. Sometimes, the symptoms can be directly attributed to brain damage, which means a disturbance to the outward brain mechanisms through which the mind conmunicates with the world. Hence the inability to communicate and act 'normally'.

But there are cases where there has neither been any accident, nor does there appear to be any other brain defect, though this does not preclude the existence of undetected biochemical or bioelectrical disorders. If this is the situation, that the brain is functioning correctly, then it means that the source of the energetic disturbance lies in the more subtle realm. But I would imagine that this disharmony must appear in some way at the level of brain function, though any detected abnormalities would be essentially secondary effects, not primary causes.

But as I have commented previously, the essential cause for everything that happens in our life lies in the seed-energy of our destiny karmas, programmed into our inner mind substance of the antashkarans. So whether we have broken a leg, 'caught' a cold or suffer from mental or emotional disturbance, the primary causative energy lies in our human mind, itself energized from within by higher aspects of mind, and by our soul.

Interestingly, there are a very few mentally subnormal children who possess the most remarkable gifts and during February 1987, BBC television showed a fascinating Q.E.D. program concerning some of them. One man, for instance, can tell you, in disrupted speech patterns, the day of the week of any date you care to mention even centuries ago, or in the future. And he does it faster than you can key the data into a computer and get a response. Yet, the possibility of his being a mathematical genius is totally precluded. He was unable to even add up 7 + 8. He insisted that the answer was 14.

Similarly, they showed a young man with a memory for intricate tunes, which he plays on the piano or guitar. This includes Bach and other complex pieces. He can hear a piece once, in small sections, and then reproduce it. His musical interpretation and finesse is lacking, but his skill in memory is greater than that of many professional musicians.

Lastly, there was the case of a boy who can make the most intricate drawings of buildings with fine pencil strokes. His manner of holding a pencil is still childlike, indicating poorly matured physical integration of brain and mind, but his ability is most remarkable. It is a skill mastered by very few normal artists. In this case, artistic interpretation and perspective were most definitely present.

Neurologists and brain specialists, of course, are quite unable to explain what is going on. As I have said, the model of mind as being of a biochemical and bioelectrical nature is so limited that it is quite unable to even integrate with psychology and the study of behaviour. For this comprehension, the multi-layered concept of subtle energies is essential.

One of the interesting points to observe in these particular cases is that in all instances the gift displays itself in a totally non-intellectual fashion. Just like a child who in his early years can learn several languages easily, rapidly and directly, without intellectual analysis, so that the ability to understand and use language remains as a spontaneous gift for the rest of his life, so do these autistic gifts find expression through a direct channel, without intellectual processes involving the logic with which we are familiar.

It simply means that the mental putty has focused on one particular skill and the mind, being the pattern for the whole of life, provides the intuitive abilities to manifest the skill.

But it is not only mentally subnormal people who have these special gifts. We are all unique, expressing totally individual characteristics. Some may have amazing athletic or gymnastic prowess, others are painters, musicians or are skilled in so many other ways. And the patterning all lies in the inner human mind, whose varieties and subtle mechanisms are almost infinite. Observe how different we all are, and have been, throughout the course of history.

In mentally handicapped people, that part of the biological vacuum state computer which permits outward expression, functions only poorly and so we have bizarre manifestations. When someone is normally adjusted and has some other great skill, we just say that they are talented. But actually, we understand that talent or indeed any aspect of human mental function, just as little as we do when it is observed in the mentally handicapped. But if the talent remains while the mechanisms of outward intelligent expression inherent in certain parts of the subtle mind function are disturbed, then we are left with a handicapped person possessing a special gift. "It's all in the mind, folks!" as Spike Milligan would say.

There is one further aspect to all of this. In India one occasionally meets or hears of those they call *mastanas*. A mastana is a mystically evolved person whose manner of outward expression is disrupted, in the normal sense. Inwardly, they are in ecstatic bliss and may often even perform miracles. Their soul flies into higher planes on a regular basis. But outwardly, they have a 'handicap' in that they cannot really express themselves normally or behave as 'normal' people. But they can and do sometimes bestow spontaneous mystic experiences on seekers whom they meet and to whom they take a fancy. Similarly, autistic people who characteristically remain absorbed in themselves and do not speak, may be spiritually in a good condition, suffering only from a disruption to that part of the mental and brain mechanisms which permit outward expression.

In fact, the inward condition of mentally handicapped and autistic people can vary tremendously. Just like everyone else, they are all different, with their own personalities and some may even have far higher spiritual aspirations than so-called normal people. Many of them have a most sweet and affectionate disposition that would advantage more than a few of the rest of us!

Hallucination and Schizophrenia

Also characteristic of schizophrenia and psychosis, hallucination is an intriguing experience when the person feels that they perceive something which is not actually there. Somewhere between awareness and the physical sense organ, an energetic oscillation slips into the system which is then appreciated as a genuine perception. Depending upon how high up within the vertical spectrum of energies this malfunction occurs, the hallucination is taken as more – or less – real.

If the brain is stimulated electrically in the visual cortex, for example, a patient will appear to perceive flashes of light and colour. But they may be simply a passive observer of the phenomenon, especially when it is not backed up by perceptions through the other senses. When one does not hear or feel anything, for example, to endorse his visual impression. But if the hallucination takes place very close to the inner centre of awareness, most probably manifesting out of the melee of subconscious mind energies, then a person is most likely to be upset by it. Especially if he is already emotionally or even schizophrenically disturbed.

Mystics, in fact, say that this physical world is like a dream or an hallucination. The entire play is intricately programmed into our antashkarans when we take birth. The roll of cine film or the pre-recorded videotape that comprises our destiny, plays itself automatically, intricately connected with the similar destinies of others, with our own inner physical and psychological constitution and with events in the so-called outer world. Thus are we all jointly deluded into taking it as real, through the close identification of our ego or ahankar with these predestined events; ego itself being an integral part of the antashkarans.

Even in meditation, there comes a time when images or impressions from the mind come before the practitioner, even of frightful or horrific appearance, or beautiful and fascinating. One is advised to observe these visions with a detached mind and to be neither attracted nor repulsed. But to those whom these experiences happen spontaneously and without control, during the normal course of a working day, they can be disturbing and in schizophrenic conditions, they will be a part of the symptoms of the patient's psychosis.

Schizophrenia can thus have a basis both in the brain biochemistry as well as in inner mental and emotional malfunction. In fact, the inner patterning of mind and pranic energies under the karmic influence would be primarily responsible for a schizophrenic tendency. Thus diet, as well as sociological and environmental factors, can be expected to modulate physiological brain function just as much in schizophrenics as with the rest of us. As in all things the inner reflects the outer and vice versa.

Thus it is understandable that the levels of certain neuro-transmitters, such as *dopamine*, found in brain cell synapses or junctions, are higher in schizophrenic types than in the rest of us, while *serotonin* levels are higher in depressive types. Dopamine is an activator of inter-neuronal signals and with one of the schizophrenics' major problems being an over-active mind and over-sensitive response to sti-muli, this is understandable. So though no doubt some relief from schizophenia can be obtained by physically blocking or reducing dopamine activity with a drug, the better treatment, if it were available, would be to reach within the higher mental energies and there perform subtle energy manipulation and rebalancing. But since the lower, molecular level, reflects the higher, changes to the lower will also affect the higher and until we have better under-standing of subtle techniques, changes to the biochemical balance, through diet, would seem a natural starting point, as I have previously suggested.

It would also, no doubt, be greatly advantageous if some of the subtle energy therapies were given a thorough trial for healing not only advanced schizophrenia and psychosis, but also all other forms of illness and disturb-ances to physical and psychological health. Because some of these therapies already possess physical techniques for influencing the subtle state.

Time and Consciousness

Actually, time is essentially something which is experi-enced only by life forms. Inert matter, itself, experiences no time, though *we* may perceive matter within a temporal context. The experience of time arises due to a differentia-tion of the observer from the observed, whose changes are then perceived within a context of time. Since the frame of reference of different observers can and does vary, time – or its *rate of change* – may therefore be perceived differently by observers in different frames of reference, as Einstein both noted and encapsulated in mathematical notation. It is almost like a Doppler effect taking place within the framework of time and space.[1]

Time first arises in the causal realm of the Universal Mind, where the soul receives its first covering of materiomental substance and therefore, first begins experiencing 'reality' as an observer, rather than as one with it. If, like God, we were at one with everything, part and parcel and within every particle, then from that point of view – no time would exist. Past, present and future would collapse into one.

Time is therefore a part of the fabric of change, together with the three spacial dimensions, and this truth can be expressed mathematically as Einsteinian space-time.

Note, however, that time and space do not cease to exist in the subtle realms. Far from it. They are, however, greatly expanded, until, with God, they reach infinite proportions. This is experienced and described by mystics, when they move into the inner realms, as the inner universes being increasingly more vast in spacial dimensions and with time, or the rate of change, being greatly slowed down.

Subtle Time, Subjective Time

It is a matter of observation that while some folk appear to achieve very little in a given span of time, others seem full of ingenuity (air) and drive (fire) accomplishing far-reaching goals in apparently no time at all. The underlying patterning, of course, is derived from the karmic energy of destiny, but impressed upon the human mind and selectively stimulating the subtle tattvic constitution through the medium or curtain of the subtle akashic state.

Since time is a measure of change as subjectively experienced by the individual, the one whose mental energy is focused more upon the airy and fiery aspects of their subtle being experiences life through a window coloured by the more rapid rate at which these two tattwas vibrate. The

---

[1] The Doppler effect is due to compression or expansion of propagating waveforms created by the relative speeds between the observer and the wave source. This is why the siren of a travelling ambulance appears to change pitch as it passes you, for example.

slower earthy and watery natures accomplish things more slowly and surely, pedantically and systematically plodding their way through the events of life. These are generalizations, of course, because, as discussed earlier, the emotional activity of the tattwas is considerably intermixed. Thus the airy nature may be frustrated by the slowness of earth, or may be harmoniously blended with it, providing well-organized practicality and rapid manifestation of the airy ideas.

The point I am moving towards is that the inner sense of being of each individual has a different appreciation of time because of their subtle energetic constitution. As with all psychology, the *feeling* is based upon the attention playing upon real energies in the subtle tattvic state. Our subjective time *is* energetically different from each other and in any relationship, the parties will always be out of step (a function of timing), unless, firstly, they are constitutionally similar, and then they permit their energies to merge into one functioning whole. That is, they work together as one.

Alternatively, two people with quite different *subjective time* can still operate well together provided that they can adapt to and totally accept that the other is perceiving things in a different subjective time scale and is therefore accomplishing their tasks in quite a different way. Just as the airy and fiery wren can accommodate twenty notes per second in his song, so too does the atmosphere of similarly constituted human beings seem to radiate a subtle vibration of compression, a dynamo of activity.

Concentration of mind is the key to all accomplishment whether by air, fire, water or earth, and the fast-moving, airy and scattered mind, whilst still filling each minute with activity, compression and busy-ness, actually achieves very little. It is here that the earthy tortoise will beat the hare. But if the hare retains its sense of concentration and purpose, the tortoise will never catch it. Indeed, what is business, but busy-ness?

Time, therefore, in addition to its outer aspects, is a genuinely energetic, subjective phenomenon, as we all experience within the limited confines of our own psychology. Boredom or waiting with an idle mind makes time drag, whereas concentration, enjoyment and involvement makes one unaware of its passage. Time is then subjectively both 'slowed down', since by concentration our mind is narrowed in its focus, and 'speeded-up' when we realize how unaware we have been of its passage, after our concentration lapses.

Interestingly, birds, with their fiery and airy tattwas expressed within a matrix of water, have a basal metabolic rate (BMR) many times higher than other species. A heavy bird like the ostrich is perhaps at the same rate as a gazelle, but a wren or a hummingbird possess both metabolic rates and a corresponding patterning in the subtle fields of their instinctive intelligence active at a speed of which we humans have no experience.

To a hummingbird or a wren, a second must be a vastly longer span of *experience* than it would be to ourselves, when one observes what they can pack into it, in terms of song, activity, observation and metabolic change.

Serotonin, LSD, Brain Drugs, Consciousness, Time and Psychosis

The debate concerning the origins of psychosis has generally speaking produced two camps: those who feel that the causes are experiential, psychological, social and environmental. And those who feel that its causes are of a biochemical nature, whilst conceding that environmental factors can also play a part.

In the context of the inner dimensional thinking of this book, it is clear that the way one perceives the cause depends entirely upon one's concept of the total human mechanism which is observed to be operating in a psychotic mode.

The understanding of an energetic model which includes both the gross physical, horizontal energies of biochemistry and bioelectricity, as well as the vertical energy spectrum that provides the energy fields which includes those of the mind and emotions, is extremely powerful. For the horizontal and the vertical spectra interact continuously, the horizontal being created from within out of the more inward field. The inward therefore affects the outward and the outward modifies the inward. The inward field of our mind and emotions, conscious and unconscious, therefore affects our biochemistry automatically and conversely our biochemistry will affect the way we feel and think.

Thus, both philosophies of schizophrenia are automatically seen as a part of just one energetic mechanism. But, as with all aspects of our human life, the primary patterning is built into our mind structure, the antashkarans, at birth, as our destiny. From there it is spun out over the course of time, as our life passes, creating the circumstances from within that we experience in our daily lives.

At the biochemical level, some interesting research has been performed on key substances that are linked to the manifestation of psychotic states. Chief among these are a family of molecules which are structurally quite similar and which include serotonin, LSD, L-dopa, dopamine, amphetamine, mescaline, noradrenaline and many others, (see figures 13-1 and 13-2). Some of these occur naturally in the body, while others are synthetic or found in various plants, especially some species of mushroom.

Serotonin is found in many parts of the body – in the blood, skin, spleen, lungs, intestines, liver, hypothalamus and pineal, as well as in the brain. In the body, it is associated with the contraction of involuntary musculature, where it is thought to be implicated in the transport of calcium ions – an essential part of the process of muscle cell contraction. The mechanisms of its action within the brain are even less understood, except that it is involved in the inhibition of nervous impulse transmission.

Hallucinogenic drugs such as LSD, L-dopa, ergot and other naturally occurring *alkaloids* seem to act, at least in part, by blocking the activity of serotonin. At the molecular level, a blocker acts like a key that fits the key-hole, but will not turn. It therefore prevents the real key from doing its job. But exactly how the energetic link from biochemistry to mind operates is a matter for some speculation and various models have already been suggested. But operate it most definitely does.

In general terms, brain drugs such as LSD and L-dopa can move the centre of attention into the more subtle physical realms by biochemically ligaturing part of the physical brain pathways, thereby forcing the attention to

Serotonin

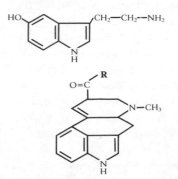

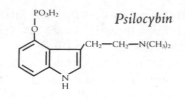 *Psilocybin*

Ergot alkaloid base
When R *is diethylamino-,*
it becomes LSD
When R *is a peptide,*
it becomes ergotoxine,
ergotamine etc.

Figure 13-1. Serotonin, LSD and the ergot alkaloids, psilocybin. Note how the same centrally-positioned double ring structure is present in all of these mind-affecting substances.

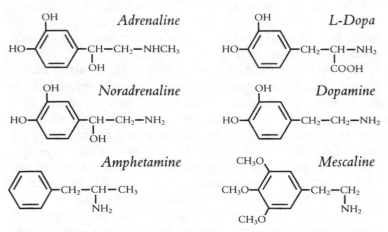

Figure 13-2. Adrenaline, noradrenaline, amphetamine, dopamine, L-dopa and mescaline. Note once again the similarities between these modifiers to central nervous system activity. Interestingly, mescaline, which has similar psychedelic effects to LSD, does not contain the serotonin double ring. Users of these psychedelic substances have reported distinct differences, as well as underlying similarities, between the subjective, psychedelic experiences induced by LSD, psilocybin and mescaline, while ergot induces temporary psychotic states. Note, too, how amphetamine, known on the drug scene as 'speed', because of its 'speeding-up' effects upon the mind, bears distinct similarities to adrenaline and noradrenaline, two naturally-produced substances inducing rapidity of response.

focus on its more inward subtle constitution. The subject then experiences a greatly expanded sense of time such that looking at a watch will make them stare with incredulity both at their appreciation of time, which has become quite different, and at the apparent slowness with which the second hand is moving.

In fact, subjects in these states can also experience their thought vibrations as *real things*, while their closer association with the mental indriyas or mental analogues of the sense organs, leads to both a heightened perceptual experience and awareness of colour, form, sound, taste, touch and smell. The likelihood of hallucination is also increased because the physical brain linkages with the sensory organs have been partially disrupted, creating the potential for schizophrenic-like states, in which thoughts become experiences.

Subconscious images from within the mind and emotional energy complex can also, therefore, impinge upon the indriyas. In the absence of solid grounding within the normal five physical senses, due to the effect of the drug, the result can be severe hallucination that is capable of arousing a tremendous emotional response, depending upon the individual's rational control and psychological constitution. The emotional response then becomes linked into the hallucination in a complex feedback loop and the patient can become locked in to symptoms and experience of severe paranoia and psychosis.

It is interesting, however, how different brain and mind-affecting drugs each produce subtley different subjective experiences and how some substances which from their molecular structure might be expected to possess psychoactive properties are apparently quite inert. We meet another old friend here, because for example, LSD, one of the most powerful of synthetic hallucinogenic substances *is only psychoactive in L-isometric form*. The D-isomer has no such effect.

Conventionally, psychosis can be considered as being of three kinds. *Organic psychoses* are those produced by anatomical changes to the central nervous system – from *syphilis*, for example. Secondly, there are those induced by toxic substances like alcohol and mind-affecting drugs. Thirdly, there are those not immediately attributable to physical causes including schizophrenia, manic depression and involutional melancholia.

Symptomatically, the appearance of the psychosis may be similar in all three categories, and it has been said, for example, that the psychosis induced by sodium bromide or foods infested with ergot are indistinguishable from pathological schizophrenia. In the case of psychoses induced by toxins, the individual usually returns to normal as soon as the source of the toxin is removed. In all such statements, however, it must be remembered that observation and interpretation of mental states and the resulting behaviour patterns depends upon the degree of awareness, the intellectual approach and the philosphical outlook of the observer, however well-trained such a person may be. So while it is clear to some that the effect of LSD or mescaline can produce quite a different inward condition to that experienced by the schizophrenic, to others who observe only the grosser aspects of outward behaviour, the similarities can seem to be remarkable.

This is not to say that there is no similarity in the biochemical changes which are integral with such states. Clearly there is. But the point to bear in mind is that the inward mental energy structure of each person is quite unique and that drugs, serotonin and many other substances will therefore affect each individual in a unique fashion.

Conversely, the mind energies will pattern the biochemistry and the bioelectrical condition according to its inward state. If then, we observe these inwardly induced changes in biochemistry and take them to be primary causes, we are missing the point. But such is the nature of all superficial and symptomatic observation to which, as humans, we are inherently prone.

In other words, the inward energetic imbalances of the psychotic condition will themselves influence the concentration and distribution of serotinin, dopamine and many other neurochemicals, just as much as these substances produce psychoactive effects. For returning once again to an old theme, we are just one integrated energy complex where the parts reflect and affect the whole, and the whole is more than just the sum of its parts.

Concluding

We are all constituted of the same five tattwas, the same senses and the same antashkarans, and we can all empathize to some degree from our own experience with the sufferings of others, whether physical or mental. Many of us do not wish to accept that we have within us the seeds of all the disturbances we may reject or criticize or fail to comprehend in others. But as we grow within ourselves, we come to understand more and more that the secret of wisdom lies inside ourselves and that the source of all knowledge and love is to be found in our own inner beings. And to that we must always hold fast, for the key to life's mysteries is within, and can never be written in a book.

Poetic Interlude

MIRACLES

Why, who makes much of a miracle?
As to me I know of nothing else but miracles,
Whether I walk the streets of Manhattan,
Or dart my sight over the roofs of houses toward the sky,
Or wade with naked feet along the beach just in the edge of the
    water,
Or stand under trees in the woods,
Or talk by day with any one I love, or sleep in bed at night with
    any one I love,
Or sit at table at dinner with the rest,
Or look at strangers opposite me riding in the car,
Or watch honey-bees busy around the hive of a summer forenoon,
Or animals feeding in the fields,
Or birds, or the wonderfulness of insects in the air,
Or the wonderfulness of the sundown, or of stars shining so quiet
    and bright,
Or the exquisite delicate thin curve of the new moon in spring;
These with the rest, one and all, are to me miracles . . .

To me every hour of the light and dark is a miracle,
Every cubic inch of space is a miracle,
Every square yard of the surface of the earth is spread with the
    same,
Every foot of the interior swarms with the same.
To me the sea is a continual miracle,
The fishes, that swim – the rocks – the motion of the waves – the
    ships with men in them,
What stranger miracles are there?

Walt Whitman

CHAPTER 14

Life Energies and Modern Physics

Schools of Thought in Modern Physics

In general outline, one could say that there are two schools of thought in modern physics. There are those who believe that mathematically and conceptually it is possible to explain away the problem of where the universe came from by deft intellectual and mathematical manoeuvering that allows 'nothing' to spontaneously come into manifestation. Thus, everything can be reduced, in this thinking, to movements of one ultimate superforce that arrived out of nowhere and may one day disappear back into non-existence. Everything therefore is physically observable either by the senses or extensions therefrom in our physical instrumentation. Life, consciousness, mind, emotion, and all human feelings and psychology, our ills and our happinesses, time, space, causality and everything else are seen in this approach as simply movements amongst subatomic particles and their resultant forces. They are considered to be ultimately reducible and understandable through mathematic formulation, and by physicists only, in a grand unified theory of the universe.

Evolution of life is simply the chance arrangement of molecules, evolving into greater and greater complexity until self-consciousness emerges by an odd twist of self-organizing, electro-physiological activity. Paranormal phenomena, telepathy, appreciation of subtle atmosphere, mystic experience and anything else that does not fit into the picture are highly suspect and thought to be the result of a disturbed mind. At best, they must be explicable in terms of physical reality and the superforce or unified, physical field.

Life, therefore, in this kind of theory, is organized chaos and has no meaning whatsoever, no inner source of itself and no intrinsic morality, ethics or code of behaviour.

Man has total free-will to do as he likes, within the laws of nature and the laws of his society.

This is the materialistic philosophy and it is, of course, clear from the context of this book that I do feel it to be the expression of a clever, but limited consciousness and mental activity. A consciousness and life that is all but unaware of itself.

There are, on the other hand, a smaller number of physicists who realize within themselves due to inner experience or deep intuition that the energy of life and consciousness is at an altogether higher and more real level. They realize that the outward manifestation of the physical universe is from a more inward reality. That is that both consciousness and matter are created from within. That the unity sought by modern physics is ultimately only to be found by inner, mystic experience at the level of Godhead, Supreme Being, Universal Consciousness or Absolute, Undifferentiated Reality – whatever name appeals to the individual's way of thinking.

To physicists such as these, it is clear that the formulations of physics will always be inherently limited and, as they presently stand, are inaccurate representations of the reality, in need of reformulation. They suggest that what is required is for the correct and experimentally verifiable concepts and descriptions to be developed, permitting an understanding that energy or matter, including all forces, is created from within itself and from a higher energetic vibration or movement.

Throughout all the ages and recorded history of mankind, this same dichotomy has existed of the materialistic versus the more mystical. The flavour has varied according to the cultural conditions and prevalent philosophies, but it is the same debate, in essence.

In more modern times, we have seen expression of the attempt to link the materialistic and the mystical in the work of such thinkers and writers as Fritjof Capra and David Bohm. Isaac Bentov in his book, *Stalking the Wild Pendulum*, and more recently Dr Inomata from Japan have also both attempted to show that 'consciousness' should be part of all fundamental physics and they have produced mathematical models in which it is included. But in these contexts 'consciousness' is often equated with self-

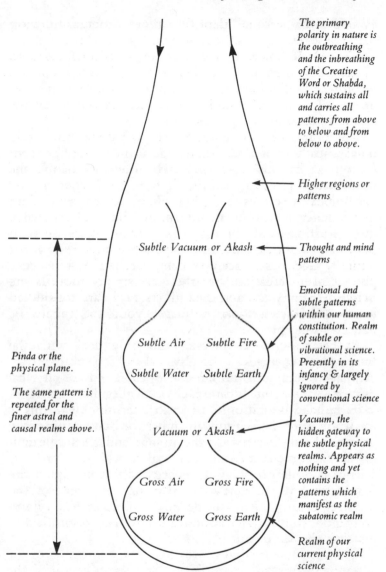

The primary polarity in nature is the outbreathing and the inbreathing of the Creative Word or Shabda, which sustains all and carries all patterns from above to below and from below to above.

Higher regions or patterns

Subtle Vacuum or Akash ← Thought and mind patterns

Emotional and subtle patterns within our human constitution. Realm of subtle or vibrational science. Presently in its infancy & largely ignored by conventional science

Subtle Air   Subtle Fire

Subtle Water   Subtle Earth

Pinda or the physical plane.

The same pattern is repeated for the finer astral and causal realms above.

Vacuum or Akash ← Vacuum, the hidden gateway to the subtle physical realms. Appears as nothing and yet contains the patterns which manifest as the subatomic realm

Gross Air   Gross Fire

Gross Water   Gross Earth

Realm of our current physical science

Figure 14-1. The physical universe, showing the energetic extent of modern science. The true Life Force is of the Shabda, which gives us consciousness and provides the pranas with their intelligent ability to weave and maintain the complex tapestry of organic life. The greater the number of subtle tattwas which are woven into the orbit of consciousness, then the higher the outwardly manifested intelligence of the creature.

awareness or personal identity – more a mental function than an expression of the true soul or consciousness within. Dr Inomata, in fact, equates consciousness with the vacuum, akash or ch'i. He has even derived mathematical formulae linking mass, energy and this vacuum state. So people also have differing concepts concerning the nature of their own consciousness.

The intuitive knowledge of such people that ultimately there is just one unified reality, has also led some of them to suppose that this Absolute is to be found just behind the fundamental physical reality. In fact, the deeper mystic cosmology describes a highly pluralistic cosmos, with many inner levels of more subtle, but still complex differentiation. And, they say, the individual can rise up in personal mystic ascent and experience this reality for himself. God is still seen as being present within every particle of his creation, but there are simply more layers between the physical and the universal than are considered in the "God consciousness just beyond the subatomic particle" concept.

At best, therefore, physics can only deal with the fundamental energies of the physical and the subtle physical that make up our human constitution and the physical universe we inhabit. It can reach no further than that. This is its built-in limitation. In Sanskrit terminology, this is the realm of *Pinda*, within which lies the human mind, the gross and subtle tattwas, the pranas and all subtle and gross phenomena of the material world. At present, science is dealing only with energy vibrations up to the first natural valve, gateway, 'sky' or zero-point of the physical vacuum. The subtle physical realm has yet (in conventional research laboratories) to be 'scientifically' discovered! (See figure 14-1).

The Subjective Nature of Reality

We talk, by convenience and by habit, as if the physical universe were 'out there'. In reality, there is no 'out there', only an 'in here'. The gross physical universe appears outside only because of the outward direction of our attention. The experiencer, our mind, is within and the world of the gross tattwas is really a reflection of what is being played from within as a movie, upon our subtle and inward tattvic screen.

Our attention, however, is outward, so we think that it is without. This is the illusion, which can be cured by reversing the direction of our attention in deep meditation. In fact, what we see does not exist in the way that we think it does. What we do not see, because we are looking in the wrong direction, is the true reality.

Our descriptions of this world, including this book, are hence essentially circular. In respect of their being ultimate explanations, they are inherently flawed. All our descriptions assume that the perceived is objective and separate from us, but this is, in fact, untrue. The physical world is a reflection of what is within us, perceived in our mind but thought to be outside because of the direction of our attention. So when we apply this thinking and illusory perception to our own brain and think that it, too, is 'out there', we run into serious difficulties. The only solution is a deep breath and a Zen-inspired 'Aa. . . .ah!'

But even this model or manner of explanation is inadequate, for the apparently external universe seems to have a reality independent of the perceiver. Things do not cease to exist, for example, when we are no longer perceiving them! Or put in another way, if you and I are both 'dreaming' our physical existence, then why are we having such similar dreams? In inward thought, feeling and interpretation, of course, we may not be. But all the same there is an apparent concreteness associated with physical existence which we both acknowledge.

Expressed in yet another fashion, this paradox again appears when we consider that although the life force, patterned by the mind and inner energies, itself becomes the blueprint of our physical bodies, yet when we die, the physical body remains behind to decay. As does the external world which that soul and mind once perceived. So it means that the 'outside' world does have some measure of differentiation from our perception and inward life.

Everything – inert or animate – is created from within. But the life force weaves the otherwise inimical and inanimate tattvic states of material substance into a physical body by patterning the vacuum matrix into the complex biochemical and bioelectronic processes which we perceive as a living body.

This differentiation is a built-in part of the mechanism of creation, under the law of karma, because souls, when incarnate in human or other physical bodies, constantly relate to each other through the medium of inert material substance, giving and taking in the endless karmic cycle of birth, death and rebirth.

Perhaps the neatest way of expressing an answer to this conundrum is to say that the akashic state would remain as an unmanifested plenum of potentiality were it not for the minds and karmas of the souls inhabiting this world. We are all shareholders, co-creators of the world we inhabit. It is all of us living creatures that have together whipped up the akashic state into manifesting our karmas to us. Remove the souls and perhaps everything would go back to the akashic state. This is part of the mechanism of pralaya or dissolution. Our minds, linked by karmic bonds, have conjointly created all that we perceive or experience, for the karmas are actually stored as potential within our own mind structure, ready to pattern our own inward subtle akashic state. This is the mystic point of view, and it is not so very different to some interpretations of the strange world of quantum physics.

But true understanding lies in mystic experience within oneself, so the best one can do is to say that under the law of karma we are all an integral part of the mechanism by which our physical universe is created and within which the Universal is ever present in His sustaining power.

Scalar Electromagnetic Theory, the Vacuum State and the Five Tattwas

No fully comprehensive model has yet been put forward in modern physics that describes the phenomena and energy fields of the physical plane as described and experienced within by generations of yogic and mystic practitioners. There have been many that talk in terms of an ether, envisaging it in a variety of different conceptual ways, but one of the best that I have encountered, and one that has been worked out in considerable mathematical detail, is called *Scalar Electromagnetic Theory* and is propounded, amongst others, by T.E. Bearden of the U.S.A. What follows is a brief outline of the fundamentals of this theory, without the mathematics, enlarged upon by a few ideas and visualizations of my own. For example, the concepts of a zero-point condition being real energy in potential, and the vacuum state being a field of *locked-in, stressed potential* – the equivalent to relativistic space-time but seen as a real energy domain – these are both derived and expanded upon from the writings of Bearden and others. The *Blip and Bud Model of Manifestation*, however, is my own attempt at a very simple graphic imagery of how our observable reality comes into being. The perception that vacuum and the gross akashic tattwa are the same, is derived from eastern mystical philosophy.

Bearden himself does not talk specifically about the tattwas, but describes physical reality only in terms of *nested levels of scalar anenergy* and *scalar waves*. In the terminology of this book, that means levels of subtle energy created from within and the patternings or waveforms therein. More specifically, it means the subtle tattwas that reach up to the level of mental thought energy. These are also seen by Bearden as higher levels of scalar wave activity.

What distinguishes Bearden's theorizing from that of other more academically acceptable theories of the vacuum state structure, is that Bearden attempts to provide a model that demonstrates how energy can exist in an inwardly tiered structure. This therefore includes the more psychic, subtle energy realms of our physical being, whilst most other models that see material substance as a web of interconnected energy patterns stop short at the vacuum state.

My description is also given in simplistic terms, rather than being discursive and involving the history of theoretical considerations of modern physics. The reason is firstly that this kind of complex intellectual discussion has been written in a number of other books. Secondly, it is largely incomprehensible to all but mathematicians and physicists.[2]

___

[2] A full discussion of these topics is given in my next book, *The Secret of the Creative Vacuum.*

Life and its understanding is the inheritance of us all and if its outward explanations become so complex that only those with a particular quality of mind can comprehend it, then it means that from the spiritual point of view it is suspect. At best, it is of value only to those particular academics in their own personal search for meaning. It becomes, therefore, an analysis that has relative value only in terms of technological achievement or the amassing of scientific knowledge. This is where the role of the expert and specialist is both appreciated and essential, whether as a physician, an engineer or a theorist.

As described in chapter one, in yogic, mystical perception and understanding, according to the Sanskrit yoga tantras, both the physical, observable universe as well as the higher or inner regions are said to be manifested out of *Prakriti*. Prakriti is primal energy or Nature, the prime cause or essence of material substance. Physical matter, in the outwardly observable, scientific sense, is its final outward expression. Prakriti is that which gives form to the creative power of the One, known as Shabda, when it reaches the realm of Universal Mind. So form is, in a sense, the result of stress and strain, manifesting within the primal prakriti, under the influence of the three gunas or modes of duality. Prakriti is, so to speak, the first form that manifests within the higher materio-mental region. All other forms are derived from it.

This understanding of Primal Energy and the formation of 'lower' vibrations and form due to stress, or locked-in potential, within the more subtle realm or dimension associated with physical reality, is at the basis of Scalar Electromagnetic (EM) Theory.

Scalar EM theory does not supplant Einsteinian relativity and quantum theory, but it does show them to be special cases, able to describe certain material phenomena, but incomplete. Much in the same way that Einstein did not make Newton's understanding obsolete or incorrect, but simply placed it in a wider context. Physicists are, of course, already well aware of the incompleteness of both relativity and quantum theories.

Scalar EM research is continuing and is capable of scientific verification through the creation of advanced devices and instrumentation that can be seen to work. In fact, Bearden claims that the Russians have been working on scalar electromagnetic instrumentation for many years and already possess a considerable armoury of such energy devices. This new research seems to me to be the most far-reaching advance in scientific understanding since the formulation of relativity during the early years of this century (1905-1915) and quantum theory in the 1920's.

Scalar Electromagnetic Theory, The Holographic Paradigm and Life

The problem with the scalar EM model and indeed with probably all mathematical expression or description is that, in a broad sense, it is still linear. Nature itself, however, is non-linear. It operates at a multitude of levels and in a myriad forms, *simultaneously* and as a *whole*. It is our logical, conceptual minds which are linear, perceiving only linear cause and effect pathways, rather than the actually self-existent, holistic, holographic and simultaneously active relationships of the whole. Even our most modern computing technology still has only one central processing or logical unit. We may combine many computers into one system, but the central processors function *separately*, not in an automatically integrated fashion, with each simultaneously knowing what the other is doing, and acting accordingly and in harmony.

For such advanced computing technology, what is required would still be a logical system but one which is based upon the holographic principle in which the 'individual' parts are automatically 'aware' of all the other parts and of the total functioning of the whole. Such a system would operate primarily, as a whole. Note that the holographic model is still logical in nature, still functioning under the primary law of cause and effect, of interconnectedness, of karma.

As we described earlier, this is how the whole body operates with its autonomous cells each linked by resonance and holography to each other and to the whole. This is reflected, for example, in the vibrating pattern of energy we call the molecule of DNA.

In the brain and central nervous system, the complexity of this linkage is immense, with each of the 10^{12} brain neurons connected by up to 100,000 others in non-linear, avalanche discharge, energetic relationships.

The more primary patterner and organizer of this effect lies quite clearly in the more subtle tattvic, pranic and mental realms where the laws of energetic relationship are inherently holographic and holistic and are thus able to cope with what appears to us as an amazing degree of complexity.

To make an advanced computing system which would model this is actually quite impossible for we could never endow it with a soul or with consciousness. It is in consciousness where the fundamental capacity for wholeness actually resides. It is there that the individual can become the Universal.

Put quite simply, we cannot make a machine and endow it with life. The best we can do is to copy only the patterning of life's outermost processes as best we may. Man's machines have always been only conscious or unconscious copies or artefacts of nature's superbly constructed processes. Without the life force of consciousness, nature's individual holographic units – souls entrapped in physical bodies, living creatures – cannot be even remotely constructed by man. With all our analytical thinking and experimental probing, we are still no nearer constructing the most simple cell or the most 'primitive' life form. This, we must be so happy to acknowledge, will never be within our power.

Vacuum and Akash

While we can readily comprehend the first four states of gross physical matter, since they are already recognized by western science, it is the akash tattwa which usually presents us with the most difficulty in understanding. As we have been discussing, the gross physical form of akash is, in fact, the vacuum or space, within which, and *from which*, all other observable material substance takes its existence. According to Bearden and others, vacuum is not 'nothing with dimensions', but is a zero-balanced point of locked-in, potential energy.

Just as:

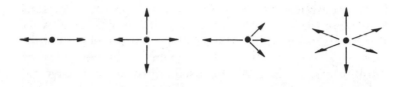

(After Bearden)

all sum to zero at the balance point and yet are comprised of real energy, (as is readily observed if one of the forces in the *substructure* changes or is removed), to outward observation the balance point *appears* as 'no thing', as zero energy or a zero point. This, however, is an illusion.

Two or more electric or magnetic fields, for example, may sum to zero, but the zero point, though absent of field effects, contains a stressed, or locked-in potential that reflects the summation of the substructure. Any 'unbalanced' variations in the constitution of this substructure will result in observable field effects and whilst conventional physics expresses this as the field itself, the new approach recognizes the importance of the potentials that have created the field. Potentials are thus regarded as 'real things', while fields are simply effects. This is a reversal of the conventional approach, where potential is generally described in terms of its effect and is not regarded as the 'real thing'.

In more specific terms, what we may think of as 'empty' vacuum is actually 'packed full' of potential, summed to zero, in a stable state, giving us the illusion of there being 'nothing there'. In scalar EM terminology, this is known as the *virtual* state of *electrostatic scalar potential*, a scalar value being one characterized by magnitude only, i.e. potential without manifestation.

Vacuum is thus a zero point in the structure of manifestation from within-out. And it is full of potential energy, as the gross akashic condition.

Actually, the concept of zero-point energy was first conceived by physicists back in the 1930's when they realized the necessity of a mathematical term arising from the calculations of quantum theory. For with the concept of an ether having lost respectability, the mathematics still required that vacuum possessed an energy. In fact, these days, theoretical calculations lead to the embarrassing conclusion that ninety-nine percent of the mass/energy of the universe is 'missing'. This energy was called zero point energy because it still remains even at temperatures of absolute zero, when all the oscillations we call thermal energy have ceased.

Paul Dirac actually showed theoretically how electron-positron (matter-antimatter) pairs could arise from it and its role in the manifestation of subatomic particles has been the subject of continuous speculation and theorizing over the last few decades. So the concept of an ether by another name has never really gone away.

In more recent thinking, the expression of zero point has also acquired an additional meaning, as a point of structured balance or zero – the sattvas guna – as I have described earlier.

The Blip and Bud Model of Manifestation

Physicists tell us that if all the subatomic particles of our planet were compressed so that there were no space or vacuum between, that it would then take up no more room than a pin head or an orange – *but with the same mass and gravitational attraction*. That is, that the entire volume of our physical reality, *including our gross physical body – all its cells, biochemistry and everything else – is* almost entirely vacuum with bits (subatomic particles) in it and forces between.[3] In the new concept, however, these bits and forces are not to be visualized like pieces of vegetable floating about in a soup, *but as being spun out of the fabric of the energy-packed vacuum itself.*

Space is (observably) three-dimensional, but let us look at it for a moment as two-dimensional, for ease of visualization. Vacuum can then be conceived of as being like a

---

[3] Physicists say that all interactions can be described in terms of just four basic, universal physical forces: electromagnetic, gravitational, weak and strong. In quantum theory, these forces are thought to arise through the interchange of short-lived, subatomic particles.

plain white sheet, stretched tight and all-pervasive. Within the *subtle*, non-physically observable substructure of this sheet arise standing waves, oscillations or vibrations, which result in a *Blip* (figure 14–2).

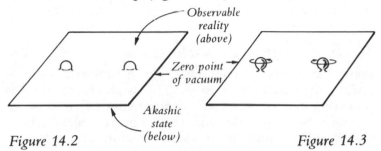

Figure 14.2   *Figure 14.3*

When this blip begins to spin, it *appears* to *Bud* off (figure 14–3). Thus the vibration or standing wave within the vacuum becomes observable as physical reality. *Mass, therefore, becomes understandable as a subtle or scalar, vacuum wave, trapped by particle spin.* And the four basic forces (eg gravity) of our physical universe are actually no more than the 'stresses' or energetic interactions and relationships within the fabric of vacuum due to the budding of subatomic particles. The 'observable' tapestry of sub-atomic particles and forces thus arise due to the energetic structure and activity within the vacuum state, itself.

Our entire physical reality is comprised of these sub-atomic particles and forces, but in all-pervasive, three dimensions, not two. In fact, according to physicists, time itself is integrated as a dimension of this fabric, as Einstein pointed out. Vacuum is thus space-time, itself. But it is to be understood as a real entity, not a theoretical concept.

Motion and polarity, of course, are at the basis of all manifestation and physicists have long been aware that the spin and movement of subatomic particles is not just a property of their existence, *but is an integral part of their existence itself.* There is, for example, no such thing as a *still* electron. Indeed, concepts such as 'spin' need to be viewed with circumspection, for particle spin has little in common with a spinning top. It is altogether a different kind of energetic movement, with no parallels to anything in our macroscopic world.

Out of these subatomic particles, then, are spun the four

conditions or octaves of matter with which we are familiar: air, fire (plasmic state), water and earth. Our apparently solid physical universe is thus no more than a vibrating dance of energy, manifested out of the locked-in, potential energy of vacuum.

Vertical Energy Spectrum

Looked at in another way, energy in manifestation has an inward or vertical dimension. The structure of space is actually possessed of more than three dimensions, but we are only able to perceive three of them. In general terms, the other dimensions are the *inward* and the *outward* directions of energy flow in the process of its materialization.

The common example used to graphically express additional spatial dimensions is that of the allegorical 'flatlanders' who perceive only two dimensions. This means that were an orange to pass through their world, they would see only a point expanding to a circle and contracting back to a point once more. They would never see its third dimension of depth.

Similarly, we are perceiving only a part of the total picture. We see only our three dimensional space. The hidden dimensions which reveal the mechanism by which matter is created are not available to our normal physical perception. So we have difficulty both in understanding how they operate or even in accepting that they exist at all.

So the mechanism of manifestation does not stop at the observable vacuum state, but is *vertically continuous*. That is to say that lower energies are spun out of the higher in a continuous spectrum, and within our human constitution the highest level of patterning energy lies in our mind. Mind, of course, in the mystic conception, is an energy field enlivened from within by soul or consciousness.

This concept of the vertical energy spectrum requires a caveat, however. As has been indicated, life is created from within. There is no 'out there' at all, it is all 'in here'. The lack of a full understanding of this reality is one of the reasons why quantum theory, while being forced almost reluctantly to admit that the 'outer' is related to the 'inner', gets itself into such a tangle, mathematically and philosophically.

The objects of our senses are not separate from the senses themselves. Perception is not objective, but subjective. What this means therefore is that the vertical energy spectrum lies *within* ourselves, *including the apparently outside world.* You cannot, for example, find subtle or thought energies by examining apparently physical, objective substance, because they – like the physical substances – are within us. Nor can you find the experience of perceiving this world.

It seems to me that modern physics will make great strides forward when it realizes and fully accepts the implications of three factors with which it is currently confused. Firstly, the vacuum state *is* a real, energetic, vibrating matrix – a real, though formative, condition of matter. In fact, many academic physicists already suspect that this is so. Secondly, the statistical aspects of quantum theory are underlain by a deterministic, but more subtle, order in which the laws of cause and effect, and polarity, are also intrinsic, but extend beyond our normal conceptions of them. To understand the laws which govern energy relationships in the subtle states will be the main drive of science in the next century.

Thirdly, the suggestion that the observer is implicated in the process of manifestation is, in fact, the primary reality. Apparently objective substance is, indeed, a part of our consciousness itself. Or stated more simply, God is everywhere and within everything – within ourselves and within material substance.

Modern physicists do already theorize concerning the existence of virtual particles which continuously form and disappear at ultra-high speeds on and off the vacuum surface. This they call the *physical vacuum*, and its nature is of great interest to them. Classical concepts, however, are so deeply engrained that interpretations are usually more classical and reductionist than truly holistic.

So the concept of 'nothing' is commonly understood to be a reality. It is this 'nothing', or *true vacuum*, 'filling' all of space, (actually it *is* space itself), which I am also suggesting is a part of the energy-rich, akashic matrix. An understanding of this will lead us into the real *space* age, where we begin to understand the inner energetic structure of space itself.

The Mysterious Vacuum and Mystic Skies

The blips and buds, then, are formed due to activity and motion, ie. to underlying energetic vibrations constituting the stresses between intrinsic polarities both within the vacuum state itself and between the vacuum state and observable manifestation.

The concept of an ether, or aether, dates back in western thought to classical and pre-classical times and has been an integral aspect of eastern philosophy for as long as recorded history. It is only in the last one hundred years or so that the idea has been rejected. I would say that this has been a diversion, a necessary one perhaps, that will soon be brought back into 'mainstream' thinking. Conventional modern physics, if such an entity exists, largely rejects the idea, but as a result has enormous difficulties in dealing with both vacuum and forces. For without an interpenetrating medium, there can be no real structure within which force is transmitted. This means that force has to be explained away as interactions between fundamental particles, moving in a sea of nothing, but which all the same appears to have properties. It is actually very unsettling for them! Even gravitation, in quantum theory, has to be reduced to a *graviton*, while electromagnetism has to be seen as a stream of particles or *photons*. For a *wave* has to have a medium in which to vibrate.

Given an ether or akashic state, however, as a real energy field, physics becomes relatively simple once again. Even Einstein's concept of space-time is essentially a geometric expression of an ether, as are the multi-dimensional models employed by currently fashionable Grand Unified Theories. Einstein himself never really rejected the possibility of an ether.

In more modern times, Paul Dirac and other physicists who have suggested an etheric or vacuum medium have variously ascribed an essential driving polarity between physically observable subatomic particles and the etheric condition. None of these physicists, however, have suggested that this ether is actually just a link in a vertical spectrum of energies, in the way that it is presented mathematically in Scalar EM theory, or philosophically and experientially in the eastern wisdom.

Rejecting Einsteinian special relativity, the physicist Harold Aspden similarly suggests a quantized ether comprised of a fine lattice of energetic focuses or quanta. He suggests that it is within this that our world of subatomic particles exists and from which the electromagnetic and gravitational forces are automatically formed.

Using this concept of a structured space and the forces between moving electrons, he goes on to derive all of the major and prevalent mathematical formulae including Newton's constant of gravitation and Einstein's, $e=mc^2$. He thus appears to have indeed unified physics. But he gives no explanation of where either the structured space or our subatomic particles originated.

The possibility of a real ether is, however, discounted by the conservative majority of physicists, largely based on philosophical considerations, popular scientific idiom and upon an experiment performed by Michelson and Morley back in 1887, which appeared to have discredited the long-held idea of an ether. Aspden, does however point out that with modern versions of the experiment, using lasers, the Doppler effect accounts precisely for the required correction used to discredit the idea of an ether and demonstrated in the original experiment.

Moreover, a second experiment performed between 1923 and 1925 by Michelson, Gale and Pearson produced results conflicting with his previous experiment, and which can be seen as a verification of the existence of an ether. An experiment which an already pre-conditioned scientific fraternity have quietly ignored.

Actually, Michelson's experiments concerning the existence of an ether were based upon the concept of an ether as a flowing substance. In fact, his concept was too simplistic. For as we have been discussing, the ether or vacuum is the structured, inwardly-dimensioned, fabric of space. Without a clearer idea of the nature of the ether and the laws by which it is governed, Michelson's experiments were at best only capable of proving or disproving whether his *concept* of the ether had any validity. Not whether the ether actually existed.

Mainstream modern physics has much to say concerning the vacuum state. Grand Unified Theories require the involvement of what they call the physical vacuum or *quantum vacuum*. In the quantum description of the universe, this vacuum becomes the dominant structure, seething with virtual particles and energetic activity. But it is conceived of as possessing probabilistic, rather than causal, 'connections'. Its potentially intense energies are also used in explanations of the Big Bang which, it is proposed, occurred at the 'start' of the Universe. And to account for where that original primal energy came from, the attempt is made to explain how the proposed state of absolute, quiescent, empty or 'true' vacuum, bootstraps itself into a seething and expanding state of 'false' vacuum containing subatomic particles, the stuff of our known universe.

The essential problem in modern physics is highlighted as soon as one comes up against the vacuum, the mysterious space or apparent 'nothing' in which all subatomic particles exist and which appears quite incongruously to possess properties, whichever way you look at it. Away from that enigmatic wall, there is agreement, by and large. The mathematical description of forces at the macroscopic and even atomic level, poses no real problem. But up against the wall of vacuum, then mathematical and philosophical complexities abound, with no final solution yet scientifically proven in the presently conventional idiom.

I have an image, here, of someone peering into a box filled with the most fascinating contents, looking deeper and deeper to see what it contains. Fundamentally, the modern experimental physicist has parted the molecules, the atoms and the subatomic particles until he is left facing the blank wall of vacuum. Mentally, he pronounces a loud, "Um!" and goes back to looking at the particles. Occasionally, but increasingly, some brave soul has a go at showing theoretically how particles and vacuum could interact, or how they can even be an integral part of each other. "Very interesting," say the experimental physicists (at best), "That's an ingenious idea", but immediately revert to designing experiments for particle accelerators.

Or you could say that akash represents the real walls of the prison of our human existence. But we are so used to being prisoners that we examine only the contents of our prison and not the confinement mechanisms themselves. We never see the walls of our jail and so never come to understand the real nature of its contents. This, indeed, is how it is intended to be.

In mystic cosmology and experience, these barriers are both understood and described as an essential part of the cosmic structure for keeping everything in place. They are the valves, gateways or zero-points separating one region from another, and one sub-region from another sub-region. They are the 'skies', the akashic medium, that we find at various points in the mystic ascent. They are the doors to which we require some special, "Open Sesame".

In our physical universe there are said to be two such major skies or levels of akash. Firstly, there is this mystifying vacuum at the gross physical level. The clear, shiny, apparently featureless wall of space which faces us on all sides. It contains, however, the patterns and energy for the manifestation of the subatomic particles which comprise the other four gross tattvic states with which we are familiar.

It is the crossroads for energy pathways from above and from below. Above it, or within it, lie the four subtle tattwas, themselves derived out of the subtle akashic state, which is the real sky of the body, in the head area, just above the eyes and above the nine sensory openings of the body.[4] Of these, the most important to us and physically the highest, too, are the two eyes and the two ears.

It is this inner sky that prevents most of us from leaving our body before the time of death and from knowing about the inner regions of the mind and soul. Just as physicists are currently prevented from perceiving beyond the physical vacuum or sky, so too is our mind kept in darkness, unable to see and travel within, through the inner and more subtle akashic veil.

The purpose of mystic practice is to pierce this inner veil. True mysticism is a deeply and naturally structured, practical science of self and God realization. There is nothing 'wishy-washy' about it. But then, there are few practitioners who have reached the inner heights of true enlightenment, although there are many who aspire, and do understand a part of the total picture.

[4] The nine outward openings are the two eyes, two ears, two nostrils, the mouth, the genital/urethral opening and the anus. The Third Eye is the one door opening inward.

In this respect, it is also interesting to note that in the neck lies the chakra associated with the administration of the akashic fields. The neck, too, is the crossroads, the point of intensive energetic interchange between the body and the brain, the point at which vocalization of language is effected. This akashic role of the valve or sky or zero point is clearly demonstrated by its size: the neck possesses the smallest diameter of all, along the spinal axis.

The five tattwas have their physical reflection upon both sides of this akashic control centre. In the lower part of the body, below the neck, we have the other four chakras and tattwas previously described, involved with the formation and administration of gross bodily function. Above the level of the throat and neck in the head, we again find the expression of the five tattwas, but this time linked more intimately to consciousness and intelligence in the form of the five senses.

The ears and hearing (akash), the eyes and sight (fire), the nose and smell (earth), the tongue and taste (water), the lips and touch (air), are all linked through to intelligent consciousness more than any other part of our body. The only exception is the skin and its sensation of touch which gives us awareness of the rest of our body and its relationship with the outside world. As we have discussed, its main focus is in the hands, where the airy, sensory and motor indriyas of touch and manipulation are highly integrated. But it also has a point of focus in the head, as the lips. And hands and mouth are closely associated, as we know.

Similarly, amongst the endocrine centres above the neck, we find the pituitary-hypothalamic centre containing biochemical linkages, reflections and resonances to all lower endocrine activity.

The addition of experiential and intelligent personal awareness as we move into the realms of subtle linkage above and within the akashic level is, as we have described, what makes the human species unique. For it is only in man that the formative akashic realm is fully linked into the consciousness of any species, giving us perceptive abilities and an expression of intelligence denied to lower creatures.

Further Considerations of Vacuum Manifestation

One of the fundamental conceptual difficulties in present day modern physics is the dichotomy of particle and wave behaviour, where electromagnetic radiation, for example, at one moment appears to behave like solid particles and at another has the properties of a wave. In fact, De Broglie and others showed, back in the 1920's, that *all* particles, whether photons of light, electrons, neutrons or whatever, exhibit both wave and particle characteristics. And this is acknowledged to be partially due to the interaction of the observer and the observed, as well as in the design of the experiment. For when we look for wave behaviour – we find it. And when we search for evidence of particles, we find them too. An understanding, however, of creation from within the vacuum state, such that our observable physical reality is seen as a manifested effect from within the vacuum substructure, permits us to perceive that this manifested, vibrating energy is *neither* particles *nor* waves. It only appears so because of our limited concepts. These concepts are then reflected in the nature of our highly complex experimentation, which are designed upon the a priori assumption that we are indeed dealing with either waves or particles. They therefore fail to demonstrate anything else.

These problems are, of course, understood by physicists. But to design experiments to look for those kind of energetic vibration or relationship for which we have no parallel in our macroscopic world is no easy matter.

A further interesting corollary of the vacuum manifestation theory is that electromagnetic radiation (eg light), rather than being a transverse Hertzian wave, is actually a longitudinal pressure wave in the vacuum space-time medium itself. It appears to our observable reality as a transverse wave, in much the same way that the ripples on a pond after a stone has been thrown in *appear* to be Hertzian and transverse in nature. But actually, they are propagated by longitudinal pressure waves within the water itself.

Furthermore, since vacuum is energy-packed and can vary in its energetic constitution or density, *it follows that* the speed of light is not a constant in vacuum, but varies according to the vibrational composition and structure of the vacuum. For light itself is an *effect*, as are subatomic particles. Light is our three dimensional perception of certain aspects and changes which are actually taking place in the more complexly dimensioned vacuum state. Interestingly enough, variations in the speed of light in vacuum is also a postulate of the eleven-dimensional models of physical existence. And experimental work conducted by American physicist, Dr Doug Torr, at the University of Alabama over the past four years has indeed shown that the velocity of light in a vacuum is variable.

Mathematically and within the current conventions of modern physics, an eleven-dimensional model is one way of conceiving how the basic forces and particles of nature are all manifested out of the same 'superforce'. The additional seven spatial dimensions are considered to be rolled up or locked into the spin and stress that we observe as subatomic particles and the basic natural forces. In fact, with an understanding of manifestation from within, the eleven dimensions then become seen as a description of modifications to space and time itself, as subatomic particles dance and spin into existence from within-out, in a continuously vertical spectrum. This provides an understanding, too, in terms of a real mechanism, of how in the subjective mystic experience, the higher and more subtle regions are often described as being 'greater in magnitude' and with time 'slowed down' or 'greatly extended'. It is an attempt to express in earthly language the different nature and perception of dimensions which are experienced in the mystic ascent.

Actually, once one realizes that energies are created from within themselves and that observable 'reality' is an immediate expression of the vacuum state, then the pressure on theoretical physics to tie everything up as a self-created and self-organized universe at the gross physical level only, relaxes. And with this knowledge in mind, the mathematics will immediately follow suit. Many of the complexities introduced to maintain what is essentially a *philosophical* rather than *scientific* position, will dissolve, leaving the mathematical simplicity and natural aesthetics that theoreticians intuitively strive for and know must exist as a true reflection of 'reality'.

In other words, the mathematical formulations may (in fact, should) contain an open-endedness, leaving space for the understanding of 'creation from within'. Then, immediately, the horrendous complexities of, for example, GUT (Grand Unified Theories) and supergravity calculations will fall away with the realization that understanding of physical reality does not need to be tied up completely in mathematical or theoretical terms, on the gross physical side of the vacuum state.

The Four Forces and the Four Tattwas

It is actually a conceivable possibility that the four subtle tattwas (excluding the formative matrix of subtle akash) are reflected in the four basic forces known to modern science, (see figure 3-1, page 66). The quality of solidity, of preservation in structure, inherent in the subtle earthy tattwa, is hence seen in the power of the strong force which holds atoms together. The sensitive and spreading matrix of the subtle watery tattwa is perceived in the tenuous but all-embracing quality of gravitation, whereby all objects are related to each other. The driving force of electricity, magnetism and electromagnetic radiation can be observed as a manifestation of the subtle fiery tattwa. And the manipulative and intricate mechanisms of the subtle airy tattwa may be noted in the activities of the weak force, which provides the ability for subatomic matter to change and adapt.

This also means, of course, that there is no direct one-to-one relationship between the subtle tattwas and their gross manifestation, but that the subtle tattvic impression upon the vacuum or akashic state from within gives rise to their representation at the gross tattvic level in a number of separate, vibrational ways.

Thus, at the immediately perceivable level we have the molecular and atomic states characterized by the solid, liquid, plasmic and airy condition, while in the more intricate mechanisms of subatomic existence, we again perceive this other manifestation of subtle tatvic activity, programming the vacuum state from within into the four basic forces of our physical universe. Whether this is true or not, I do not know. This little section was really put in as a passing thought.

Actually, recent experimentation suggests that gravity may be comprised of two forces – one attractant and the other repellent. It is the sum of the two that we have been describing as gravitational attraction, all these years. This brings gravity into line with other forces such as electricity and magnetism which exhibit the yin and yang principle of duality in their positive and negative electrical charge or in north and south poles.

This suggestion also underlines the point that classical science is largely concerned only with effects or forces – not with real energies, per se. When two forces interact and add or subtract from each other, it is conventionally considered that what really exists is the sum of the two forces. If the sum is zero, then it is mathematically considered that nothing exists, though common sense indicates otherwise. This is observable with two equally matched teams playing tug-of-war. Mathematically, the centre of the rope is a zero-point, but the real nature of the outwardly zero-balanced situation is immediately seen if one side simply lets go!

Scalar Wave and Vacuum State Engineering

Scalar electromagnetic theory does more than provide an understanding of mechanisms by which manifestation may take place. For, being a true scientific theory, it contains the mathematics and physics required to *engineer the virtual state*, in order to create effects at the gross physical or observable level. Using relativistic concepts, but seen in the light of the new approach, it describes how, by summing electric and magnetic fields to zero, the conservation of energy principle results in a 'bleed off' into certain aspects of the gravitational field, through the medium of the virtual condition. In other words, by manipulating the electromagnetic effects of the virtual substructure, this substructure can itself be *deterministically* and *quantifiably* altered resulting in changes in the observable, physical 'reality'. Note that in the terminology of this writing, the virtual state and the vacuum state are more or less synonymous.

Such scalar electromagnetic engineering is already the subject of experimentation and provides, too, a theoretical basis for genuine 'free energy' machines. The concept of 'free energy' has conventionally been laughed off the stage because it apparently violates the laws of energy conservation by assuming that one can get something for nothing. This is, of course, correct, but the new approach allows one to both perceive and mathematically formulate that if the locked-in potential of the virtual or subtle state can be engineered into manifestation, then the apparent gain in energy at the observable level is counterbalanced by the release of stress or loss of potential in the virtual. The laws of energy conservation are thus satisfied.

Note that such virtual substructure engineering theoretically permits both materialization and dematerialization of not only electromagnetic phenomena, but also of mass, charge, spin etc., i.e. 'objects'. For mass itself is conceived of as a standing scalar wave in the virtual state, trapped by particle spin, as already described. The scalar wave or pattern in the virtual condition being set up by internal resonance within the mass due to an essential driving polarity between the vacuum and 'real' states. It is therefore theoretically possible to dematerialize objects and rematerialize them elsewhere by engineering their physical existence into the virtual state and then 'releasing the tension' and permitting re-materialization at another location, simply by modulating the spatial parameters of material existence.

In fact, there are a number of private laboratories who claim to have preliminary 'free energy' devices working, have achieved scalar transmutation of chemical elements, have lifted heavy weights by antigravity and so on. Unfortunately, I have no personal verification of these and similar statements, although I am presently researching the reports of such devices, to be discussed in a forthcoming book, *The Secret of the Creative Vacuum*. But some of these reports do appear to be quite convincing and understandable.

Scalar waves, longitudinal pressure waves in the potential energy of the virtual state, may be generated by a number of methods including both electromagnetic and mechanical stress. When two such scalar waves are deterministically created and beamed such that, like two searchlights, they overlap at a distance from their source, then the interaction or interference of these two virtual waves can produce observable energy at that point by a process Bearden calls by the imaginatively expressive word *kindling*. Anenergy is 'kindled' into observable energy – electromagnetic, subatomic particles, mass and so on. This technique is known as *scalar wave interferometry*, and again, Bearden suggests that the Russians are experts in this technology.

Systems which can transform electromagnetic energy into subtle energy or scalar waves and vice versa, Bearden calls *translators* and they include, he says, plasmas, ionized gases, stressed crystals, Pulsors, Reich's orgone boxes, scalar interferometers, some semi-conductive materials, dielectric capacitors and so on.

In fact, Bearden also suggests, as I have commented upon in earlier chapters, that the two halves of the human cerebrum act as scalar wave generators and detectors, with electrical brain waves being just the 'residue' or reflection of scalar wave activity. He points out, too, that all activity in the nervous system is essentially scalar in origin and that the neuronal synaptic system is ideal for scalar wave generation. For if nature had really intended the nervous system to be primarily a conductor of electricity, we would surely have been endowed with straight wire conductors or their equivalent!

Amongst other species, whiskers and antenna, composed of keratin, which possesses piezo-electric properties, are also seen to have scalar wave detection capabilities in the new terminology. The same will be true of the 'sixth sense' and indeed all vibrational awareness found in both humans and lower species. Since scalar waves pass through all substances at the gross physical level, sensory apparatus on the exterior of the body is not necessarily required and one imagines that the brain and central nervous system themselves are tuned for scalar wave detection.

Electromagnetism and Molecules

There are many aspects to this understanding of the way in which energies are manifested from within, many of which are discussed in my books, *Subtle Energy* and

The Secret of the Creative Vacuum, for it provides us with a scientific basis for comprehending all physical phenomena, gross or subtle.

The subtle, vibrational atmosphere of a place, for example, is a subtle encoding of the virtual energy patterns which still sum together in the same way, producing the same outwardly observable phenomena, whilst being different in their inner or infolded substructure. And from the viewpoint of observable physical 'reality', this new physics explains how mass, charge, spin, subatomic particles, electric fields, magnetic fields, the speed of light, gravitation and all the basic forces and phenomena of our physical world are directly related to and arise from variations and patternings in the virtual state.

Electromagnetism, for example, is a product or an effect caused by activity within the vacuum or virtual state. Conversely, manipulating these electric and magnetic fields will affect the polarities, harmony and energy flow in the subtle condition (for better or worse). Thus, an understanding of how electro-acupuncture, magnetic healing, MORA therapy and many similar therapeutic techniques function, can be derived.

Similarly, the electric and magnetic fields of the brain and body can be understood simply as a residue or lower harmonic of subtle state activity reflecting this subtle functioning. Modulated electric and magnetic fields can therefore be used to modify the subtle energy fields of the body and mind by reverse pressure, from without-in. This, for example, is the basis of psychotronic devices such as the Soviet Woodpecker signal, where an electromagnetic patterning can affect mind and emotional functioning. And could perhaps be used to transmit vibrational patterns that relate to physical disease, too.

Within the context of this thinking, molecules are seen, (as indeed the whole of biochemistry), as an energetic vibration formed out of and directly related to the subtle state. Molecules are simply complex patterns on the three-dimensional 'surface' of vacuum. The specific hormones of the major endocrine glands can thus be seen as vibrational, lower harmonics of the chakras, which each have a particular tattvic resonance or association. And I have attempted to draw attention to many of these parallels, in this book.

The organs and systems of the body are, therefore, simply a holographic complex, an outward projection of tattvic vibrations, each having a preponderance of one or more tattwas in its subtle and gross constitution, the organizing and life-giving role being played by the pranas.

The New Medicine

Considered in this manner, medicine or healing simply becomes an understanding of techniques that will re-arrange these energy patterns into a harmonious whole, whilst constrained by the higher constitutional patterning of the patient's own mind or destiny. The more subtle the level at which healing is applied, then the less are the other effects (also called, erroneously, 'side'-effects). As we have previously discussed, dis-ease is just that – lack of balance and free flow of the energies within our beings. And the patternings of our human mind are clearly seen as the ultimate shaper of our condition of health or illness, harmony or disease.

All forms of medicine, therefore, are energy medicine, in the wider sense, for there is nothing but energy. Even a drug (a molecule) is a vibrating energy complex. The question is, how harmonious to the total energy system of our physical form is any particular therapeutic technique? So the application of energy (at any level) to the human system in order to bring about healing, will have the greatest positive results when the manner of integrated functioning within both our human mind-emotion-body complex and the outer universe, is understood. And when the full implications of any healing method on this human energy system are fully appreciated.

In simple words, we can make a therapy work when we know *exactly* what we are doing and what the problems are. This is indeed the case with any detailed engineering. But for the attainment of this ideal, we still have far to travel, for at present we barely understand the mechanisms at the molecular level, let alone in the electrobiological, the subatomic and the subtle domains.

But a direct appreciation of harmony in the energy fields of our human constitution, of their creation from within themselves and of techniques which permit their deterministic observation and modification will almost certainly constitute the advanced healing technology of the twenty-first century. For theoretically, it can be seen that intricate vacuum state substructure engineering can be used to heal or ameliorate disease, within the context, constraints and higher patterning of the individual's karmas.

There are many, many sides to all of this, as we experience in our daily lives, and it is a road of understanding which I personally find both intriguing and evolutionary, in terms of inner development. For ultimately, it is the spiritual and mystic side of life which provides us with its real meaning.

Epilogue

Throughout all of history, the mistreatment of mystics and visionaries by materialistic authority has been a constant theme. It is a characteristic of the human mind, held in the grip of unconsciousness, to react with devastating emotion to ideas which threaten the shaky edifice of its mundane intellect and lack of human, let alone divine, understanding. The calm authority of Christ was enough to enrage the bigots amongst the Jewish religion, until they saw that messenger of spiritual love die in (to them) great agony. And many other mystics in Eastern countries have suffered similar fates.

The zealots of the inquisition wiped out entire communities of human beings simply because they thought differently. They were, they thought, purging the world of evil. In psychological terms, they were doing no more than projecting the negativity in their own hearts and minds onto those whose goodness, integrity, inner freedom or simple difference, enraged their ignorance and excited their lust for destruction.

This quality of attacking or distrusting what is alien to us is a natural human defence mechanism which permits us to continue in our own way without having to look within ourselves. Habit of thought is a primary factor in mental and emotional life. The aim of all true yoga and spiritual science is to lift the mind out of the distress of ignorance by freeing it from its attachment to the world of the senses and from its own inner energetic patterns of action and reaction.

It is not an easy process to look deep within one's own self, to realize that what we criticize or attack in others is a reflection of what is within our own selves. It takes time and often brings suffering in its train, as we begin to struggle with our own minds. Shankarcharya, one of the most respected of the ancient Hindu, yogic philosophers is said to have commented: "If someone came to me and told me that they could drink up all the water in the oceans of the world, I know it is impossible, but just for a moment I might believe him. If someone came to me and said that they could fly right around the world and return in as much time as it takes to snap one's fingers, I know that is impossible, but I might for a moment think that perhaps there was someone who possessed such a power. But if someone were to come to me and say that they had controlled their own mind, then I would know that such a one was not telling the truth."

The human mind is so powerful that despite the examples of history, we do the same things, not realizing just what we are doing. Often, we would rather commit the grossest crimes against humanity than look within our own hearts. Similarly, with all new ideas. An old, habituated and ego-centric mind – whether in a young body or an old one – can never accept the possibility of something outside its ken. As surely as an apple will fall, the energies of a closed mind will find arguments to refute an idea that may shed some light on its own workings.

Similarly, while the true mystic or yogi is never heard to rant and rave or attempt to demean others – because his understanding encompasses a comprehension of humankind that does not permit him to hurt the feelings or attack the lives of others – the closed, subconscious mind has no compunction in using his intellect or even physical means to silence the originators of mystical and spiritual ideas. He has no understanding of it, though he may call it names or use his mind to refute it, and yet there are a multitude of phenomena (including life itself) for which he has no real or complete place of understanding in his scheme of things.

And yet, a philosophy and practice that has a place for everything is attacked instinctively and emotionally – perhaps with a veneer of rationality to make it acceptable both to the individual himself and to others. The motivating instinct, however, is buried deep in the subconscious.

The underlying philosophy expressed in this book and in *Subtle Energy* contains an appreciation of, and a place for, all aspects of life and human endeavour. This is the hallmark of mystical philosophy, when truly understood. Yet many openly materialistic scientists describe mystical ideas as "dangerous", "fantasy" or "an illusion". They have, I assume, fully studied mystical literature, met a suitable teacher and followed the highly scientific yogic practices taught to them. Without this, their refutation of mysticism is without foundation, for under true open-minded scientific thinking, they have not studied the subject, and are thus in no position to judge . . .

A belief or understanding of the mystical does not mean a refutation of the logical and the rational. Quite the reverse, in fact. The power behind what have become major world religions has almost always been of a mystical nature. Imagine the power of such experience that even millenia after the death of the 'founder', the message is still relevant to the hearts of human beings. Can we claim the same for science? Where theories come and go in just a few centuries, or even decades. Inklings of the mystical are found in the writings of so many great personalities of the world, in all walks of life. In recent western history we can count Einstein, Yeats, Tennyson, William Blake, Carl Jung and many more. Deep thought is always inspired from within. If we do not comprehend it, we should at least be honest rather than rejectionist. You see, this life is so big that we should expand into it, not cut ourselves off from it. It is so grand and beautiful when seen with a truer eye.

Actually, a study of the energies within the human constitution is not, strictly speaking, mysticism. Though it is seen as such by materially-minded and even some spiritually-minded people who do not realize the sheer height to which the soul can aspire.

True mysticism really only starts above the eye centre, from where the soul, accompanied to begin with by the higher aspects of mind, may fly to inner realms, ultimately reaching the Supreme Being, the Source of Life, Consciousness, Bliss and Love, Himself.

Bibliography and Further Reading

Biomagnetism and Bioelectricity

Blueprint for Immortality, Harold S. Burr; Spearman, 1952.

The Cycles of Heaven, Guy Lyon Playfair and Scott Hill; Souvenir, 1978.

Electrographic Imaging in Medicine and Biology, Dumitrescu and Kenyon; Spearman, 1983.

Electromagnetic Fields and Life, A.S. Presman; Plenum, 1970.

Electromagnetism and Life, Robert O. Becker and A. Marino; State University of New York, 1982.

The Geomagnetic Field and Life, A.P. Dubrov; Plenum, 1978.

Healing by Biomagnetism, Bruce Copen; Academic Publications, 1960.

The Magnetic Blueprint of Life, Davis and Rawls; Exposition Press, 1979.

Magnetism and Its Effects on The Living System, Davis and Rawls; Exposition Press, 1974.

The Magnetic Effect, Davis and Rawls; Exposition Press, 1983.

Magnetic Guidance of Organisms, Richard Frankel. Annual Review of Biophysics and Bioengineering, Vol. 13; Annual Reviews Inc., 1984.

Mind, Body and Electromagnetism, John Evans; Element, 1986.

Mora Therapy: A Revolution in Electro-Magnetic Medicine, Geoffrey Foulkes and Anthony Scott-Morley; Journal of Alternative Medicine, July 1984.

New Wave Magnetic Field Therapy, Anthony Scott-Morley; Journal of Alternative Medicine, August 1985.

Radiation – What It Is, What It Does To Us and What We Can Do About It, John Davidson M.A. Cantab; C.W. Daniel, 1986.

Brain Anatomy and Function

The Cerebral Cortex of Man, Wilder Penfield; Macmillan, 1957

Electric Fields of The Brain, Paul L Nunez, Ph.D; Oxford University Press, 1981.

The Human Brain, Gilling and Brightwell; Orbis, 1982.

Injuries of the Brain and Spinal Cord, edited by Samuel Brock; Cassell and Co, 1960.

The Living Brain, W.G. Walter; Duckworth, 1953.

Man on His Nature, Sir Charles Sherrington; Cambridge University Press, 1951.

The Mystery of the Mind, Wilder Penfield; Princetown University Press, 1975.

Speech and Brain Mechanisms, Wilder Penfield; Princetown University Press, 1959.

The Understanding of the Brain, John C. Eccles; McGraw-Hill, 1977.

Embryology

Embryogenesis, Richard Grossinger; North Atlantic Books, 1986.

Human Embryology, Beck, Moffat and Davies; Blackwell, 1985.

Endocrinology

The Bitter Pill, Dr Ellen Grant; Elm Tree Books, 1985.

Endocrinology, C.R.W. Edwards; Heinemann, 1986.

Essential Endocrinology, Laycock and Wise; Oxford University Press, 1983.

Hormones, The Messengers of Life, Lawrence Crapo; Freeman, 1985.

The Pineal Organ, Lutz Vollrath; Springer-Verlag, 1981.

The Thymus Gland, Marion D. Kendall (Ed); Academic Press, 1981.

Evolution

Adam and Evolution, Michael Pitman; Hutchinson, 1985.

In The Minds Of Men, Ian T. Taylor; TFE Publishing, 1984.

Miscellaneous

Biotypes, Joan Arehart-Treichel; W.H. Allen, 1981.

A Harmony of Science and Nature – Ways of Staying Healthy in A Modern World, John and Farida Davidson; Wholistic Research Company, 1986.

Ideas and Opinions, Albert Einstein; Souvenir Press, 1973.

Introduction to Submolecular Biology, Szent Gyorgi; 1960.

Lamark, The Founder of Evolution, A.S. Packard; Longmans, Green and Co, 1901.

Laser Focus on Fast Chemistry, David Andrews; New Scientist, March 12th 1987.

The Lost World of The Kalahari, Laurens van der Post; Hogarth Press, 1958.

Self-Organization in Non-equilibrium Systems, Prigogine; Wiley and Sons, 1977.

Tuning In To Nature, Philip Callahan, Devin-Adair, 1975.

Morphogenesis

The Chemical Basis of Morphogenesis, A.M. Turing; Philosophical Translations of the Royal Society, 1952.

Mind, Body and Electromagnetism, John Evans; Element, 1986.

A New Science of Life, Rupert Sheldrake; Blond and Briggs, 1981.

Mystic and Yogic Philosophy

Autobiography of a Yogi, Paramhamsa Yogananda; Rider, 1950

Living With The Himalayan Masters, Swami Rama; Himalayan International Institute of Yoga Science and Philosophy of the U.S.A., 1978.

The Master Answers, Maharaj Charan Singh Ji; Radha Soami Satsang Beas, 1966.

The Mystic Bible, Dr Randolph Stone; Radha Soami Satsang Beas, 1956.

Nagas and the Magical Cosmology of Buddhism, Andrew Rawlinson Ph.D.; Religion 16, 1986.

The Path of the Masters, Dr. Julian Johnson; Radha Soami Satsang Beas, 1939.

The Serpent Power, Sir John Woodroffe; Ganesh, 1931.

Shakti and Shakta, Sir John Woodroffe; Ganesh, 1920.
Spiritual Gems, Maharaj Sawan Singh Ji; Radha Soami Satsang Beas, 1965.
The Textbook of Yoga Psychology, Rammurti S. Mishra, M.D.; Lynebird Press, 1972.
The Way of Mysticism, (An Anthology), Joseph James; Jonathan Cape, 1950.
The Yoga-Sutra of Patanjali, Georg Feverstein; Dawson, 1979.

Mysticism and Physics

Stalking The Wild Pendulum, Isaac Bentov; Fontana, 1979.
The Tao of Physics, Fritjof Capra; Fontana, 1984.

The New Physics

Directions in Physics, Paul Dirac; John Wiley and Sons, 1978.
The Life of Nicola Tesla, John J.O'Neil; Spearman, 1968.
The Particle Play, J.C. Polkinghorne; Freeman, 1979.
Physics Unified, Harold Aspden; Sabberton Publications, 1980.
Superforce, Paul Davies; Unwin, 1984.
The World of Elementary Particles, K.W. Ford; Blaisdell Publishing Co., 1958.

Physics and The New Energy Science

Cohering The Zero Point Energy, Moray B. King; privately published paper, 1986.
The Emerging Energy Science, T.E. Bearden and Andrew Michrowski; Planetary Association For Clean Energy, 1985.
The Energy Machine Of Joseph Newman, Joseph Newman; Joseph Newman Publishing Co., 1987.
The Holistic Paradigm, Moray B. King; privately published paper, 1986.
The Secret of The Creative Vacuum, John Davidson; C.W. Daniel Co. To be published, 1988.
Revolution In Technology, Medicine And Society, Dr Hans A. Nieper; MIT Verlag, 1985.

Toward A New Electromagnetism, Thomas Bearden; Tesla Book Company, 1983.

Psychology and Psychiatry

Alchemical Studies, C.G. Jung; Routledge and Kegan Paul, 1967.

Astrology, Psychology and The Four Elements, Stephen Arroyo, M.A.; CRCS, 1975.

Awakening The Heart, John Welwood; Shambhala, 1983.

The Biochemical Basis of Psychoses, The Serotonin Hypothesis about Mental Disease, D.W. Woolley; Wiley and Sons, 1962.

The Divided Self, R.D. Laing; Penguin, 1965.

An Introduction To Jung's Psychology, Frieda Fordham, Penguin, 1953.

Modern Man In Search of a Soul, C.G. Jung; Routledge and Kegan Paul, 1978.

The Psychology of The Transference, C.G. Jung; Routledge and Kegan Paul, 1983.

Psychological Reflections, C.G. Jung; Routledge and Kegan Paul, 1953.

Sybil, F.R. Schreiber; Penguin, 1975.

States Of Consciousness

Altered States of Consciousness, Charles Tart, John Wiley and Sons, 1969.

The Projection of The Astral Body, S.V. Muldoon; Rider and Co, 1929.

Subtle Energy and Therapeutic Techniques

Ayurveda, The Science of Self-Healing, Dr Vasant Lad; Lotus Press, 1984.

Breakthrough to Creativity, Shafica Karagulla, De Vorss, 1967.

Chakras – Rays and Radionics, David Tansley; C.W. Daniel, 1984.

Chinese Tonic Herbs, Ron Teeguarden; Japan Publications, 1984.

Esoteric Healing, Alice Bailey; Lucis, 1953.

The Etheric Double, A.E. Powell; Theosophical Publishing House, 1925.

Geopathic Stress: The Reason Why Therapies Fail? Anthony Scott-Morley; Journal of Alternative Medicine, May 1985.

Health Building, The Conscious Art of Living Well, Dr Randolph Stone; CRCS, 1985.

Inner Bridges, A Guide To Body Energies, Frederick Smith M.D.; Humanics, 1986.

The Pattern of Health, Aubrey Westlake; Shambala, 1973.

Polarity Therapy – The Complete Collected Works, Dr Randolph Stone D.O., D.C.; CRCS, P.O. Box 1460, Sebastopol, Calif. 95472, USA. 1986.

The Principles and Art of Cure by Homoeopathy, Herbert A. Roberts M.D.; Health Science Press (now C.W. Daniel), 1979.

Pulsor, Miracle of Micro-Crystals, Dr George Yao; Gyro Industries, 1986.

Radionics and The Subtle Anatomy of Man, David V. Tansley D.C.; C.W. Daniel, 1972.

The Raiment of Light, David Tansley; Routledge and Kegan Paul, 1984.

The Rainbow in Your Hands, Davis and Rawls; Exposition Press, 1976.

The Soul and Its Mechanism, Alice A. Bailey; Lucis, 1950.

Subtle Energy, John Davidson; C.W. Daniel, 1987.

Index

Further Information

The author is very interested to hear from anyone researching along these lines. He may be contacted through:

**Wholistic Research Company,
Bright Haven,
Robin's Lane,
Lolworth,
Cambridge CB3 8HH.
England**

Wholistic Research Company make available a range of health and environmental products, including some of the books listed in the bibliography. Please send £1.95 (£5 or $10 if overseas) for a large and full information pack, including their 72pp book/catalogue: *A Harmony of Science and Nature – Ways of Staying Healthy in A Modern World*, by John and Farida Davidson.

The author also holds occasional seminars on the understanding of subtle and life energies for use as a basis in the healing arts. *Visits by appointment only, please.*